CALORIES
AND CARBOHYDRATES

THE BOOK THAT MAKES IT EASY
TO TRIM DOWN—
AND STAY THAT WAY

Whether you aim to lose five pounds or fifty, the only safe, healthy way is to eat an adequate, well-balanced diet, choosing your calories from many different kinds of foods in order to ensure that you're getting sufficient vitamins, minerals, and other nutrients. *Calories and Carbohydrates* contains the most accurate and dependable calorie and carbohydrate counts for practically everything you will eat and drink—thousands and thousands of brand names and basic foods (such as your favorites, from Jack-in-the-Box to White Castle).

SO DIET WITH EASE—
AND LOSE AS
NEVER BEFORE!

Barbara Kraus

CALORIES
AND
CARBOHYDRATES

TENTH REVISED EDITION

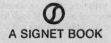

A SIGNET BOOK

SIGNET
Published by the Penguin Group
Penguin Books USA Inc., 375 Hudson Street,
New York, New York 10014, U.S.A.
Penguin Books Ltd, 27 Wrights Lane,
London W8 5TZ, England
Penguin Books Australia Ltd, Ringwood,
Victoria, Australia
Penguin Books Canada Ltd, 10 Alcorn Avenue,
Toronto, Ontario, Canada M4V 3B2
Penguin Books (N.Z.) Ltd, 1823-190 Wairau Road,
Auckland 10, New Zealand

Penguin Books Ltd, Registered Offices:
Harmondsworth, Middlesex, England

Published by Signet, an imprint of New American Library, a division of
Penguin Books USA Inc. Also published in a Plume edition.

First Signet Printing, August, 1973
Second Revised Edition (Seventh Printing), July, 1975
Third Revised Edition (Fourteenth Printing), March, 1979
Fourth Revised Edition (Nineteenth Printing), May, 1981
Fifth Revised Edition (Twenty-fourth Printing), May, 1983
Sixth Revised Edition (Twenty-seventh Printing), June, 1985
Seventh Revised Edition (Thirty-fourth Printing), April, 1987
Eighth Revised Edition (Thirty-seventh Printing), March, 1989
Ninth Revised Edition (Forty-second Printing), March, 1991
Tenth Revised Edition (Forty-third Printing), March, 1993
51   50   49   48   47   46   45   44

In memory of Daniel A. Brennie

In memory of Daniel A. Brown

Contents

Introduction

This dictionary of foods lists several thousand brand-name products and basic foods with their caloric and carbohydrate content. The calorie yield of your diet versus the amount of energy you expend is the key to whether you maintain your ideal weight, gain too many pounds or lose weight.

Because of the relationship of weight to health, many individuals are "counting calories" at every meal. Interest has also been directed to the carbohydrate content of the diet in relation to weight control. Comprehensive information on these values in basic foods and brand-name products is not readily available in any one source. Nor is the information regularly supplied in single-serving portions. (For example, the United States Department of Agriculture supplies counts primarily in bulk-sized portions.) To compound the problem, hundreds of new food items appear in our stores every year.

Analyses of foods to provide information on nutritive values are extremely expensive to conduct. Many small companies have not been able to afford to have their products analyzed and thus were unable to provide data for this book or were able to provide only the calories or only the carbohydrates. Other companies have simply never gotten around to having the analyses done. Other companies simply refuse to supply nutritional information. New requirements for labeling nutritive values of products may provide information on additional items in the future. Therefore, wherever data for carbohydrates were unavailable, blank spaces were left which may be filled in by the reader at a later time.

Arrangement of This Book

Foods are listed alphabetically by brand name or by the name of the food. The singular form is used for most entries that is, Blackberry instead of Blackberries. Most items are listed individually though a few are grouped under the general food category. For example, all candies are listed together so that if you are looking for *Mars* bar, you look first under Candy, then under *M* in alphabetical order; but, if you are looking for a breakfast food such as oatmeal, you will find it under *O* in the main alphabet. Other foods that are grouped include Baby Food, Gravy, Ice Cream, Marinade Mix, Pie, Sauce, Soft Drinks, Soup, and "Vegetarian Foods." Many cross references are included to assist in finding items called by different names.

Under the main headings, it was often not possible or even desirable to follow an alphabetical arrangement. For basic foods such as apricots, for example, the first entries are for the fresh product weighed with seeds as it is purchased in the store, then the fruit in small portions as they may be eaten or measured. These entries are followed by the processed products, canned (although it may actually be a bottle or jar), dehydrated, dried and frozen. This basic plan, with adaptations where necessary, was followed for fruits, vegetables and meats.

In almost all entries where data were available the U.S. Department of Agriculture figures are shown first. The Department values represent averages from several manufacturers and are shown for comparison with the values from individual companies or for use where particular brands are not available.

All brand-name products have been italicized and company names appear in parentheses.

Portions Used

The portion column is a most important one to read and note. Common household measures are used insofar as possible. For some items, the amounts given are those commonly purchased in the store, such as 1 pound of meat. These quantities can be divided into the number of servings used in the home, and the nutritive values available to each person served can then be readily determined. Of course, any ingredients added when preparing such products must also be taken into account.

The smaller portions given are for foods as served or measured in moderate amounts, such as ½ cup of juice reconstituted, or 4 ounces of meat. Be sure to adjust the calories and carbohydrates to the actual portions you use. For example, if you serve 1 cup of juice instead of ½ cup, multiply the calories and carbohydrates shown for the smaller amount by 2.

Don't fool yourself about the size of portions you use. If you are serious about controlling the calories and carbohydrates in your diet, weigh your foods until you can accurately gauge the weight visually. Remember, the calories and carbohydrates go up with any increase in the weight of foods. Remember, too, that 4 ounces by weight may be very different from 4 fluid ounces or ½ cup. Ounces in the table are always ounces by weight unless specified as fluid ounces, or fractions of a cup or other volumetric measure. Foods that are fluffy in texture, such as flaked coconut and bean sprouts, vary greatly in weight per cup depending on how tightly they are packed into the cup. Such foods as canned green beans also vary when weighed with or without liquid; for example, canned green beans with liquid weigh 4.2 ounces for ½ cup, but drained beans weigh 2.5 ounces for the same ½ cup. Check the weights of your serving portions regularly. Bear in mind that you can cut calories and carbohydrates by cutting the serving size.

It was impossible to convert all the portions to a uniform basis. Some sources were only able to report data in terms of weights with no information on cup or other volumetric measures. I have shown small portions in quantities that might reasonably be expected to be served or measured in the home. Package sizes are useful to show the composition of products as they are purchased and may be divided into the number of serving portions prepared from the entire product, taking into account any added ingredients.

You will find in the portion column the phrases "weighed with bone," or "weighed with skin and seeds" or other inedible parts. These descriptions apply to the products as you purchase them in the markets, but the caloric values and the carbohydrate content as shown are for the amount of edible food after you discard the bone, skin, seed or other inedible part. The weight given in the "measure or quantity" column is to the nearest gram or fraction of an ounce.

Data on the composition of foods are constantly changing for many reasons. Better sampling and analytical methods, improvements in marketing procedures and changes in formulas of mixed products, all may alter values for carbohydrates and other nutrients as well as caloric values. Weights of packaged foods are frequently changed. It is essential to read label information to be informed about these matters and to make intelligent use of food tables.

This book, along with the individual calorie annual guide (*The Barbara Kraus 1992 Calorie Guide to Brand Names and Basic Foods*), is constantly revised and updated to help keep you as up-to-date as possible.

Calories

What is a calorie? It is not a nutrient nor is it a good guide to the nutritive value of food. It is more like a yardstick to measure the energy that a food will yield in the body. You need energy for your body functions as well as for exercise. If your diet contains more calories than your body uses for these purposes, the extra "energy" will be stored as fat.

If your plan is to cut down on calories, the easiest way to do so is to consult the calorie column of this counter and keep an accurate count of your total intake of food and beverages for a period of seven days. If you have not gained or lost weight during that week divide that number by seven and you'll have your maintenance diet expressed in calories. To lose weight, you must reduce your daily or weekly intake of calories below this maintenance level. (To gain, increase the intake.)

One pound of fat is equal to 3,500 calories. Add this number of calories to those you need to balance your energy requirements and you will gain one pound; subtract it, and you will lose a pound.

Carbohydrates

The carbohydrate column shows the amount of this nutrient in grams for the quantities of foods indicated in the portion column. Some dietitians are giving special attention to this nutrient at present in connection with weight control. Carbohydrates include sugars, starches, some acids and other nutrients.

Other Nutrients

Do not forget that other nutrients are extremely important in diet planning – protein, fat, minerals and vitamins. Calories yielded by alcohol must also be taken into consideration. From a nutrition viewpoint, perhaps the best advice that can be given to the dieter is to eat a varied diet with all classes of foods represented. Meat, fish, chicken, fats and oils, milk, vegetables, fruits and grain products are all important sources of essential nutrients and some foods from each of these classes of foods should be included in the diet every day. With the great abundance and variety of foods on the grocer's shelves, there is no reason why the dieter should not enjoy a tasty, nutritious and attractive diet. Just eat in moderation and there is no need to eliminate any one food altogether, except in special conditions under a doctor's directions. Choose wisely and eat well.

Sources of Data

Values in this dictionary are based on publications issued by the U.S. Department of Agriculture and on data submitted by manufacturers and processors. The U.S. Department of Agriculture issues basic tables on food composition for use in the United States. The commercial products from USDA publications represent average values obtained on products of more than one company. The figures designated "home recipe" are based on recipes on file with the Department of Agriculture. Data on commercial products listed by brand name in this publication are based on values supplied by manufacturers and processors for their own individual products. Very few supermarket brand names, such as Safeway or private labels, were included in this book because they are not usually analyzed under these trade names. Every care has been taken to interpret the data and the descriptions supplied by the companies as fully and accurately as possible. Many values have been recalculated to different portions from those submitted in order to bring about greater uniformity among similar items.

Calories in these different sources are not always on a

strictly uniform basis. In the Department of Agriculture, calories are calculated using specific factors, which make allowances for losses in digestion and metabolism. The technical explanation of these factors is given in Handbook 74 of the USDA. Most manufacturers use average factors of 4, 9 and 4 for calories yielded by each gram of protein, fat and carbohydrate respectively; a factor of 7 is used as an average value to calculate the calories from one gram of alcohol. These differences in procedure will give somewhat different results for products of similar composition. Some manufacturers have adopted the values from U.S. Department of Agriculture publications as representative of their own products. In these cases, it will be apparent in the table that the data from the companies match exactly those from USDA publications.

Bear in mind that small differences in calorie values on similar products of the same weight are not important in diet planning. They may be due to different methods of calculating the calories or to small differences in the nutritive values of the samples analyzed because no two foods ever have exactly the same composition. Some differences may also be due to the way the food was measured, as noted in the case of green beans earlier.

Carbohydrates in this book are usually total carbohydrates by difference. A few manufacturers reported only "available carbohydrates." These values were omitted.

Abbreviations and Symbols

(USDA) = United States Department
     of Agriculture
(HHS/FAO) = Health and Human
     Services/Food
     and Agriculture
     Organization
* = prepared as package directs[1]
< = less than
& = and
" = inch
canned = bottles or jars
     as well as cans
dia. = diameter

fl. = fluid
liq. = liquid
lb. = pound
med. = medium
oz. = ounce
pkg. = package
pt. = pint
qt. = quart
sq. = square
T. = tablespoon
Tr. = trace
tsp. = teaspoon
wt. = weight

italics or name in parentheses = registered trademark,®
The letters DNA indicate that data are not available.

Equivalents

By Weight
1 pound = 16 ounces
1 ounce = 28.35 grams
3.52 ounces = 100 grams

By Volume
1 quart = 4 cups
1 cup = 8 fluid ounces
1 cup = ½ pint
1 cup = 16 tablespoons
2 tablespoons = 1 fluid ounce
1 tablespoon = 3 teaspoons

[1]If the package directions call for whole or skim milk, the data given here are for whole milk, unless otherwise stated.

CALORIES
AND
CARBOHYDRATES

Food and Description	Measure or Quantity	Calories	Carbo-hydrates (grams)
A			
ABALONE (USDA):			
Raw, meat only	4 oz.	111	3.9
Canned	4 oz.	91	2.6
AC'CENT	¼ tsp.	3	0.
ACEROLA, fresh fruit	¼ lb. (weighed with seeds)	52	12.6
AGNOLETTI, frozen (Buitoni):			
Cheese filled	2-oz. serving	196	33.4
Meat filled	2-oz. serving	206	31.7
ALBACORE, raw, meat only (USDA)	4 oz.	201	0.
ALCOHOL (See **DISTILLED LIQUOR**)			
ALE (See **BEER**)			
ALFALFA SEEDS (USDA) sprouted	1 cup	10	1.0
ALLSPICE (French's)	1 tsp.	6	1.3
ALMOND:			
Fresh (USDA):			
In shell	10 nuts	60	2.0
Shelled, raw, natural, with skins	1 oz.	170	5.5
Roasted:			
Dry (Planters)	1 oz.	170	6.0

(USDA) = United States Department of Agriculture
(HHS/FAO) = Health and Human Services/Food and Agriculture Organization
* = prepared as package directs

Food and Description	Measure or Quantity	Calories	Carbo-hydrates (grams)
Honey roast (Eagle)	1 oz.	150	10.0
Oil:			
(Fisher)	1 oz.	178	5.5
(Tom's)	1 oz.	180	6.0
ALMOND BUTTER (Hain):			
Raw, natural	1 T.	95	1.5
Toasted, blanched	1 T.	105	1.5
ALMOND DELIGHT, cereal (Ralston/Purina)	¾ cup (1 oz.)	110	23.0
ALMOND EXTRACT (Virginia Dare) pure	1 tsp.	10	0.
ALPHA-BITS, cereal (Post)	1 cup (1 oz.)	113	24.6
AMARANTH, raw, trimmed (USDA)	4 oz.	41	7.4
AMARETTO DI SARONNO **LIQUEUR,** 28% alcohol	1 fl. oz.	82	9.0
ANCHOVY, PICKLED, canned:			
(USDA) flat or rolled, not heavily salted, drained	2-oz. can	79	.1
(Granadaisor)	2-oz. can	80	Tr.
ANISE EXTRACT (Virginia Dare) 76% alcohol	1 tsp.	22	0.
ANISE SEEDS (USDA)	1 T.	21	3.0
ANISETTE:			
(DeKuyper)	1 fl. oz.	95	11.4
(Mr. Boston)	1 fl. oz.	87	10.8
APPLE:			
Fresh (USDA):			
Eaten with skin	2½″ dia. (4.1 oz.)	61	15.3
Eaten without skin	2½″ dia. (4.1 oz.)	53	13.9
Canned:			
(Comstock):			
Rings, drained	1 ring (1.1 oz.)	30	7.0
Sliced	⅙ of 21-oz. can	45	10.0

Food and Description	Measure or Quantity	Calories	Carbo-hydrates (grams)
(White House):			
Rings, spiced	.7-oz. ring	11	8.0
Sliced	½ cup (4 oz.)	54	14.0
Dried:			
(Sun-Maid/Sunsweet) chunks	2-oz. serving	150	42.0
(Town House)	2-oz. serving	150	40.0
(Weight Watchers):			
Chips	¾-oz. pkg.	70	19.0
Snacks	.5-oz. pkg.	50	13.0
Frozen (USDA), sweetened, slices	10-oz. pkg.	264	68.9
APPLE BROWN BETTY, home recipe (USDA)	1 cup	325	63.9
APPLE BUTTER:			
(Empress) regular or spiced	1 T.	37	9.0
(Home Brands)	1 T.	51	13.5
(Piedmont)	1 T.	37	7.5
(White House)	1 T.	38	9.0
APPLE CHERRY BERRY DRINK, canned (Lincoln)	6 fl. oz.	90	23.0
APPLE-CHERRY JUICE COCKTAIL, canned:			
Musselman's	8 fl. oz.	110	28.0
(Red Cheek)	6 fl. oz.	113	28.0
APPLE CIDER:			
Canned:			
(Johanna Farms)	½ cup	56	14.5
(Mott's) sweet	½ cup	59	14.6
(Town House)	6 fl. oz.	90	23.0
(Tree Top)	6 fl. oz.	90	22.0
*Frozen (Tree Top)	6 fl. oz.	90	22.0
*Mix:			
Country Time	8 fl. oz.	98	24.5
(Hi-C)	6 fl. oz.	72	18.0

(USDA) = United States Department of Agriculture
(HHS/FAO) = Health and Human Services/Food and Agriculture Organization
* = prepared as package directs

Food and Description	Measure or Quantity	Calories	Carbo-hydrates (grams)
APPLE-CRANBERRY JUICE, canned (Lincoln)	6 fl. oz.	100	25.0
APPLE CRISP, frozen (Pepperidge Farm)	4¾-oz. serving	250	43.0
APPLE DRINK, canned:			
Capri Sun, natural	6¾ fl. oz.	90	22.7
(Hi-C)	6 fl. oz.	92	23.0
(Johanna Farms) *Ssips*	8.45-fl.-oz. container	130	32.0
APPLE DUMPLINGS, frozen (Pepperidge Farm)	1 dumpling (3.1 oz.)	260	33.0
APPLE, ESCALLOPED:			
Canned (White House)	½ cup (4.5 oz.)	163	39.0
Frozen (Stouffer's)	4-oz. serving	130	27.0
APPLE-GRAPE JUICE:			
Canned:			
(Mott's)	8.45-fl.-oz. container	128	32.0
(Mott's)	9½-fl.-oz. can	139	37.0
(Red Cheek)	6 fl. oz.	109	27.0
(Tree Top)	6 fl. oz.	100	25.0
*Frozen (Tree Top)	6 fl. oz.	100	25.0
APPLE JACKS, cereal (Kellogg's)	1 cup (1 oz.)	110	26.0
APPLE JAM (Smucker's)	1 T.	53	13.5
APPLE JELLY:			
Sweetened (Smucker's)	1 T. (.7 oz.)	54	12.0
Dietetic:			
(Featherweight; Louis Sherry)	1 T. (.6 oz.)	6	0.
(Diet Delight)	1 T. (.6 oz.)	12	3.0
(Estee)	1 T. (.6 oz.)	6	0.
APPLE JUICE:			
Canned:			
(Ardmore Farms)	6 fl. oz.	90	22.2
(Borden) *Sippin' Pak*	8.45-fl.-oz. container	110	28.0
(Land O' Lakes)	6 fl. oz.	90	22.0

Food and Description	Measure or Quantity	Calories	Carbo-hydrates (grams)
(Minute Maid)	8.45-fl.-oz. container	128	31.9
(Mott's)	6 fl. oz.	88	22.0
(Ocean Spray)	6 fl. oz.	90	23.0
(Red Cheek)	6 fl. oz.	97	24.0
(Town House)	6 fl. oz.	90	23.0
(Tree Top) any type	6 fl. oz.	90	22.0
(White House)	6 fl. oz.	87	22.0
Chilled (Minute Maid):			
Regular	6 fl. oz.	91	22.7
On the Go	10-fl.-oz. bottle	152	37.8
*Frozen:			
(Minute Maid)	6 fl. oz.	91	22.7
(Sunkist)	6 fl. oz.	59	14.5
(Tree Top)	6 fl. oz.	90	22.0
APPLE JUICE DRINK, canned:			
Squeezit (General Mills)	6¾-fl.-oz. bottle	110	27.0
(Sunkist)	8.45 fl. oz.	140	34.0
APPLE NECTAR, canned:			
(Libby's)	6 fl. oz.	100	25.0
APPLE-PEAR JUICE, canned or *frozen (Tree Top)	6 fl. oz.	90	22.0
APPLE PUNCH DRINK, canned (Red Cheek)	6 fl. oz.	113	28.0
***APPLE RAISIN CRISP**, cereal (Kellogg's)	⅔ cup (1 oz.)	130	32.0
APPLE PIE (See PIE, Apple)			
APPLE-RASPBERRY DRINK, canned (Mott's)	10-fl.-oz. container	158	40.0

(USDA) = United States Department of Agriculture
(HHS/FAO) = Health and Human Services/Food and Agriculture Organization
* = prepared as package directs

Food and Description	Measure or Quantity	Calories	Carbo-hydrates (grams)
APPLE-RASBERRY JUICE:			
Canned, regular pack:			
(Mott's)	8.45-fl.-oz. container	124	31.0
(Mott's)	9½-fl.-oz. container	134	35.0
(Red Cheek)	6 fl. oz.	113	28.0
(Tree Top)	6 fl. oz.	80	21.0
*Frozen (Tree Top)	6 fl. oz.	80	21.0
APPLE SAUCE, canned:			
Regular:			
(Hunt's) *Snack Pack*:			
Regular	4¼ oz.	80	19.0
Natural	4¼ oz.	50	12.0
Raspberry	4¼ oz.	80	21.0
Strawberry	4¼ oz.	80	20.0
(Mott's):			
Regular, jarred:			
Plain	6 oz.	150	36.0
Chunky	6 oz.	86	21.0
Cinnamon	6 oz.	152	36.0
Single-serve cups:			
Regular	4 oz.	100	24.0
Cherry	3¾ oz.	72	17.0
Cinnamon	4 oz.	101	24.0
Peach	3¾ oz.	75	18.0
Pineapple	3¾ oz.	86	21.0
Strawberry	3¾ oz.	76	18.0
(Town House)	½ cup	85	23.5
(Tree Top):			
Cinnamon or original	½ cup	80	20.0
Natural	½ cup	60	14.0
(White House)	½ cup (5 oz.)	80	22.0
Dietetic:			
(Country Pure)	4 oz.	50	12.0
(Del Monte, Lite; Diet Delight)	½ cup	50	13.0
(Mott's):			
Jarred	6 oz.	80	20.0
Single-serve cups	4 oz.	53	15.0
(S&W) *Nutradiet*, white or blue label	½ cup	55	14.0
(White House):			
Regular	½ cup (4.7 oz.)	50	12.0

Food and Description	Measure or Quantity	Calories	Carbo-hydrates (grams)
Apple juice added	½ cup (4.7 oz.)	50	13.0
APRICOT:			
Fresh (USDA):			
Whole	1 lb. (weighed with pits)	217	54.6
Whole	3 apricots (about 12 per lb.)	55	13.7
Halves	1 cup (5½ oz.)	79	19.8
Canned, regular pack, solids & liq.:			
(USDA):			
Juice pack	4 oz.	61	15.4
Extra heavy syrup	4 oz.	115	29.5
(Stokely-Van Camp)	½ cup (4.6 oz.)	110	27.0
(Town House) unpeeled, halves	½ cup	110	28.0
Canned, dietetic, solids & liq.:			
(Country Pure) halves	½ cup	60	15.0
(Diet Delight):			
Juice pack	½ cup (4.4 oz.)	60	15.0
Water pack	½ cup (4.3 oz.)	35	9.0
(Featherweight):			
Juice pack	½ cup	50	12.0
Water pack	½ cup	35	9.0
(Libby's) Lite	½ cup (4.4 oz.)	60	15.0
(S&W) *Nutradiet:*			
Halves, white or blue label	½ cup	35	9.0
Whole, juice pack	½ cup	28	7.0
Dried (Town House)	2-oz. serving	140	35.0
APRICOT, CANDIED (USDA)	1 oz.	96	24.5
APRICOT, STRAINED, canned (Larsen) no salt added	½ cup	55	14.5
APRICOT LIQUEUR (DeKuyper) 60 proof	1 fl. oz.	82	8.3

(USDA) = United States Department of Agriculture
(HHS/FAO) = Health and Human Services/Food and Agriculture Organization
* = prepared as package directs

Food and Description	Measure or Quantity	Calories	Carbo-hydrates (grams)
APRICOT NECTAR, canned:			
(Ardmore Farms)	6 fl. oz.	94	24.2
(Town House)	6 fl. oz.	100	26.0
APRICOT-PINEAPPLE NECTAR, canned, dietetic			
(S&W) *Nutradiet,* blue label	6 oz.	35	12.0
APRICOT & PINEAPPLE PRESERVE OR JAM:			
Sweetened (Smucker's)	1 T. (.7 oz.)	53	13.5
Dietetic:			
(Diet Delight; Louis Sherry)	1 T. (.6 oz.)	6	3.0
(Featherweight)	1 T.	6	1.0
(S&W) *Nutradiet,* red label	1 T.	12	3.0
(Tillie Lewis) *Tasti Diet*	1 T.	12	3.0
APRICOT PRESERVE, dietetic			
(Estee)	1 T.	6	0.
ARBY'S:			
Bac'n Cheddar Deluxe	1 sandwich	561	36.0
Beef & Cheddar sandwich	1 sandwich	490	51.0
Chicken breast sandwich	7¼-oz. sandwich	592	56.0
Croissant:			
Bacon & egg	1 order	420	32.0
Butter	1 piece	220	28.0
Chicken salad	1 order	460	16.0
Ham & swiss	1 order	330	33.0
Mushroom & swiss	1 order	340	34.0
Sausage & egg	1 order	530	31.0
French fries	1½-oz. serving	211	33.0
Ham 'N Cheese	1 sandwich	353	33.0
Potato cakes	2 pieces	201	22.0
Potato, stuffed:			
Broccoli & cheese	1 potato	541	72.0
Deluxe	1 potato	648	59.0
Mushroom & cheese	1 potato	506	61.0
Taco	1 potato	619	73.0
Roast Beef:			
Regular	5-oz. sandwich	353	32.0
Junior	3-oz. sandwich	218	22.0
King	6.7-oz sandwich	467	44.0
Super	8.3-oz. sandwich	501	50.0

Food and Description	Measure or Quantity	Calories	Carbo- hydrates (grams)
Shake:			
Chocolate	10.6-oz. serving	314	62.0
Jamocha	10.8-oz. serving	424	76.0
Vanilla	8.8-oz. serving	295	44.0
Turkey deluxe	7-oz. sandwich	375	32.0
ARTICHOKE:			
Fresh (USDA):			
Raw, whole	1 lb. (weighed untrimmed)	85	19.2
Boiled, without salt, drained	15-oz. artichoke	187	42.1
Canned (Cara Mia) marinated, drained	6-oz. jar	175	12.6
Frozen (Birds Eye) hearts, deluxe	⅓ pkg. (3 oz.)	33	6.6
ASPARAGUS:			
Fresh (USDA):			
Raw, spears	1 lb. (weighed untrimmed)	66	12.7
Boiled, without salt, drained	1 spear (½" dia. at base)	3	.5
Canned, regular pack, solids & liq.:			
(Green Giant) cuts or spears	½ cup (4 oz.)	20	3.0
(Le Sueur) green spears	½ of 8-oz. can	30	4.0
(Town House) cut or spears	½ cup	20	3.0
Canned, dietetic pack (USDA) drained solids, cut	1 cup (8.3 oz.)	47	7.3
Canned, dietetic pack, solids & liq.:			
(Diet Delight)	½ cup	16	2.0
(S&W) *Nutradiet*, green label	½ cup	17	3.0
Frozen:			
(USDA) cuts & tips, boiled, drained	1 cup (6.3 oz.)	40	6.3
(Birds Eye):			
Cuts	⅓ pkg. (3.3 oz.)	22	3.8
Spears	⅓ pkg. (3.3 oz.)	23	3.9
(Frosty Acres)	3.3-oz. serving	25	4.0

(USDA) = United States Department of Agriculture
(HHS/FAO) = Health and Human Services/Food and Agriculture Organization
* = prepared as package directs

Food and Description	Measure or Quantity	Calories	Carbo-hydrates (grams)
ASPARAGUS PILAF, frozen (Green Giant) microwave *Garden Gourmet*	9½-oz. pkg.	190	37.0
ASPARAGUS PUREE, canned (Larsen) no salt added	½ cup (4.4 oz.)	22	3.5
AUNT JEMIMA SYRUP (See **SYRUP**)			
AVOCADO, all varieties (USDA):			
Whole	1 fruit (10.7 oz.)	378	14.3
Cubed	1 cup (5.3 oz.)	251	9.5
AVOCADO PUREE (Calavo)	½ cup (8.1 oz.)	411	15.9
***AWAKE** (Birds Eye)	6 fl. oz. (6.5 oz.)	84	20.5

Food and Description	Measure or Quantity	Calories	Carbohydrates (grams)

B

BABY FOOD:

Food and Description	Measure or Quantity	Calories	Carbohydrates (grams)
Advance (*Similac*)	1 fl. oz.	15	1.5
Apple & apricot (Beech-Nut):			
Junior	7¾-oz. jar	93	24.4
Strained	4¾-oz. jar	57	14.0
Apple-apricot juice (Gerber) strained	4.2 oz.	60	15.0
Apple-banana juice (Gerber) strained	4.2 fl. oz.	70	16.0
Apple-betty (Beech-Nut):			
Junior	7¾-oz. jar	173	41.4
Strained	4¾-oz. jar	106	25.4
Apple-blueberry (Gerber):			
Junior	7½-oz. jar	110	24.0
Strained	4½-oz. jar	60	14.0
Apple-cherry juice:			
Strained:			
(Beech-Nut)	4⅕ fl. oz.	50	14.0
(Gerber)	4.2 fl. oz.	60	15.0
Toddler (Gerber)	4 fl. oz.	52	12.7
Apple-cranberry juice (Beech-Nut) strained	4½ fl. oz.	55	13.6
Apple dessert, Dutch (Gerber):			
Junior	7½-oz. jar	160	36.0
Strained	4½-oz. jar	100	21.0
Apple-grape juice:			
Strained:			
(Beech-Nut)	4⅕ fl. oz.	56	13.9
(Gerber)	4.2 fl. oz.	60	15.0
Toddler (Gerber)	4 fl. oz.	60	15.0
Apple juice:			
Strained:			
(Beech-Nut)	4⅕ fl. oz.	54	13.6

(USDA) = United States Department of Agriculture
(HHS/FAO) = Health and Human Services/Food and Agriculture Organization
* = prepared as package directs

Food and Description	Measure or Quantity	Calories	Carbo-hydrates (grams)
(Gerber)	4.2 fl. oz.	60	15.0
Toddler (Gerber)	4 fl. oz.	60	15.0
Apple-peach juice, strained:			
(Beech-Nut)	4⅕ fl. oz.	59	14.6
(Gerber)	4.2 fl. oz.	60	14.0
Apple-pineapple juice (Gerber) strained	4.2 fl. oz.	60	15.0
Apple-plum juice (Gerber) strained	4.2 fl. oz.	60	15.0
Apple-prune juice (Gerber) strained	4.2 fl. oz.	70	17.0
Applesauce:			
Junior:			
(Beech-Nut)	7¾-oz. jar	97	24.1
(Gerber)	7½-oz. jar	100	23.0
Strained:			
(Beech-Nut)	4¾-oz. jar	60	14.8
(Gerber):			
Regular	4½-oz. jar	60	14.0
First Foods	2½-oz. jar	30	7.0
Applesauce & apricots (Gerber):			
Junior	7½-oz. jar	110	24.0
Strained	4½-oz. jar	70	15.0
Applesauce & bananas (Beech-Nut) strained	4¾-oz. jar	63	15.4
Applesauce & cherries (Beech-Nut):			
Junior	7¾-oz. jar	115	28.4
Strained	4¾-oz. jar	61	15.1
Applesauce with pineapple (Gerber) strained	4½-oz. jar	60	14.0
Applesauce & raspberries (Beech-Nut):			
Junior	7¾-oz. jar	102	24.6
Strained	4¾-oz. jar	61	15.1
Apricot with tapioca:			
Junior:			
(Beech-Nut)	7½-oz. jar	113	27.9
(Gerber)	7¾-oz. jar	160	39.0
Strained (Gerber)	4½-oz. jar	90	20.0
Apricot with tapioca & apple juice (Beech-Nut) strained	4¾-oz. jar	72	17.6
Banana (Gerber) *First Foods*	2½-oz. jar	60	15.0

Food and Description	Measure or Quantity	Calories	Carbo-hydrates (grams)
Banana-apple dessert (Gerber):			
Junior	7½-oz. jar	150	34.0
Strained	4½-oz. jar	90	21.0
Banana dessert (Beech-Nut)			
Junior	7½-oz. jar	165	40.1
Banana with pineapple & tapioca (Gerber):			
Junior	7½-oz. jar	110	25.0
Strained	4½-oz. jar	70	15.0
Banana & pineapple with tapioca & apple juice (Beech-Nut):			
Junior	7¾-oz. jar	109	26.6
Strained	4¾-oz. jar	67	16.3
Banana with tapioca:			
Junior:			
(Beech-Nut)	7½-oz. jar	72	27.5
(Gerber)	7½-oz. jar	160	39.0
Strained:			
(Beech-Nut)	4¾-oz. jar	72	16.9
(Gerber)	4½-oz. jar	100	24.0
Bean, green:			
Junior (Beech-Nut)	7¼-oz. jar	62	13.0
Strained:			
(Beech-Nut)	4½-oz. jar	38	8.1
(Gerber):			
Regular	4½-oz. jar	50	8.0
First Foods	2½-oz. jar	20	5.0
Bean, green, creamed (Gerber)			
Junior	7½-oz. jar	100	20.0
Beef (Gerber):			
Junior	3½-oz. jar	110	1.0
Strained	3½-oz. jar	100	0.
Beef & beef broth (Beech-Nut):			
Junior	7½-oz. jar	235	.4
Strained	4½-oz. jar	152	.3
Beef dinner, high meat, with vegetables (Gerber):			
Junior	4½-oz. jar	130	10.0
Strained	4½-oz. jar	120	8.0

(USDA) = United States Department of Agriculture
(HHS/FAO) = Health and Human Services/Food and Agriculture Organization
* = prepared as package directs

Food and Description	Measure or Quantity	Calories	Carbo-hydrates (grams)
Beef & egg noodle (Beech-Nut):			
Junior	7½-oz. jar	122	17.0
Strained	4½-oz. jar	72	9.9
Beef & egg noodle with vegetables (Gerber) toddler, chunky	6-oz. jar	130	16.0
Beef with vegetables & cereal, high meat (Beech-Nut):			
Junior	4½-oz. jar	132	8.0
Strained	4½-oz. jar	132	8.1
Beef liver (Gerber) strained	3½-oz. jar	100	3.0
Beet (Gerber) strained	4½-oz. jar	50	11.0
Carrot:			
Junior:			
(Beech-Nut)	7½-oz. jar	67	13.8
(Gerber)	7½-oz. jar	60	12.0
Strained:			
(Beech-Nut)	4½-oz. jar	40	8.3
(Gerber):			
Regular	4½-oz. jar	40	7.0
First Foods	2½-oz. jar	30	5.0
Cereal, dry:			
Barley:			
(Beech-Nut)	½-oz. serving	54	9.9
(Gerber)	4 T. (½ oz.)	60	11.0
High protein:			
(Beech-Nut)	½-oz. serving	55	7.1
(Gerber)	4 T. (½ oz.)	50	5.0
High protein with apple & orange (Gerber)	4 T. (½ oz.)	60	4.0
Mixed:			
(Beech-Nut)	½-oz. serving	55	9.9
(Gerber)	4 T. (½ oz.)	50	10.0
Mixed with banana (Gerber)	4 T. (½ oz.)	60	11.0
Oatmeal:			
(Beech-Nut)	½-oz. serving	56	9.7
(Gerber)	4 T. (½ oz.)	50	9.0
Oatmeal & banana (Gerber)	4 T. (½ oz.)	60	10.0
Oat rings, toasted (Gerber) toddler	½ oz. serving	60	10.0
Rice:			
(Beech-Nut)	½-oz. serving	49	9.9
(Gerber)	4 T. (½ oz.)	60	11.0
Rice with banana (Gerber)	4 T. (½ oz.)	56	10.7

Food and Description	Measure or Quantity	Calories	Carbo-hydrates (grams)
Cereal or mixed cereal:			
With applesauce & banana:			
Junior (Gerber)	7½-oz. jar	131	26.4
Strained:			
(Beech-Nut)	4½-oz. jar	80	17.3
(Gerber)	4½-oz. jar	100	22.0
With egg yolks & bacon (Beech-Nut):			
Junior	7½-oz. jar	163	14.9
Strained	4½-oz. jar	113	8.9
Oatmeal with applesauce & banana (Gerber):			
Junior	7½-oz. jar	119	23.0
Strained	4½-oz. jar	100	21.0
Rice with applesauce & banana, strained:			
(Beech-Nut)	4¾-oz. jar	96	21.4
(Gerber)	4¾-oz. jar	100	23.0
Cherry vanilla pudding (Gerber):			
Junior	7½-oz. jar	150	35.0
Strained	4½-oz. jar	87	18.9
Chicken (Gerber):			
Junior	3½-oz. jar	140	0.
Strained	3½-oz. jar	140	1.0
Chicken & chicken broth (Beech-Nut):			
Junior	7½-oz. jar	228	.4
Strained	4½-oz. jar	128	.3
Chicken & noodle:			
Junior:			
(Beech-Nut)	7½-oz. jar	86	16.6
(Gerber)	7½-oz. jar	120	18.0
Strained:			
(Beech-Nut)	4½-oz. jar	59	10.5
(Gerber)	4½-oz. jar	80	12.0
Chicken & rice (Beech-Nut) strained	4½-oz. jar	72	12.0
Chicken soup, cream of (Gerber) strained	4½-oz. jar	70	11.0

(USDA) = United States Department of Agriculture
(HHS/FAO) = Health and Human Services/Food and Agriculture Organization
* = prepared as package directs

Food and Description	Measure or Quantity	Calories	Carbo-hydrates (grams)
Chicken stew (Gerber) toddler	6-oz. jar	145	12.3
Chicken sticks (Gerber) toddler	2½-oz. jar	120	1.0
Chicken with vegetables, high meat (Gerber):			
Junior	4½-oz. jar	130	8.0
Strained	4½-oz. jar	140	8.0
Chicken with vegetables & cereal (Beech-Nut):			
Junior	7½-oz. jar	150	14.9
Strained	4½-oz. jar	90	8.9
Cookie (Gerber):			
Animal-shaped	6½-gram piece	25	4.0
Arrowroot	5½-gram piece	25	4.0
Corn, creamed:			
Junior:			
(Beech-Nut)	7½-oz. jar	142	30.9
(Gerber)	7½-oz. jar	130	27.0
Strained:			
(Beech-Nut)	4½-oz. jar	85	18.5
(Gerber)	4½-oz. jar	80	17.0
Cottage cheese with pineapple juice (Beech-Nut):			
Junior	7¾-oz. jar	178	32.1
Strained	4¾-oz. jar	111	22.3
Custard:			
Apple (Beech-Nut):			
Junior	7½-oz. jar	132	27.7
Strained	4½-oz. jar	79	16.6
Chocolate (Gerber) strained	4½-oz. jar	110	3.0
Vanilla:			
Junior:			
(Beech-Nut)	7½-oz. jar	166	29.0
(Gerber)	7½-oz. jar	190	38.0
Strained:			
(Beech-Nut)	4½-oz. jar	92	15.7
(Gerber)	4½-oz. jar	100	22.0
Egg yolk (Gerber):			
Junior	3⅓-oz. jar	184	.2
Strained	3⅓-oz. jar	190	1.0
Fruit dessert:			
Junior:			
(Beech-Nut):			
Regular	7¾-oz. jar	162	40.3
Tropical	7¾-oz. jar	137	34.1
(Gerber)	7½-oz. jar	160	38.0

Food and Description	Measure or Quantity	Calories	Carbo-hydrates (grams)
Strained:			
(Beech-Nut)	4½-oz. jar	97	24.0
(Gerber)	4½-oz. jar	100	22.0
Fruit juice, mixed:			
Strained:			
(Beech-Nut)	4⅕ fl. oz.	59	14.5
(Gerber)	4.2 fl. oz.	70	15.0
Toddler (Gerber)	4 fl. oz.	60	14.0
Fruit, mixed with yogurt:			
Junior (Beech-Nut)	7½-oz. jar	120	27.3
Strained:			
(Beech-Nut)	4¾-oz. jar	76	17.3
(Gerber)	4½-oz. jar	100	21.6
Guava (Gerber) strained	4½-oz. jar	84	19.9
Guava & tapioca (Gerber) strained	4½-oz. jar	90	20.0
Ham (Gerber):			
Junior	3½-oz. jar	120	0.
Strained	3½-oz. jar	110	1.0
Ham & ham broth (Beech-Nut) strained	4½-oz. jar	143	.3
Ham with vegetables, high meat (Gerber):			
Junior	4½-oz. jar	110	10.0
Strained	4½-oz. jar	100	9.0
Ham with vegetables & cereal (Beech-Nut):			
Junior	4½-oz. jar	126	7.9
Strained	4½-oz. jar	126	7.9
Hawaiian Delight (Gerber):			
Junior	7½-oz. jar	190	42.0
Strained	4½-oz. jar	120	25.0
Isomil (*Similac*) ready-to-feed	1 fl. oz.	20	1.9
Lamb (Gerber):			
Junior	3½-oz. jar	100	0.
Strained	3½-oz. jar	100	1.0
Lamb & lamb broth (Beech-Nut):			
Junior	7½-oz. jar	265	.4
Strained	4½-oz. jar	157	.2

(USDA) = United States Department of Agriculture
(HHS/FAO) = Health and Human Services/Food and Agriculture
              Organization
* = prepared as package directs

Food and Description	Measure or Quantity	Calories	Carbo- hydrates (grams)
Macaroni alphabets with beef & tomato sauce (Gerber) toddler, chunky	6¼-oz. jar	130	20.0
Macaroni & cheese (Gerber):			
Junior	7½-oz. jar	135	18.8
Strained	4½-oz. jar	90	12.0
Macaroni & tomato with beef:			
Junior:			
(Beech-Nut)	7½-oz. jar	117	16.4
(Gerber)	7½-oz. jar	130	22.0
Strained:			
(Beech-Nut)	4½-oz. jar	81	10.7
(Gerber)	4½-oz. jar	80	12.0
Mango with tapioca (Gerber) strained	4¾-oz. jar	90	21.0
MBF (Gerber):			
Concentrate	1 fl. oz. (2 T.)	39	3.7
Concentrate	15 fl. oz. can	598	56.6
*Diluted, 1 to 1	1 fl. oz. (2 T.)	20	1.9
Meat sticks (Gerber) toddler	2½-oz. jar	110	1.0
Noodle & chicken with carrots & peas (Gerber) toddler, chunky	6-oz. jar	100	15.0
Orange-apple juice, strained:			
(Beech-Nut)	4½ fl. oz.	55	13.5
(Gerber)	4.2 fl. oz.	70	14.0
Orange-apricot juice (Beech-Nut) strained	4.2 fl. oz.	60	13.2
Orange-banana juice (Beech-Nut) strained	4⅕ fl. oz.	58	13.9
Orange juice, strained:			
(Beech-Nut)	4⅕ fl. oz.	56	13.2
(Gerber)	4.2 fl. oz.	70	14.0
Orange-pineapple dessert (Beech-Nut) strained	4¾-oz. jar	107	26.4
Orange-pineapple juice (Beech-Nut) strained	4⅕ fl. oz.	57	13.6
Orange pudding (Gerber) strained	4½-oz. jar	110	24.0
Pea:			
Junior:			
(Beech-Nut)	7¼-oz. jar	114	19.1
(Gerber)	7½-oz. jar	110	20.0
Strained:			
(Beech-Nut)	4½-oz. jar	67	11.2

Food and Description	Measure or Quantity	Calories	Carbo-hydrates (grams)
(Gerber)	4½-oz. jar	60	10.0
Pea & carrot (Beech-Nut) strained	4½-oz. jar	61	11.1
Peach:			
Junior:			
(Beech-Nut)	7¾-oz. jar	97	22.9
(Gerber)	7½-oz. jar	140	32.0
Strained:			
(Beech-Nut)	4¾-oz. jar	59	14.0
(Gerber):			
Regular	4½-oz. jar	90	19.0
First Foods	2½-oz. jar	30	7.0
Peach & apple with yogurt (Beech-Nut):			
Junior	7½-oz. jar	113	25.1
Strained	4½-oz. jar	68	15.1
Peach cobbler (Gerber):			
Junior	7½-oz. jar	160	38.0
Strained	4½-oz. jar	100	23.0
Peach melba (Beech-Nut):			
Junior	7¾-oz. jar	161	39.4
Strained	4¾-oz. jar	99	24.2
Pear:			
Junior:			
(Beech-Nut)	7½-oz. jar	106	26.2
(Gerber)	7½-oz. jar	120	27.0
Strained:			
(Beech-Nut)	4½-oz. jar	64	15.7
(Gerber):			
Regular	4½-oz. jar	80	16.0
First Foods	2½-oz. jar	40	11.0
Pear & pineapple:			
Junior:			
(Beech-Nut)	7½-oz. jar	121	29.6
(Gerber)	7½-oz. jar	109	25.4
Strained:			
(Beech-Nut)	4½-oz. serving	73	17.8
(Gerber)	4½-oz. jar	80	16.0
Pineapple dessert (Beech-Nut) strained	4¾-oz. jar	107	26.4

(USDA) = United States Department of Agriculture
(HHS/FAO) = Health and Human Services/Food and Agriculture Organization
* = prepared as package directs

Food and Description	Measure or Quantity	Calories	Carbohydrates (grams)
Pineapple with yogurt (Beech-Nut):			
Junior	7½-oz. jar	133	30.0
Strained	4¾-oz. jar	84	19.0
Plum with tapioca (Gerber):			
Junior	7½-oz. jar	160	37.0
Strained	4¾-oz. jar	100	22.0
Plum with tapioca & apple juice (Beech-Nut):			
Junior	7¾-oz. jar	120	29.3
Strained	4⅜-oz. jar	73	17.9
Pork (Gerber) strained	3½-oz. jar	110	0.
Potato & ham (Gerber) toddler, chunky	6-oz. jar	110	15.0
Pretzel (Gerber)	6-gram piece	25	5.0
Prune-orange juice (Beech-Nut) strained	4⅕ fl. oz.	66	15.7
Prune with tapioca:			
Junior (Beech-Nut)	7¾-oz. jar	174	40.5
Strained:			
(Beech-Nut)	4¾-oz. jar	107	24.8
(Gerber)	4¾-oz. jar	100	21.0
Rice & beef & tomato sauce (Gerber) toddler, chunky	6-oz. jar	150	20.0
Rice, saucy, & chicken (Gerber) toddler, chunky	6-oz. jar	110	17.0
Similac:			
Ready-to-feed or concentrated liquid, with or without added iron	1 fl. oz.	20	2.0
*Powder, regular or with iron	1 fl. oz.	20	2.0
Spaghetti, tomato & beef (Beech-Nut) junior	7½-oz. jar	131	19.4
Spaghetti with tomato sauce & beef (Gerber) junior	7½-oz. jar	140	25.0
Spinach, creamed (Gerber) strained	4½-oz. jar	60	9.0
Split pea & ham, junior:			
(Beech-Nut)	7½-oz. jar	149	23.4
(Gerber)	7½-oz. jar	150	24.0
Squash:			
Junior:			
(Beech-Nut)	7½-oz. jar	57	11.7
(Gerber)	7½-oz. jar	70	13.0

Food and Description	Measure or Quantity	Calories	Carbo- hydrates (grams)
Strained:			
(Beech-Nut)	4½-oz. jar	34	7.0
(Gerber):			
Regular	4½-oz. jar	40	8.0
First Foods	2½-oz. jar	20	4.0
Sweet potato:			
Junior:			
(Beech-Nut)	7¾-oz. jar	118	27.5
(Gerber)	7½-oz. jar	140	30.0
Strained:			
(Beech-Nut)	4½-oz. jar	68	15.9
(Gerber)	4½-oz. jar	80	18.0
Turkey (Gerber):			
Junior	3½-oz. jar	130	0.
Strained	3½-oz. jar	130	0.
Turkey & rice (Beech-Nut):			
Junior	7½-oz. jar	83	16.6
Strained	4½-oz. jar	59	12.0
Turkey & turkey broth (Beech-Nut) strained	4½-oz. jar	140	.2
Turkey with vegetables & cereal (Beech-Nut) high meat:			
Junior	4½-oz. jar	112	8.9
Strained	4½-oz. jar	112	8.9
Turkey sticks (Gerber) toddler	2½-oz. jar	120	1.0
Veal (Gerber):			
Junior	3½-oz. jar	100	0.
Strained	3½-oz. jar	100	0.
Veal & veal broth (Beech-Nut) strained	4½-oz. jar	143	.2
Veal & vegetables (Gerber):			
Junior	4½-oz. jar	110	10.0
Strained	4½-oz. jar	100	9.0
Vegetable, mixed:			
Junior:			
(Beech-Nut)	7½-oz. jar	79	17.0
(Gerber)	7½-oz. jar	90	17.0
Strained:			
(Beech-Nut):			

(USDA) = United States Department of Agriculture
(HHS/FAO) = Health and Human Services/Food and Agriculture
                    Organization
* = prepared as package directs

Food and Description	Measure or Quantity	Calories	Carbo-hydrates (grams)
Regular	4½-oz. jar	55	12.0
Garden	4½-oz. jar	66	12.5
(Gerber):			
Regular	4½-oz. jar	50	10.0
Garden	4½-oz. jar	50	8.0
Vegetable & bacon:			
Junior:			
(Beech-Nut)	7½-oz. jar	141	18.9
(Gerber)	7½-oz. jar	180	21.0
Strained:			
(Beech-Nut)	4½-oz. jar	83	9.9
(Gerber)	4½-oz. jar	100	11.0
Vegetable & beef:			
Junior:			
(Beech-Nut)	7½-oz. jar	123	18.1
(Gerber)	7½-oz. jar	140	20.0
Strained:			
(Beech-Nut)	4½-oz. jar	79	10.9
(Gerber)	4½-oz. jar	80	11.0
Vegetable & chicken:			
Junior:			
(Beech-Nut)	7½-oz. jar	89	15.9
(Gerber)	7½-oz. jar	120	18.0
Strained:			
(Beech-Nut)	4½-oz. jar	58	9.9
(Gerber)	4½-oz. jar	80	12.0
Vegetable & ham:			
Junior (Gerber)	4½-oz. jar	110	10.0
Strained:			
(Beech-Nut)	4½-oz. jar	75	10.9
(Gerber)	4½-oz. jar	80	11.0
Vegetable & lamb with rice & barley (Beech-Nut):			
Junior	7½-oz. jar	120	17.0
Strained	4½-oz. jar	74	10.0
Vegetable & liver (Gerber):			
Junior	7½-oz. jar	90	16.4
Strained	4½-oz. jar	60	11.0
Vegetable & liver with rice & barley (Beech-Nut):			
Junior	7½-oz. jar	91	16.8
Strained	4½-oz. jar	58	9.8
Vegetable & turkey:			
Junior (Gerber)	7½-oz. jar	120	19.0

Food and Description	Measure or Quantity	Calories	Carbo- hydrates (grams)
Strained:			
(Beech-Nut)	4½-oz. jar	77	12.1
(Gerber)	4½-oz. jar	70	10.0
Vegetable & turkey casserole			
(Gerber) toddler	6¼-oz. jar	147	14.2
BACON, broiled:			
(USDA):			
Medium slice	1 slice (7½ grams)	43	.1
Thick slice	1 slice (12 grams)	64	.2
Thin slice	1 slice (5 grams)	30	.2
(Hormel):			
Black Label	1 slice	30	0.
Range Brand	1 slice	55	0.
(Oscar Mayer):			
Center cut	1 slice (4 grams)	25	.1
Lower salt	1 slice	32	.1
Regular slice	6-gram slice	35	.1
Thick slice	1 slice (11 grams)	64	.2
BACON, CANADIAN,			
unheated:			
(USDA)	1 oz.	61	Tr.
(Eckrich)	1-oz. slice	35	1.0
(Hormel):			
Regular	1 oz	45	0.
Light & Lean	1 slice	17	0.
(Oscar Mayer):			
Thin	.7-oz. slice	30	0.
Thick	1-oz. slice	35	.1
BACON, SIMULATED,			
cooked:			
(Oscar Mayer) *Lean 'N Tasty:*			
Beef	1 slice (.4 oz.)	48	.2
Pork	1 slice (.4 oz.)	54	.1

(USDA) = United States Department of Agriculture
(HHS/FAO) = Health and Human Services/Food and Agriculture Organization
* = prepared as package directs

Food and Description	Measure or Quantity	Calories	Carbo-hydrates (grams)
(Swift's) *Sizzlean*:			
Beef	1 strip (4 oz.)	25	Tr.
Pork	1 strip	35	0.
BACON BITS:			
Bac*Os (Betty Crocker)	1 tsp.	12	1.0
(French's) imitation	1 tsp.	6	Tr.
(McCormick) imitation	1 tsp.	9	.7
(Oscar Mayer) real	1 tsp.	7	.1
BAGEL:			
(USDA):			
Egg	3″-dia. bagel, 1.9 oz.	162	28.3
Water	3″-dia. bagel, (1.9 oz.)	163	30.5
(Lender's):			
Plain	2-oz. bagel	150	30.0
Bagelettes	.9-oz. bagel	70	13.0
Egg	2-oz. bagel	150	29.0
Onion	1 bagel	160	31.0
Raisin & honey	2½-oz. bagel	200	40.0
Wheat & raisin with honey	2½-oz. bagel	190	39.0
BAKING POWDER:			
(USDA):			
Phosphate	1 tsp. (3.8 grams)	5	1.1
SAS	1 tsp. (3 grams)	4	.9
Tartrate	1 tsp. (2.8 grams)	2	.5
(Calumet)	1 tsp. (3.6 grams)	2	1.0
(Davis)	1 tsp. (3 grams)	7	1.7
(Featherweight) low sodium, cereal free	1 tsp.	8	2.0
BALSAMPEAR, fresh			
(HEW/FAO):			
Whole	1 lb. (weighed with cavity contents)	69	16.3
Flesh only	4 oz.	22	5.1

Food and Description	Measure or Quantity	Calories	Carbo-hydrates (grams)
BAMBOO SHOOTS:			
Raw, trimmed (USDA)	4 oz.	31	5.9
Canned, drained:			
(Chun King)	8½-oz. can	65	12.5
(La Choy)	¼ cup	6	1.0
BANANA (USDA):			
Common yellow:			
Fresh:			
Whole	1 lb. (weighed with skin)	262	68.5
Small size	5.9-oz. banana (7¾″ × 1¹¹/₃₂″)	81	21.1
Medium size	6.3-oz. banana (8¾″ × 1¹³/₃₂″)	101	26.4
Large size	7-oz. banana (9¾″ × 1⁷/₁₆″)	116	30.2
Mashed	1 cup (about 2 med.)	191	50.0
Sliced	1 cup (about 1¼ med.)	128	33.3
Dehydrated flakes	½ cup (1.8 oz.)	170	44.3
Red, fresh, whole	1 lb. (weighed with skin)	278	72.2
BANANA EXTRACT (Durkee) imitation	1 tsp.	15	DNA
BANANA NECTAR, canned (Libby's)	6 fl. oz.	110	26.0
BANANA PIE (See **PIE,** Banana)			
BARBECUE SAUCE (See **SAUCE,** Barbecue)			
BARBECUE SEASONING (French's)	1 tsp. (.1 oz.)	6	1.0

(USDA) = United States Department of Agriculture
(HHS/FAO) = Health and Human Services/Food and Agriculture Organization
* = prepared as package directs

Food and Description	Measure or Quantity	Calories	Carbohydrates (grams)
BARBERA WINE (Louis M. Martini) 12½% alcohol	3 fl. oz.	65	.2
BARDOLINO WINE (Antinori) 12% alcohol	3 fl. oz.	84	6.3
BARLEY, pearl, dry:			
Light (USDA)	¼ cup (1.8 oz.)	174	39.4
Pot or Scotch:			
(USDA)	2 oz.	197	43.8
(Quaker) Scotch	¼ cup (1.7 oz.)	172	36.3
BASIL:			
Fresh (HEW/FAO) sweet, leaves	½ oz.	6	1.0
Dried (French's)	1 tsp.	3	.7
BASS (USDA):			
Black Sea:			
Raw, whole	1 lb. (weighed whole)	165	0.
Baked, stuffed, home recipe	4 oz.	294	12.9
Smallmouth & largemouth, raw:			
Whole	1 lb. (weighed whole)	146	0.
Meat only	4 oz.	118	0.
Striped:			
Raw, whole	1 lb. (weighed whole)	205	0.
Raw, meat only	4 oz.	119	0.
Oven-fried	4 oz.	222	7.6
White, raw, meat only	4 oz.	111	0.
BATMAN, cereal (Ralston Purina)	1 cup (1 oz.)	110	25.0
BAY LEAF (French's)	1 tsp.	5	1.0
***B & B* LIQUEUR,** 86 proof	1 fl. oz.	94	5.7
B.B.Q. SAUCE & BEEF, frozen (Banquet) *Cookin' Bag,* sliced	4-oz. pkg.	100	11.0

Food and Description	Measure or Quantity	Calories	Carbo-hydrates (grams)
BEAN, BAKED:			
(USDA):			
With pork & molasses sauce	1 cup (9 oz.)	382	53.8
With pork & tomato sauce	1 cup (9 oz.)	311	48.5
With tomato sauce	1 cup (9 oz.)	306	58.7
Canned:			
(Allen's) *Wagon Master*	1 cup	260	48.0
(B&M) *Brick Oven:*			
Barbecue style	8 oz.	310	48.0
Pea bean with pork in brown sugar sauce	8 oz.	300	42.0
Red kidney or yellow eye bean in brown sugar sauce	8 oz.	290	42.0
Vegetarian	8 oz.	250	42.0
(Campbell's):			
Home style	8-oz. can	220	48.0
With pork & tomato sauce	8-oz. can	270	49.0
Old fashioned, in molasses & brown sugar sauce	8-oz. can	230	49.0
& pork, in tomato suace	8-oz. can	200	43.0
Vegetarian	7¾-oz. can	170	40.0
(Furman's) & pork, in tomato sauce	8-oz. serving	245	46.4
(Grandma Brown's) home baked	8-oz. serving	289	54.1
(Hunt's) & pork	8-oz. serving	280	52.0
(Town House) & pork	1 cup	260	48.0
BEAN, BARBECUE			
(Campbell's)	7⅞-oz. can	210	43.0
BEAN, BLACK OR BROWN:			
Dry (USDA)	1 cup	678	122.4
Canned (Goya)	1 cup	250	42.0
BEAN, CANNELLINI,			
canned (Progresso)	1 cup	160	38.0

(USDA) = United States Department of Agriculture
(HHS/FAO) = Health and Human Services/Food and Agriculture
                        Organization
* = prepared as package directs

Food and Description	Measure or Quantity	Calories	Carbo-hydrates (grams)
BEAN, FAVA, canned (Progresso)	4 oz. serving	90	15.5
BEAN, GARBANZO (See **CHICK-PEAS**)			
BEAN, GREEN:			
Fresh (USDA):			
Whole	1 lb. (weighed untrimmed)	128	28.3
French style	½ cup (1.4 oz.)	13	2.8
Boiled (USDA):			
Whole, drained	½ cup (2.2 oz.)	16	3.3
Boiled, 1½″ to 2″ pieces, drained	½ cup (2.4 oz.)	17	3.7
Canned, regular pack:			
(USDA):			
Whole, solids & liq.	½ cup (4.2 oz.)	22	5.0
Whole, drained solids	4 oz.	27	5.9
Cut, drained solids	½ cup (2.5 oz.)	17	3.6
Drained liquid only	4 oz.	11	2.7
(Allen's) solids & liq:			
Whole	½ cup (4.2 oz.)	21	4.0
Cut	½ cup (4 oz.)	25	4.0
French	½ cup (4.1 oz.)	25	4.0
(Green Giant) french or whole, solids & liq.	½ cup	20	4.0
(Larsen) *Freshlike*, solids & liq.	½ cup	20	4.0
(Town House) cut or french style	½ cup	20	4.0
Canned, dietetic or low calorie:			
(USDA):			
Solids & liq.	4 oz.	18	4.1
Drained solids	4 oz.	25	5.4
(Diet Delight) solids & liq.	½ cup (4.2 oz.)	20	3.0
(Featherweight) solids & liq.	½ cup (4 oz.)	25	5.0
(Larsen) *Fresh-Lite*, water pack	½ cup (4.2 oz.)	20	4.0
(S&W) *Nutradiet*, green label, solids & liq.	½ cup	20	4.0
Frozen:			
(Bel-Air):			
Cut or whole	3 oz.	25	6.0

Food and Description	Measure or Quantity	Calories	Carbo-hydrates (grams)
French style:			
Plain	3 oz.	25	6.0
With toasted almonds	3 oz.	45	10.0
Italian	3 oz.	35	7.0
(Birds Eye):			
Cut:			
Plain	¼ of 12-oz. pkg.	25	5.8
With mushrooms	5-oz. serving	70	9.4
French:			
Plain	⅓ of 9-oz. pkg.	26	6.0
With toasted almonds	⅓ of 9-oz. pkg.	52	8.4
Petite, deluxe	⅓ of 8-oz. pkg.	20	4.6
Whole	⅓ of 9-oz. pkg.	23	5.1
(Frosty Acres)	3-oz. serving	25	6.0
(Green Giant):			
Cut or french, with butter sauce	½ cup	30	4.0
Cut, *Harvest Fresh*	½ cup	16	4.0
With mushroom in cream sauce	½ cup	80	10.0
Polybag	½ cup	14	4.0
(Larsen)	3 oz.	25	6.0

BEAN, GREEN, & MUSHROOM CASSEROLE,
frozen (Stouffer's) — ½ of 9½-oz. pkg. — 160 — 13.0

BEAN, GREEN, PUREE,
canned (Larsen) no salt added — ½ cup (4.4 oz.) — 35 — 7.5

BEAN, ITALIAN:

Food and Description	Measure or Quantity	Calories	Carbo-hydrates (grams)
Canned (Del Monte) cut, solids & liq.	4 oz.	25	6.0
Frozen:			
(Birds Eye)	⅓ of pkg. (3 oz.)	31	7.2
(Frosty Acres)	3-oz. serving	30	7.0
(Larsen)	3 oz.	30	7.0

(USDA) = United States Department of Agriculture
(HHS/FAO) = Health and Human Services/Food and Agriculture Organization
* = prepared as package directs

Food and Description	Measure or Quantity	Calories	Carbo-hydrates (grams)
BEAN, KIDNEY OR RED:			
(USDA):			
Dry	½ cup (3.3 oz.)	319	57.6
Cooked	½ cup (3.3 oz.)	109	19.8
Canned, regular pack, solids & liq.:			
(Allen's)	½ cup (4.1 oz.)	110	20.0
(Furman's) red, fancy, light	½ cup (4½ oz.)	121	21.2
(Goya):			
Red	½ cup	115	20.0
White	½ cup	100	18.5
(Hunt's):			
Regular	½ cup (3.5 oz.)	80	16.0
Small red	4 oz.	120	21.0
(Progresso) red	½ cup	100	21.0
(Town House) dark or light	½ cup	110	20.0
Canned, dietetic (S&W) *Nutradiet*, low sodium, green label	½ cup	90	16.0
BEAN, LIMA:			
Raw (USDA):			
Young, whole	1 lb. (weighed in pod)	223	40.1
Mature, dry	½ cup (3.4 oz.)	331	61.4
Young, without shell	1 lb. (weighed shelled)	558	100.2
Boiled (USDA) drained	½ cup	94	16.8
Canned, regular pack:			
(USDA):			
Solids & liq.	4 oz.	81	15.2
Drained solids	4 oz.	109	20.8
(Allen's):			
Regular	½ cup	60	9.0
Butter, large	½ cup	105	19.0
(Furman's)	½ cup	92	16.7
(Larsen) *Freshlike*, solids & liq.	½ cup (4 oz.)	80	16.0
(Town House) butter	½ cup	100	18.0
Canned, dietetic, solids & liq.:			
(Featherweight)	½ cup	80	16.0
(Larsen) *Fresh-Lite*, water pack, no salt added	½ cup (4.4 oz.)	80	16.0

Food and Description	Measure or Quantity	Calories	Carbo-hydrates (grams)
Frozen:			
(Birds Eye):			
Baby	⅓ of 10-oz. pkg.	126	24.1
Fordhook	⅓ of 10-oz. pkg.	99	18.5
(Frosty Acres):			
Baby	3.3 oz.	130	24.0
Butter	3.3 oz.	140	26.0
Fordhook	3.3 oz.	100	19.0
(Green Giant):			
In butter sauce	½ cup	83	20.4
Harvest Fresh, or polybag	½ cup	60	15.0
(Larsen) baby	3.3 oz.	130	24.0
BEAN, MUNG (USDA) dry	½ cup (3.7 oz.)	357	63.3
BEAN, PINK, canned			
(Goya) solids & liq.	½ cup	115	20.5
BEAN, PINTO:			
Dry (USDA)	4 oz.	396	72.2
Canned:			
(Gebhardt)	½ of 15-oz. can	370	67.0
(Goya):			
Regular	½ cup (4 oz.)	100	18.0
Butter	½ cup	105	17.5
(Green Giant)	½ cup	100	21.0
(Old El Paso)	½ cup	100	19.0
(Progresso)	½ cup (4 oz.)	82	16.5
(Town House)	½ cup	105	18.5
Frozen (McKenzie)	3.2-oz. serving	160	29.0
BEAN, REFRIED, canned:			
(Gebhardt):			
Regular	4 oz.	130	20.0
Jalapeño	4 oz.	110	18.0
Little Pancho (Borden) & green chili	½ cup	80	15.0
(Old El Paso):			
Plain	½ cup	110	16.0
With bacon	½ cup	208	24.0

(USDA) = United States Department of Agriculture
(HHS/FAO) = Health and Human Services/Food and Agriculture Organization
* = prepared as package directs

Food and Description	Measure or Quantity	Calories	Carbo-hydrates (grams)
With cheese	½ cup	72	8.0
With green chili	½ cup	98	16.0
With jalapeños	½ cup	62	8.0
With sausage	½ cup	360	16.0
Spicy	½ cup	70	10.0
Vegetarian	½ cup	140	30.0
(Rosarita):			
Regular	4 oz.	130	20.0
Bacon	4 oz.	132	19.6
With beans & onion	4 oz.	125	20.0
With green chilis	4 oz.	116	18.5
With nacho cheese & onion	4 oz.	135	21.1
Spicy	4 oz.	120	18.7
Vegetarian	4 oz.	120	18.7
BEAN, ROMAN, canned, solids & liq:			
(Goya)	½ cup (2.3 oz.)	81	15.0
(Progresso)	½ cup	110	18.0
BEAN, YELLOW OR WAX:			
Raw, whole (USDA)	1 lb. (weighed untrimmed)	108	24.0
Boiled (USDA) 1″ pieces, drained	½ cup (2.9 oz.)	18	3.7
Canned, regular pack, solids & liq.:			
(Comstock)	½ cup (4.2 oz.)	20	4.0
(Larsen) *Freshlike*, cut, solids & liq.	½ cup (4.2 oz.)	25	5.0
Canned, dietetic, (Featherweight) cut stringless, solids & liq.	½ cup (4 oz.)	25	5.0
(Larsen) *Fresh-Lite*, cut, water pack, no salt added	½ cup (4.2 oz.)	18	4.0
Frozen:			
(Frosty Acres)	3 oz.	25	5.0
(Larsen) cut	3 oz.	25	5.0
BEANS 'N FIXIN'S, canned (Hunt's) *Big John's*:			
Beans	3 oz.	100	21.0
Fixin's	1 oz.	50	7.0

Food and Description	Measure or Quantity	Calories	Carbo-hydrates (grams)
BEAN & FRANKFURTER, canned:			
(USDA)	1 cup (9 oz.)	367	32.1
(Hormel) *Short Orders,* 'n wieners	7½-oz. can	280	39.0
BEAN & FRANKFURTER DINNER, frozen:			
(Banquet)	10-oz. dinner	520	57.0
(Morton)	10-oz. dinner	350	46.0
(Swanson) 3-compartment	10½-oz. dinner	440	53.0
BEAN SALAD, canned (Green Giant) three bean, solids & liq.	¼ of 17-oz. can	70	15.0
BEAN SOUP (See **SOUP,** Bean)			
BEAN SPROUT:			
Fresh (USDA):			
Mung, raw	½ lb.	80	15.0
Mung, boiled, drained	¼ lb.	32	5.9
Soy, raw	½ lb.	104	12.0
Soy, boiled, drained	¼ lb.	43	4.2
Canned, drained:			
(Chun King)	4 oz.	40	5.9
(La Choy)	⅔ cup (2 oz.)	6	1.4
BEAR CLAWS (Dolly Madison):			
Cherry	2¾-oz. piece	270	36.0
Cinnamon	2¾-oz. piece	290	39.0

BEEF. Values for beef cuts are given below for "leans and fat" and for "lean only." Beef purchased by the consumer at the retail store usually is trimmed to about one-half-inch layer of fat. This is the meat described as "lean

Food and Description	Measure or Quantity	Calories	Carbo- hydrates (grams)
and fat." If all the fat that can be cut off with a knife is removed, the remainder is the "lean only." These cuts still contain flecks of fat known as "marbling" distrib- uted through the meat. Cooked meats are medium done. Choice grade cuts (USDA):			
Brisket:			
Raw	1 lb. (weighed with bone)	1284	0.
Braised:			
Lean & fat	4 oz.	467	0.
Lean only	4 oz.	252	0.
Chuck:			
Raw	1 lb. (weighed with bone)	984	0.
Braised or pot-roasted:			
Lean & fat	4 oz.	371	0.
Lean only	4 oz.	243	0.
Dried (See **BEEF, CHIPPED**)			
Fat, separable, cooked	1 oz.	207	0.
Filet mignon. There is no data available on its composition. For dietary estimates, the data for sirloin steak, lean only, afford the closest approximation.			
Flank:			
Raw	1 lb.	653	0.
Braised	4 oz.	222	0.
Foreshank:			
Raw	1 lb. (weighed with bone)	531	0.
Simmered:			
Lean & fat	4 oz.	310	0.
Lean only	4 oz.	209	0.
Ground:			
Lean:			
Raw	1 lb.	812	0.
Raw	1 cup (8 oz.)	405	0.
Broiled	4 oz.	248	0.
Regular:			
Raw	1 lb.	1216	0.
Raw	1 cup (8 oz.)	606	0.

Food and Description	Measure or Quantity	Calories	Carbo-hydrates (grams)
Broiled	4 oz.	324	0.
Heel of round:			
Raw	1 lb.	966	0.
Roasted:			
Lean & fat	4 oz.	296	0.
Lean only	4 oz.	204	0.
Hindshank:			
Raw	1 lb. (weighed with bone)	604	0.
Simmered:			
Lean & fat	4 oz.	409	0.
Lean only	4 oz.	209	0.
Neck:			
Raw	1 lb. (weighed with bone)	820	0.
Pot-roasted:			
Lean & fat	4 oz.	332	0.
Lean only	4 oz.	222	0.
Plate:			
Raw	1 lb. (weighed with bone)	1615	0.
Simmered:			
Lean & fat	4 oz.	538	0.
Lean only	4 oz.	252	0.
Rib roast:			
Raw	1 lb. (weighed with bone)	1673	0.
Roasted:			
Lean & fat	4 oz.	499	0.
Lean only	4 oz.	273	0.
Round:			
Raw	1 lb. (weighed with bone)	863	0.
Broiled:			
Lean & fat	4 oz.	296	0.
Lean only	4 oz.	214	0.
Rump:			
Raw	1 lb. (weighed with bone)	1167	0.

(USDA) = United States Department of Agriculture
(HHS/FAO) = Health and Human Services/Food and Agriculture Organization
* = prepared as package directs

Food and Description	Measure or Quantity	Calories	Carbo-hydrates (grams)
Roasted:			
Lean & fat	4 oz.	393	0.
Lean only	4 oz.	236	0.
Steak, club:			
Raw	1 lb. (weighed without bone)	1724	0.
Broiled:			
Lean & fat	4 oz.	515	0.
Lean only	4 oz.	277	0.
One 8-oz. steak (weighed without bone before cooking) will give you:			
Lean & fat	5.9 oz.	754	0.
Lean only	3.4 oz.	234	0.
Steak, porterhouse:			
Raw	1 lb. (weighed with bone)	1603	0.
Broiled:			
Lean & fat	4 oz.	527	0.
Lean only	4 oz.	254	0.
One 16-oz. steak (weighed with bone before cooking) will give you:			
Lean & fat	10.2 oz.	1339	0.
Lean only	5.9 oz.	372	0.
Steak, ribeye, broiled:			
One 10-oz. steak (weighed before cooking without bone) will give you:			
Lean & fat	7.3 oz.	911	0.
Lean only	3.8 oz.	258	0.
Steak, sirloin, double-bone:			
Raw	1 lb. (weighed with bone)	1240	0.
Broiled:			
Lean & fat	4 oz.	463	0.
Lean only	4 oz.	245	0.
One 12-oz. steak (weighed before cooking with bone) will give you:			
Lean & fat	6.6 oz.	767	0.
Lean only	4.4 oz.	268	0.
One 16-oz. steak (weighed before cooking with			

Food and Description	Measure or Quantity	Calories	Carbo-hydrates (grams)
bone) will give you:			
Lean & fat	8.9 oz.	1028	0.
Lean only	5.9 oz.	359	0.
Steak, sirloin, hipbone:			
Raw	1 lb. (weighed with bone)	1585	0.
Broiled:			
Lean & fat	4 oz.	552	0.
Lean only	4 oz.	272	0.
Steak, sirloin, wedge & round-bone:			
Raw	1 lb. (weighed with bone)	1316	0.
Broiled:			
Lean & fat	4 oz.	439	0.
Lean only	4 oz.	235	0.
Steak, T-bone:			
Raw	1 lb. (weighed with bone)	1596	0.
Broiled:			
Lean & fat	4 oz.	536	0.
Lean only	4 oz.	253	0.
One 16-oz. steak (weighed before cooking with bone) will give you:			
Broiled:			
Lean & fat	4 oz.	463	0.
Lean only	4 oz.	245	0.
BEEFAMATO COCKTAIL, canned (Mott's)	6 fl. oz.	80	19.0
BEEF BOUILLON:			
(Borden) *Lite-Line*	1 tsp.	12	2.0
(Herb-Ox):			
Cube	1 cube	6	.7
Packet	1 packet	8	.9
(Knorr)	1 cube	15	.5
(Wyler's)	1 cube	6	1.0
Low sodium (Featherweight)	1 tsp.	18	2.0

(USDA) = United States Department of Agriculture
(HHS/FAO) = Health and Human Services/Food and Agriculture Organization
* = prepared as package directs

Food and Description	Measure or Quantity	Calories	Carbo-hydrates (grams)
BEEF, CHIPPED:			
Cooked, creamed, home recipe			
(USDA)	½ cup (4.3 oz.)	188	8.7
Frozen, creamed:			
(Banquet)	4-oz. pkg.	100	9.0
(Stouffer's)	5½-oz. serving	230	9.0
BEEF DINNER OR ENTREE:			
*Canned (Hunt's) *Entree Maker*, oriental	7.6-oz. serving	271	14.0
Frozen:			
(Armour):			
Classic Lite, Steak Diane	10-oz. meal	290	25.0
Dining Lite, teriyaki	9-oz. meal	270	36.0
Dinner Classics:			
Sirloin roast	10.4-oz. meal	190	21.0
Sirloin tips	10¼-oz. meal	230	20.0
(Banquet):			
Dinner, chopped	11-oz. dinner	420	14.0
Dinner, *Extra Helping*	16-oz. dinner	870	50.0
Platter	10-oz. meal	460	20.0
(Chun King) Szechuan	13-oz. entree	340	57.0
(Healthy Choice) sirloin tips	11¾-oz. meal	290	33.0
(La Choy) *Fresh & Lite*, & broccoli, with rice	11-oz. meal	260	42.0
(Le Menu):			
Chopped sirloin	12¼-oz. dinner	430	28.0
Sirloin tips	11½-oz. dinner	400	29.0
(Morton) sliced	10-oz. dinner	220	20.0
(Stouffer's):			
Lean Cuisine:			
Oriental, with vegetable & rice	8⅝-oz. meal	250	28.0
Szechuan, with noodles & vegetables	9¼-oz. meal	260	22.0
Right Course:			
Dijon, with pasta & vegetables	9½-oz. meal	290	31.0
Fiesta, with corn & pasta	8⅞-oz. meal	270	23.0
Ragout, with rice pilaf	10-oz. meal	300	38.0
(Swanson):			
4-compartment dinner:			
Regular	11¼-oz. dinner	310	38.0
In barbecue sauce	11-oz. dinner	460	51.0
Chopped sirloin	10¾-oz. dinner	340	28.0

Food and Description	Measure or Quantity	Calories	Carbo- hydrates (grams)
Homestyle Recipe, sirloin tips	7-oz. meal	160	16.0
Hungry Man:			
Chopped	16¾-oz. dinner	640	41.0
Sliced	15¼-oz. dinner	450	49.0
(Weight Watchers):			
London broil in mushroom suace	7.4-oz. meal	140	9.0
Sirloin tips & mushrooms in wine sauce	7½-oz. meal	250	23.0
BEEF, DRIED, packaged:			
(Carl Buddig) smoked	1 oz.	38	Tr.
(Hormel) sliced	1 oz.	45	0.
BEEF GOULASH (Hormel)			
Short Orders	7½-oz. can	230	17.0
BEEF, GROUND, SEASON- ING MIX:			
*(Durkee):			
Regular	1 cup	653	9.0
With onion	1 cup	659	6.5
(French's) with onion	1⅛-oz. pkg.	100	24.0
BEEF HASH, ROAST:			
Canned, *Mary Kitchen* (Hormel):			
Regular	7½-oz. serving	350	18.0
Short Orders	7½-oz. can	360	18.0
Frozen (Stouffer's)	10-oz. meal	380	16.0
BEEF, PACKAGED:			
(Carl Buddig) smoked	1 oz.	38	Tr.
(Hormel)	1 oz.	50	0.
(Safeway)	1 oz.	60	1.0
BEEF, PEPPER, ORIENTAL:			
Canned (La Choy)	¾ cup	90	10.0

(USDA) = United States Department of Agriculture
(HHS/FAO) = Health and Human Services/Food and Agriculture Organization
* = prepared as package directs

Food and Description	Measure or Quantity	Calories	Carbo-hydrates (grams)
Frozen:			
(Chun King)	13-oz. entree	310	53.0
(La Choy)	12-oz. dinner	250	45.0
BEEF PIE, frozen:			
(Banquet)	7-oz. pie	510	39.0
(Empire Kosher)	8-oz. pie	540	51.0
(Morton)	7-oz. pie	430	27.0
(Stouffer's)	10-oz. pie	500	33.0
(Swanson):			
Regular	7-oz. pie	370	36.0
Hungry Man	16-oz. pie	610	58.0
BEEF, POTTED (USDA)	1 oz.	70	0.
BEEF, SHORT RIBS, frozen:			
(Armour) *Dinner Classics,* boneless	9¾-oz. meal	380	34.0
(Stouffer's) boneless, with gravy	9-oz. entree	350	12.0
BEEF SOUP (See **SOUP,** Beef)			
BEEF SPREAD, ROAST, canned:			
(Hormel)	1 oz.	62	0.
(Underwood)	½ of 4¾-oz. can	140	Tr.
BEEF STEW:			
Home recipe, made with lean beef chuck	1 cup (8.6 oz.)	218	15.2
Canned, regular pack:			
Dinty Moore (Hormel):			
Regular	⅓ of 24-oz. can	220	15.0
Short Orders	7½-oz. can	180	14.0
(Libby's)	7½-oz. serving	160	18.0
Canned, dietetic:			
(Estee)	7½-oz. serving	210	15.0
(Featherweight)	7½-oz. serving	220	24.0
Frozen (Banquet) *Family Entree*	2-lb. pkg.	560	72.0
Mix (Lipton) *Microeasy,* hearty	¼ pkg.	70	14.1

Food and Description	Measure or Quantity	Calories	Carbo-hydrates (grams)
BEEF STEW SEASONING MIX:			
*(Durkee)	1 cup	379	16.7
(French's)	1⅛-oz. pkg.	150	30.0
BEEF STOCK BASE (French's)	1 tsp (.13 oz.)	8	2.0
BEEF STROGANOFF, frozen:			
(Le Menu)	10-oz. dinner	430	28.0
(Stouffer's) with parsley noodles	9¾-oz. pkg.	390	28.0
(Weight Watchers)	9-oz. meal	320	27.0
BEER & ALE:			
Regular:			
Anheuser	12 fl. oz.	167	15.4
Black Label	12 fl. oz.	136	11.2
Blatz	12 fl. oz.	142	11.8
Budweiser: Busch Bavarian	12 fl. oz.	142	11.1
C. Schmidt's	12 fl. oz.	136	11.2
Michelob, regular	12 fl. oz.	152	13.6
Old Milwaukee	12 fl. oz.	142	13.4
Old Style	12 fl. oz.	147	12.1
Pearl Premium	12 fl. oz.	148	12.3
(Schlitz)	12 fl. oz.	150	13.2
Light or low carbohydrate:			
Budweiser Light	12 fl. oz.	110	6.7
LA	12 fl. oz.	112	15.8
Natural Light	12 fl. oz.	110	6.0
Michelob Light	12 fl. oz.	134	11.5
Old Milwaukee	12 fl. oz.	120	9.2
Pearl Light	12 fl. oz.	68	2.3
Schmidt Light	12 fl. oz.	96	3.2
BEER, NEAR:			
Goetz Pale	12 fl. oz.	78	3.9
(Metbrew)	12 fl. oz.	73	13.7
BEET:			
Raw (USDA):			

(USDA) = United States Department of Agriculture
(HHS/FAO) = Health and Human Services/Food and Agriculture Organization
* = prepared as package directs

Food and Description	Measure or Quantity	Calories	Carbohydrates (grams)
Whole	1 lb. (weighed with skins, without tops)	137	31.4
Diced	½ cup (2.4 oz.)	29	6.6
Boiled (USDA) drained:			
Whole	2 beets (2″ dia., 3.5 oz.)	32	7.2
Diced	½ cup (3 oz.)	27	6.1
Sliced	½ cup (3.6 oz.)	33	7.3
Canned, regular pack, solids & liq.:			
(Larsen) *Freshlike:*			
Pickled	½ cup (4.3 oz.)	100	25.0
Sliced or whole	½ cup (4.7 oz.)	40	9.0
(Town House):			
Regular	½ cup	35	8.0
Pickled	½ cup	80	19.0
Canned, dietetic, solids & liq.:			
(Del Monte) no salt added	½ cup (4 oz.)	35	8.0
(Featherweight) sliced	½ cup	45	10.0
(Larsen) *Fresh-Lite*, sliced, water pack, no salt added	½ cup (4.3 oz.)	40	9.0
(S&W) *Nutradiet*, sliced, green label	½ cup	35	9.0
BEET GREENS (USDA):			
Raw, whole	1 lb. (weighed untrimmed)	61	11.7
Boiled, halves & stems, drained	½ cup (2.6 oz.)	13	2.4
BEET PUREE, canned (Larsen) no salt added	½ cup (4.7 oz.)	45	10.0
BÉNÉDICTINE LIQUEUR (Julius Wile) 86 proof	1 fl. oz.	112	10.3
BERRY BEARS, *Fruit Corners* (General Mills)	.9-oz. pouch	100	22.0
BERRY DRINK, MIXED:			
Canned (Johanna Farms) *Ssips*	8.45-fl.-oz. container	130	32.0
*Mix, *Crystal Light* (General Foods)	8 fl. oz.	3	Tr.

Food and Description	Measure or Quantity	Calories	Carbo-hydrates (grams)
BIGG MIXX, cereal (Kellogg's):			
Plain	½ cup (1 oz.)	110	24.0
Raisin	½ cup (1.3 oz.)	140	31.0
BIG MAC (See **McDONALD'S**)			
BISCUIT DOUGH (Pillsbury):			
Baking powder, *1869 Brand*	1 piece	100	12.0
Butter	1 piece	50	10.0
Buttermilk:			
Regular	1 piece	50	10.0
Ballard Ovenready	1 piece	50	10.0
Big Country	1 piece	100	14.0
1869 Brand	1 piece	100	12.0
Heat 'n Eat	1 piece	85	13.5
Hungry Jack:			
Extra rich	1 piece	50	9.0
Flaky	1 piece	80	12.0
Fluffy	1 piece	90	12.0
Tender layer	1 piece	60	9.0
Butter Tastin':			
Big Country	1 piece	100	14.0
1869 Brand	1 piece	100	12.0
Country	1 piece	50	10.0
Flaky, *Hungry Jack:*			
Regular	1 piece	80	12.0
Butter Tastin'	1 piece	90	11.0
Honey	1 piece	90	13.0
Fluffy, *Good 'n Buttery*	1 piece	90	11.0
Heat 'n Eat, Big Premium	1 piece	140	16.0
Ovenready, Ballard	1 piece	50	10.0
Southern style, *Big Country*	1 piece	100	14.0
BITTERS (Angostura)	1 tsp.	14	2.1
BLACKBERRY:			
Fresh (USDA) includes boysenberry, dewberry, youngsberry:			

(USDA) = United States Department of Agriculture
(HHS/FAO) = Health and Human Services/Food and Agriculture Organization
* = prepared as package directs

Food and Description	Measure or Quantity	Calories	Carbo-hydrates (grams)
With hulls	1 lb. (weighed untrimmed)	250	55.6
Hulled	½ cup (2.6 oz.)	41	9.4
Canned, regular pack (USDA) solids & liq.:			
Juice pack	4-oz. serving	61	13.7
Light syrup	4-oz. serving	82	19.6
Heavy syrup	½ cup (4.6 oz.)	118	28.9
Extra heavy syrup	4-oz. serving	125	30.7
Frozen (USDA):			
Sweetened, unthawed	4-oz. serving	109	27.7
Unsweetened, unthawed	4-oz. serving	55	12.9
BLACKBERRY JELLY:			
Sweetened (Smucker's)	1 T. (.7 oz.)	54	12.0
Dietetic:			
(Diet Delight)	1 T. (.6 oz.)	12	3.0
(Featherweight) imitation	1 T.	16	4.0
BLACKBERRY LIQUEUR			
(Bols)	1 fl. oz.	95	8.9
BLACKBERRY PRESERVE OR JAM:			
Sweetened (Smucker's)	1 T. (.7 oz.)	54	12.0
Dietetic:			
(Estee, Louis Sherry)	1 T. (.6 oz.)	6	0.
(Featherweight)	1 T.	16	4.0
(S&W) *Nutradiet*, red label	1 T.	12	3.0
BLACKBERRY WINE (Mogen David)	3 fl. oz.	135	18.7
BLACK-EYED PEAS:			
Canned, with pork, solids & liq:			
(Allen's) regular	½ cup	100	16.0
(Goya)	½ cup	105	19.5
(Green Giant)	½ cup	90	18.0
(Town House)	½ cup	105	19.5
Frozen:			
(Frosty Acres; McKenzie; Seabrook Farms)	⅓ of pkg. (3.3 oz.)	130	23.0
(Southland)	⅕ of 16-oz. pkg.	120	21.0

Food and Description	Measure or Quantity	Calories	Carbo-hydrates (grams)
BLINTZE, frozen:			
(Empire Kosher):			
Apple	2½ oz.	100	24.0
Blueberry or cherry	2½ oz.	110	25.0
Cheese	2½ oz.	110	20.0
Potato	2½ oz.	130	21.0
(King Kold) cheese	2½ oz.	132	21.4
BLOODY MARY MIX:			
Dry (Bar-Tender's)	1 serving	26	5.7
Liquid:			
(Holland House) *Smooth N' Spicy*	1 fl. oz.	3	<1.0
(Libby's)	6 fl. oz.	40	9.0
Tabasco	6 fl. oz.	56	5.0
BLUEBERRY:			
Fresh (USDA):			
Whole	1 lb. (weighed untrimmed)	259	63.8
Trimmed	½ cup (2.6 oz.)	45	11.2
Canned, solids & liq.:			
(USDA):			
Syrup pack, extra heavy	½ cup (4.4 oz.)	126	32.5
Water pack	½ cup (4.3 oz.)	47	11.9
(Thank You Brand):			
Heavy syrup	½ cup (4.3 oz.)	102	25.4
Water pack	½ cup (4.2 oz.)	48	12.0
Frozen (USDA):			
Sweetened, solids & liq.	½ cup (4 oz.)	120	30.2
Unsweetened, solids & liq.	½ cup (2.9 oz.)	45	11.2
BLUEBERRY PIE (See **PIE,** Blueberry)			
BLUEBERRY PRESERVE OR JAM:			
Sweetened (Smucker's)	1 T.	54	12.0
Dietetic (Estee, Louis Sherry)	1 T.	6	0.

(USDA) = United States Department of Agriculture
(HHS/FAO) = Health and Human Services/Food and Agriculture Organization
* = prepared as package directs

Food and Description	Measure or Quantity	Calories	Carbo-hydrates (grams)
BLUEBERRY SQUARES, cereal (Kellogg's)	½ cup (1 oz.)	90	23.0
BLUEFISH (USDA):			
Raw:			
Whole	1 lb. (weighed whole)	271	0.
Meat only	4 oz.	133	0.
Baked or broiled	4.4-oz. piece (3½″ × 3″ × ½″)	199	0.
Fried	5.3-oz. piece (3½″ × 3″ × ½″)	308	7.0
BODY BUDDIES, cereal (General Mills) natural fruit flavor	1 cup (1 oz.)	110	24.0
BOLOGNA:			
(Eckrich):			
Beef:			
Regular	1 oz.	90	2.0
Smorgas Pak:	¾-oz. slice	70	1.0
Thick slice	1½-oz. slice	140	2.0
Thin slice	1 slice	55	1.0
Garlic	1-oz. slice	90	2.0
German Brand, sliced or chub	1-oz. slice	80	1.0
Lunch chub	1-oz. serving	100	2.0
Meat:			
Regular	1-oz. slice	90	2.0
Thick slice	1.7-oz. slice	160	3.0
Thin slice	1 slice	55	1.0
Ring or sandwich	1-oz. slice	90	2.0
Hebrew National, beef	1 oz.	90	<1.0
(Hormel):			
Beef:			
Regular	1 slice	85	.5
Coarse grind	1 oz.	80	.5
Meat:			
Regular	1 slice	90	0.
Light & Lean:			
Regular	1 slice	70	1.0
Thin slice	1 slice	35	.5

Food and Description	Measure or Quantity	Calories	Carbo-hydrates (grams)
(Ohse):			
Beef	1 oz.	85	1.0
Chicken, 15%	1 oz.	90	1.0
Chicken, beef & pork	1 oz.	75	3.0
(Oscar Mayer):			
Beef	.5-oz. slice	48	.5
Beef	1-oz. slice	90	.6
Beef Lebanon	.8-oz. slice	47	.3
Meat	1-oz. slice	90	.7
(Smok-A-Roma):			
Beef	1-oz. slice	90	1.0
Galric	1-oz. slice	70	1.0
German	1-oz. slice	80	1.0
Meat:			
Regular	1 slice	90	1.0
Thick sliced	1 slice	180	2.0
15% chicken	1-oz. slice	90	1.0
Turkey	1-oz. slice	60	1.0
BOLOGNA & CHEESE:			
(Eckrich)	.7-oz. slice	90	2.0
(Oscar Mayer)	.8-oz. slice	74	.6
BONITO:			
Raw (USDA) meat only	4 oz.	191	0.
Canned (Star-Kist):			
Chunk	6½-oz. can	605	0.
Solid	7-oz. can	650	0.
BOO*BERRY, cereal			
(General Mills)	1 cup (1 oz.)	110	24.0
BORSCHT:			
Regular:			
(Gold's)	8-oz. serving	100	21.0
(Manischewitz) with beets	8-oz. serving	80	20.0
(Rokeach)	1 cup (8 oz.)	96	21.5

(USDA) = United States Department of Agriculture
(HHS/FAO) = Health and Human Services/Food and Agriculture Organization
* = prepared as package directs

Food and Description	Measure or Quantity	Calories	Carbohydrates (grams)
Dietetic or low calorie:			
(Gold's)	8-oz. serving	20	5.0
(Manischewitz)	8-oz. serving	20	4.0
(Rokeach):	8-oz. serving	27	6.7
Diet	1 cup (8 oz.)	15	4.0
Unsalted	1 cup (8 oz.)	103	23.0

BOURBON (See **DISTILLED LIQUOR**)

BOSCO (See **SYRUP**)

BOYSENBERRY:

Fresh (See **BLACKBERRY**)			
Frozen (USDA) sweetened	10-oz. pkg.	273	69.3

BOYSENBERRY JELLY:

Sweetened (Smucker's)	1 T. (.7 oz.)	54	12.0
Dietetic (S&W) *Nutradiet*, red label	1 T.	12	3.0

BOYSENBERRY JUICE,

canned (Smucker's)	8 fl. oz.	120	30.0

BRAINS, all animals

(USDA) raw	4 oz.	142	.9

BRAN:

Crude (USDA)	1 oz.	60	17.5
Miller's (Elam's)	1 T. (.2 oz.)	17	2.8

BRAN BREAKFAST CEREAL:

(Kellogg's):			
All Bran or *Bran Buds*	⅓ cup (1 oz.)	70	22.0
Cracklin' Oat Bran	½ cup (1 oz.)	110	20.0
40% bran flakes	¾ cup (1 oz.)	90	23.0
Fruitful Bran	¾ cup (1 oz.)	110	27.0
Raisin Bran	¾ cup	110	30.0
(Loma Linda)	1 oz.	90	19.0
(Malt-O-Meal):			
40% bran	⅔ cup (1 oz.)	93	22.5
Raisin	¾ cup (1.4 oz.)	129	29.7
(Post):			
40% bran flakes	⅔ cup (1 oz.)	88	23.0
With raisins	½ cup (1 oz.)	122	32.0

Food and Description	Measure or Quantity	Calories	Carbo-hydrates (grams)
(Ralston Purina):			
Bran Chex	⅔ cup (1 oz.)	90	24.0
Bran News	¾ cup (1 oz.)	100	23.0
Oat	1 cup	130	32.0
(Safeway):			
40% branflakes	⅔ cup	90	23.0
Raisin	¾ cup	110	29.0

BRANDY (See DISTILLED LIQUOR)

BRANDY, FLAVORED (Mr. Boston) 35% alcohol:
Apricot	1 fl. oz.	94	8.9
Blackberry	1 fl. oz.	92	8.6
Cherry	1 fl. oz.	87	8.4
Coffee	1 fl. oz.	72	10.6
Ginger	1 fl. oz.	72	3.5
Peach	1 fl. oz.	94	8.9

BRAUNSCHWEIGER:
(Eckrich) chub	1 oz.	70	1.0
(Hormel)	1 oz.	80	0.
(Oscar Mayer):			
German Brand	1-oz. serving	94	.5
Sliced	1-oz. slice	96	.6
Tube	1-oz. serving	96	.9
(Swift) 8-oz. chub	1 oz.	109	1.4

BRAZIL NUT:
Raw (USDA):
Whole, in shell	1 cup (4.3 oz.)	383	6.4
Shelled	½ cup (2.5 oz.)	458	7.6
Shelled	4 nuts (.6 oz.)	114	1.9
Roasted (Fisher) salted	1 oz. (¼ cup)	193	3.1

BREAD:
Apple cinnamon (Pritikin)	1-oz. slice	80	14.0

(USDA) = United States Department of Agriculture
(HHS/FAO) = Health and Human Services/Food and Agriculture Organization
* = prepared as package directs

Food and Description	Measure or Quantity	Calories	Carbo-hydrates (grams)
Autumn grain (Interstate Brands) *Merita*	1-oz. slice	75	14.0
Barbecue, *Millbrook*	1.23-oz. slice	100	17.0
Black (Mrs. Wright's)	1 slice	60	11.0
Boston brown:			
(USDA)	3″ × ¾″ slice (1.7 oz.)	101	21.9
Canned, plain or raisin:			
(B&M)	½″ slice (1.6 oz.)	80	18.0
(Friend's)	½″ slice	80	18.0
Bran (Roman Meal):			
5 Bran	1-oz. slice	65	13.0
Oat, light	.8-oz. slice	42	9.6
Rice, honey or honey nut	1-oz. slice	71	12.3
Butter & egg (Mrs. Wright's) regular or sesame	1 slice	70	13.0
Buttermilk, *Butternut*	1-oz. slice	80	13.0
Cinnamon (Pepperidge Farm)	1 slice	90	15.0
Cracked wheat:			
(Pepperidge Farm) thin sliced	.9-oz. slice	70	13.0
(Roman Meal)	1-oz. slice	67	12.6
Crispbread, *Wasa*:			
Mora	3.2-oz. slice	333	70.5
Rye:			
Golden	.3-oz. slice	37	7.8
Lite	.3-oz. slice	30	6.2
Sesame	.5-oz. slice	50	10.6
Sport	.4-oz. slice	42	9.1
Date nut roll (Dromedary)	1-oz. slice	80	13.0
Egg, *Millbrook*	1-oz. slice	70	14.0
Flatbread, *Ideal*:			
Bran	.2-oz. slice	19	4.1
Extra thin	.1-oz. slice	12	2.5
Whole grain	.2-oz. slice	19	4.0
French:			
(Arnold) *Francisco*	1/16 of loaf (1 oz.)	70	12.0
(Interstate Brands):			
Eddy's, sour	1.5-oz. slice	110	19.0
Sweetheart, regular	1-oz. slice	70	14.0
(Mrs. Wright's) unsliced	.7-oz. slice	60	10.5

Food and Description	Measure or Quantity	Calories	Carbo- hydrates (grams)
(Pepperidge Farm):			
Fully baked, hearth	1 oz.	75	14.0
Twin	1 oz.	80	15.0
Garlic (Arnold)	1-oz. slice	80	10.0
Hi-fibre (Monks')	1-oz. slice	50	13.0
Hillbilly, Holsum	1-oz. slice	70	13.0
Hollywood:			
Dark	1-oz. slice	72	12.5
Light	1-oz. slice	71	13.1
Honey bran (Pepperidge Farm)	1 slice (1.2 oz.)	90	18.0
Honey & molasses graham (Mrs. Wright's)	1 slice	100	19.0
Hunter's grain (Interstate Brands) *Country Farms*	1.5-oz. slice	120	22.0
Italian (Arnold) *Francisco*	1 slice	70	12.0
Low sodium (Eddy's)	1-oz. slice	80	13.0
Mountain oat (Interstate Brands) *Country Farms*	1.5-oz. slice	130	23.0
Multi-grain:			
(Arnold) *Milk & Honey*	1-oz. slice	70	14.0
(Pritikin)	1-oz. slice	70	12.0
(Weight Watchers)	¾-oz. slice	40	9.4
Natural grains (Arnold)	.8-oz. slice	60	11.0
Oat (Arnold):			
Brannola	1.3-oz. slice	90	14.0
Milk & Honey	1-oz. slice	80	15.0
Oat bran (Roman Meal):			
Honey	1-oz. slice	69	12.7
Honey nut	1-oz. slice	72	12.1
Oatmeal:			
(Mrs. Wright's)	1 slice	80	15.0
(Pepperidge Farm):			
Regular	1 slice	90	17.0
Light	1 slice	49	9.0
Thin sliced	1 slice	40	8.0
Olympian meal (Interstate Brands) *Holsum*	1-oz. slice	70	13.0
Onion dill (Pritikin)	1-oz. slice	70	12.0
Potato (Interstate Brands) *Sweetheart*	1-oz. slice	70	14.0

(USDA) = United States Department of Agriculture
(HHS/FAO) = Health and Human Services/Food and Agriculture Organization
* = prepared as package directs

Food and Description	Measure or Quantity	Calories	Carbo-hydrates (grams)
Pita, Sahara (Thomas'):			
White:			
Regular	2-oz. piece	160	31.0
Mini	1-oz. piece	80	16.0
Large	3-oz. piece	240	48.0
Whole wheat:			
Regular	2-oz. piece	150	28.0
Mini	1-oz. piece	80	14.0
Poulsbo (Interstate Brands) *Eddy's*	1-oz. slice		
Pumpernickel:			
(Arnold)	1.1-oz. slice	80	14.0
(Levy's)	1.1-oz. slice	80	14.0
(Pepperidge Farm):			
Regular	1.1-oz. slice	80	15.0
Party	.2-oz. slice	15	3.0
Raisin:			
(Arnold) tea	.9-oz. slice	70	13.0
(Interstate Brands) *Butternut*	1-oz. slice	80	15.0
(Monk's) & cinnamon	1-oz. slice	70	10.0
(Pepperidge Farm)	1 slice	90	16.0
(Pritikin)	1-oz. slice	70	13.0
Sun-Maid (Interstate Brands)	1-oz. slice	80	15.0
Round top (Roman Meal)	1-oz. slice	69	13.4
Rye:			
(Arnold):			
Jewish	1.1-oz. slice	80	14.0
Melba Thin	.7-oz. slice	40	8.0
(Levy's) real	1.1-oz. slice	80	14.5
(Mrs. Wright's):			
Regular, with or without seeds	1 slice	60	11.0
Bavarian	1 slice	60	11.0
Dill, *Grainbelt*	1 slice	100	19.0
Jewish	1 slice	60	9.0
Swedish	1-oz. slice	80	15.0
(Pepperidge Farm):			
Dijon:			
Regular	1 slice	50	9.0
Hearty	1 slice	70	15.0
Family, with or without seeds	1 slice	80	16.0
Party	1 slice	15	3.0
(Pritikin)	1-oz. slice	70	12.0
(Weight Watchers)	¾-oz. slice	39	9.5

Food and Description	Measure or Quantity	Calories	Carbo-hydrates (grams)
Salt Rising (USDA)	.9-oz. slice	67	13.0
Sesame seed (Mrs. Wright's)	1 slice	70	14.0
7-Grain, Home Pride	1-oz. slice	72	12.8
Sourdough, Di Carlo	1-oz. slice	70	13.6
Split top (Interstate Brands) Merita	1-oz. slice	70	12.0
Sunflower & bran (Monk's)	1-oz. slice	70	12.0
Sun grain (Roman Meal)	1-oz. slice	70	12.6
Texas toast (Interstate Brands) Holsum	1.4-oz. slice	90	17.0
Wheat (See also Cracked Wheat or Whole Wheat): America's Own, cottage (Arnold):	1-oz. slice	70	13.0
Brannola: Dark	1.3-oz. slice	80	13.0
Hearty	1.3-oz. slice	90	13.0
Brick Oven	.8-oz. slice	60	9.0
Brick Oven	1.1-oz. slice	90	14.0
Country	1.3-oz. slice	80	13.0
Less or Liteway	.8-oz. slice	40	7.0
Milk & Honey	1-oz. slice	80	15.0
Very thin	.5-oz. slice	40	6.0
Fresh Horizons	1-oz. slice	54	9.6
Fresh & Natural	1-oz. slice	77	13.6
Home Pride	1-oz. slice	73	13.1
(Pepperidge Farm): Regular	1 slice	90	18.0
Family	1 slice	70	13.0
Light	1 slice	45	19.0
Very thin slice	1 slice	35	7.0
(Safeway)	1-oz. slice	70	13.0
(Wonder) family	1-oz. slice	75	13.6
Wheatberry, Home Pride: Honey	1-oz. slice	74	13.3
Regular	1-oz. slice	70	12.5
White: America's Own, cottage	1-oz. slice	70	15.0

(USDA) = United States Department of Agriculture
(HHS/FAO) = Health and Human Services/Food and Agriculture Organization
* = prepared as package directs

Food and Description	Measure or Quantity	Calories	Carbo- hydrates (grams)
(Arnold):			
Brick Oven	.8-oz. slice	60	11.0
Brick Oven	1.1-oz. slice	90	14.0
Country	1.3-oz. slice	100	18.0
Less or Liteway	.8-oz. slice	40	7.0
Milk & Honey	1-oz. slice	80	15.0
Very thin	.5-oz. slice	40	7.0
Fresh Horizons	1-oz. slice	54	10.0
Home Pride	1-oz. slice	72	13.1
(Interstate Brands):			
Butternut	1-oz. slice	70	14.0
Cookbook	1-oz. slice	75	14.0
Holsum	1-oz. slice	70	14.0
(Monk's)	1-oz. slice	60	10.0
(Pepperidge Farm):			
Family	1 slice	70	13.0
Hearty country	1 slice	95	19.0
Sandwich	1 slice	65	12.0
Thin sliced	1 slice	70	13.0
Toasting	1 slice	90	17.0
Very thin slice	1 slice	40	8.0
(Roman Meal) light	.8-oz. slice	40	10.2
Whole wheat:			
(Arnold):			
Brick Oven	.8-oz. slice	60	9.5
Stone ground	.8-oz. slice	50	8.0
Home Pride	1-oz. slice	70	12.2
(Monk's) 100% stone ground	1-oz. slice	70	13.0
(Pepperidge Farm):			
Thin slice	.9-oz. slice	65	12.0
Very thin slice	.6-oz. slice	40	7.5
BREAD CRUMBS:			
(Contadina) seasoned	½ cup (2.1 oz.)	211	40.6
(4C):			
Plain	4 oz.	405	85.2
Seasoned	4 oz.	384	77.3
(Progresso):			
Plain or Italian style	1 T.	30	5.5
Onion	1 T.	27	5.5

Food and Description	Measure or Quantity	Calories	Carbo-hydrates (grams)
*BREAD DOUGH:			
Frozen (Rich's):			
French	¹/₂₀ of loaf	59	11.0
Italian	¹/₂₀ of loaf	60	11.0
Raisin	¹/₂₀ of loaf	66	12.3
Wheat	.5-oz. slice	60	10.5
White	.8-oz. slice	56	9.4
Refrigerated (Pillsbury)			
Poppin' Fresh:			
French	1" slice	60	11.0
Wheat	1" slice	80	12.0
White	1" slice	80	13.0
*BREAD MIX:			
Home Hearth:			
French	³/₈" slice	85	14.5
Rye	³/₈" slice	75	14.0
White	³/₈" slice	75	14.5
(Pillsbury):			
Banana	¹/₁₂ of loaf	170	27.0
Blueberry nut	¹/₁₂ of loaf	150	26.0
Cherry nut	¹/₁₂ of loaf	180	29.0
Cranberry	¹/₁₂ of loaf	160	30.0
Date	¹/₁₂ of loaf	160	32.0
Nut	¹/₁₂ of loaf	170	28.0
BREAD PUDDING, with raisins, home recipe (USDA)	1 cup (9.3 oz.)	496	75.3
BREAD STICK (Stella D'oro):			
Regular:			
Plain	1 piece	40	7.0
Onion or wheat	1 piece	40	6.0
Pizza	1 piece	45	7.0
Sesame	1 piece	50	6.0
Dietetic:			
Regular	1 piece	45	7.0
Sesame	1 piece	60	7.0

(USDA) = United States Department of Agriculture
(HHS/FAO) = Health and Human Services/Food and Agriculture Organization
* = prepared as package directs

Food and Description	Measure or Quantity	Calories	Carbo-hydrates (grams)
*BREAD STICK DOUGH (Pillsbury) soft	1 piece	100	17.0
BREAKFAST WITH BARBIE, cereal (Ralston Purina)	1 cup (1 oz.)	110	25.0
BREAKFAST DRINK:			
(Lucerne):			
Chocolate	1 envelope	130	26.0
Coffee, strawberry or vanilla	1 envelope	130	28.0
*(Pillsbury):			
Chocolate	8 fl. oz.	290	38.0
Strawberry	8 fl. oz.	290	39.0
Vanilla	8 fl. oz.	300	41.0
BRIGHT & EARLY	6 fl. oz.	90	20.8
BRITOS, frozen (Patio):			
Beef & bean	½ of 7¼-oz. pkg.	250	33.0
Chicken, spicy	½ of 7¼-oz. pkg.	250	33.0
Chili:			
Green	½ of 7¼-oz. pkg.	250	33.0
Red	½ of 7¼-oz. pkg.	240	31.0
Nacho beef	½ of 7¼-oz. pkg.	270	30.0
Nacho cheese	½ of 7¼-oz. pkg.	250	32.0
BROCCOLI:			
Raw (USDA):			
Whole	1 lb. (weighed untrimmed)	69	16.3
Large leaves removed	1 lb.	113	20.9
Boiled (USDA):			
½" pieces, drained	½ cup (2.8 oz.)	20	3.5
Whole, drained	1 med. stalk (6.3 oz.)	47	8.1
Frozen:			
(Bel Air):			
Chopped	3.3 oz.	25	5.0
Cuts:			
Plain	3.3 oz.	25	5.0
Cheese sauce	3.3 oz.	45	6.0
Spears, cut or whole	3.3 oz.	25	5.0
(Birds Eye):			
With almonds & selected seasonings	⅓ of pkg. (3.3 oz.)	62	5.7

Food and Description	Measure or Quantity	Calories	Carbo-hydrates (grams)
In cheese sauce	⅓ of pkg. (3.3 oz.)	87	8.4
Chopped, cuts or florets	⅓ of pkg. (3.3 oz.)	26	4.9
Spears:			
Regular	⅓ of pkg. (3.3 oz.)	26	5.0
In butter sauce	⅓ of pkg. (3.3 oz.)	58	5.3
Deluxe	⅓ of pkg. (3.3 oz.)	29	5.0
& water chestnuts with selected seasonings	⅓ of pkg. (3.3 oz.)	35	5.8
(Frosty Acres)	3.3-oz. serving	25	5.0
(Green Giant):			
In cream sauce	3.3 oz.	0	7.4
Cuts, *Harvest Fresh*	3 oz.	16	3.0
Cuts, polybag	½ cup	12	3.0
Spears:			
In butter sauce, regular	3⅓ oz.	40	6.0
Harvest Fresh	3 oz.	19	4.0

BROWNIE (See **COOKIE**)

BROWNIE MIX (See **COOKIE MIX**)

BRUSSELS SPROUT:

Raw (USDA) trimmed	1 lb.	204	37.6
Boiled (USDA) drained	3-4 sprouts	28	4.9
Frozen:			
(USDA) boiled, drained	4 oz.	37	7.4
(Bel-Air)	3.3 oz.	35	7.0
(Birds Eye):			
Regular	⅓ of 10-oz. pkg.	37	7.3
In butter sauce	⅓ of 10-oz. pkg.	59	7.2
Baby, with cheese sauce	⅓ of 10-oz. pkg.	84	8.7
Baby, deluxe	⅓ of 10-oz. pkg.	49	7.3
(Frosty Acres)	3-oz. serving	30	7.0

(USDA) = United States Department of Agriculture
(HHS/FAO) = Health and Human Services/Food and Agriculture Organization
* = prepared as package directs

Food and Description	Measure or Quantity	Calories	Carbo-hydrates (grams)
(Green Giant):			
In butter sauce	3.3 oz.	40	8.0
Polybag	½ cup	25	6.0
(Larsen)	3.3-oz. serving	35	7.0
BUCKWHEAT:			
Flour (See **FLOUR**)			
Groats (Pocono):			
Brown, whole	1 oz.	104	19.4
White, whole	1 oz.	102	20.1
*BUC*WHEATS*, cereal			
(General Mills)	1 oz. (¾ cup)	110	24.0
BULGUR (form of hard red winter wheat) (USDA):			
Dry	1 lb.	1605	343.4
Canned:			
Unseasoned	4-oz. serving	191	39.7
Seasoned	4-oz. serving	206	37.2
BURGER KING:			
Apple pie	1 serving	311	44.0
Breakfast bagel sandwich:			
Plain	1 serving	387	46.0
Bacon	1 serving	438	46.0
Ham	1 serving	418	46.0
Sausage	1 serving	621	46.0
Breakfast Croissan'wich:			
Bacon	1 serving	355	20.0
Ham	1 serving	335	20.0
Sausage	1 serving	538	20.0
Cheeseburger:			
Regular	1 serving	304	27.0
Double:			
Plain	1 serving	464	27.0
Bacon	1 serving	510	27.0
Condiments:			
Ketchup	1 serving on sandwich	11	3.0
Mustard	1 serving on sandwich	2	0.
Pickles	1 serving on sandwich	0	0.

Food and Description	Measure or Quantity	Calories	Carbo-hydrates (grams)
Chicken specialty sandwich:			
Plain	1 serving	492	54.0
Condiments:			
Lettuce	1 serving on sandwich	2	0.
Mayonnaise	1 serving on sandwich	194	2.0
Chicken Tenders	1 piece	34	1.7
Coffee, regular	1 serving	2	0.
Danish, great	1 piece	500	40.0
Egg platter, scrambled:			
Bacon	1 serving	68	0.
Croissant	1 serving	187	18.0
Eggs	1 serving	119	2.0
Hash browns	1 serving	162	13.0
Sausage	1 serving	234	0.
French fries	1 regular order	227	24.0
French toast sticks	1 serving	499	49.0
Ham & cheese specialty sandwich:			
Plain	1 sandwich	365	41.0
Condiments:			
Lettuce	1 serving on sandwich	3	1.0
Mayonnaise	1 serving on sandwich	97	1.0
Tomato	1 serving on sandwich	6	1.0
Hamburger:			
Plain	1 burger	262	26.0
Condiments:			
Ketchup	1 serving on burger	11	3.0
Mustard	1 serving on burger	2	0.
Pickles	1 serving on burger	0	0.
Milk:			
2% low fat	1 serving	121	12.0
Whole	1 serving	157	11.0

(USDA) = United States Department of Agriculture
(HHS/FAO) = Health and Human Services/Food and Agriculture Organization
* = prepared as package directs

Food and Description	Measure or Quantity	Calories	Carbo-hydrates (grams)
Onion rings	1 serving	274	28.0
Orange juice	1 serving	82	20.0
Salad:			
Chef	1 serving	180	7.0
Chicken	1 serving	140	8.0
Garden	1 serving	90	7.0
Side	1 serving	20	4.0
Salad dressing:			
Regular:			
Bleu cheese	1 serving	156	2.0
House	1 serving	130	3.0
1000 Island	1 serving	117	4.0
Dietetic, Italian	1 serving	14	2.0
Shakes:			
Chocolate	1 shake	374	60.0
Vanilla	1 shake	334	51.0
Soft drink:			
Sweetened:			
Pepsi-Cola	1 regular size	159	40.0
7UP	1 regular	144	38.0
Dietetic, *Pepsi*	1 regular size	1	0.
Whaler:			
Plain sandwich	1 sandwich	353	43.0
Condiments:			
Lettuce	1 serving on sandwich	1	0.
Tartar sauce	1 serving on sandwich	134	2.0
Whopper:			
Regular:			
Plain	1 burger	452	38.0
With cheese	1 burger	535	39.0
Condiments:			
Ketchup	1 serving on burger	17	4.0
Lettuce	1 serving on burger	1	0.
Mayonnaise	1 serving on burger	146	2.0
Onion	1 serving on burger	5	1.0
Pickle	1 serving on burger	1	0.
Tomato	1 serving on burger	6	1.0

Food and Description	Measure or Quantity	Calories	Carbo-hydrates (grams)
Junior:			
Plain	1 burger	262	26.0
With cheese	1 burger	305	27.0
Condiments:			
Ketchup	1 serving on burger	8	2.0
Lettuce	1 serving on burger	1	0.
Mayonnaise	1 serving on burger	48	1.0
Pickle	1 serving on burger	0	0.
Tomato	1 serving on burger	3	1.0
BURGUNDY WINE:			
(Carlo Rossi)	3 fl. oz.	69	1.2
(Louis M. Martini) 12½% alcohol	3 fl. oz.	60	.2
(Paul Masson) 12% alcohol	3 fl. oz.	70	2.2
(Taylor) 12½% alcohol	3 fl. oz.	75	3.3
BURGUNDY WINE, SPARKLING:			
(B&G) 12% alcohol	3 fl. oz.	69	2.2
(Great Western) 12% alcohol	3 fl. oz.	82	5.1
(Taylor) 12% alcohol	3 fl. oz.	78	4.2
BURRITO:			
*Canned (Old El Paso)	1 burrito	299	36.0
Frozen:			
(Fred's Frozen Foods) *Little Juan:*			
Bean & cheese	5-oz. serving	331	46.9
Beef & bean, spicy	10-oz. serving	814	92.2
Beef & potato	5-oz. serving	389	48.9

(USDA) = United States Department of Agriculture
(HHS/FAO) = Health and Human Services/Food and Agriculture Organization
* = prepared as package directs

Food and Description	Measure or Quantity	Calories	Carbo-hydrates (grams)
Chili:			
Green	10-oz. serving	741	87.6
Red	10-oz. serving	799	96.4
Chili dog	5-oz. serving	313	31.4
Red hot	5-oz. serving	433	47.7
(Old El Paso):			
Regular:			
Bean & cheese	1 piece	340	43.0
Beef & bean:			
Hot	1 piece	340	41.0
Medium	1 piece	330	41.0
Mild	1 piece	330	40.0
Dinner, festive, beef & bean	11-oz. dinner	470	72.0
(Patio):			
Beef & bean:			
Regular	5-oz. serving	370	43.0
Green chili	5-oz. serving	330	43.0
Red chili	5-oz. serving	340	44.0
Red hot	5-oz. serving	360	43.0
(Weight Watchers):			
Beefsteak	7.62-oz. meal	310	36.0
Chicken	7.62-oz. meal	310	34.0
BURRITO SEASONING MIX			
(Lawry's)	1½-oz. pkg.	132	23.3
BUTTER, salted or unsalted:			
Regular:			
(USDA)	¼ lb.	812	.5
(USDA)	1 T. (.5 oz.)	102	.1
(USDA)	1 pat (5 grams)	36	Tr.
(Breakstone)	1 T.	100	Tr.
(Land O' Lakes)	1 tsp.	35	0.
(Meadow Gold)	1 tsp.	35	0.
Whipped (Breakstone)	1 T.	67	Tr.
BUTTERFISH, raw (USDA):			
Gulf:			
Whole	1 lb. (weighed whole)	220	0.
Meat only	4 oz.	108	0.
Northern:			
Whole	1 lb. (weighed whole)	391	0.

Food and Description	Measure or Quantity	Calories	Carbo-hydrates (grams)
Meat only	4 oz.	192	0.
BUTTERSCOTCH MORSELS (Nestlé)	1 oz.	150	19.0
BUTTER SUBSTITUTE:			
Butter Buds:			
Dry	⅛ oz.	12	3.0
Liquid	1 fl. oz.	12	3.0
Sprinkles	1 tsp.	14	2.0
Molly McButter, sprinkles	½ tsp.	4	1

(USDA) = United States Department of Agriculture
(HHS/FAO) = Health and Human Services/Food and Agriculture Organization
* = prepared as package directs

Food and Description	Measure or Quantity	Calories	Carbo-hydrates (grams)

C

CABBAGE:
  White (USDA):
    Raw:

Food and Description	Measure or Quantity	Calories	Carbo-hydrates (grams)
Whole	1 lb. (weighed untrimmed)	86	19.3
Finely shredded or chopped	1 cup (3.2 oz.)	22	4.9
Coarsely shredded or sliced	1 cup (2.5 oz.)	17	3.8
Wedge	3½" × 4½"	24	5.4
Boiled:			
Shredded, in small amount of water, short time drained	½ cup (2.6 oz.)	15	3.1
Wedges, in large amount of water, long time, drained	½ cup (3.2 oz.)	17	3.7
Dehydrated	1 oz.	87	20.9
Red:			
Raw (USDA) whole	1 lb. (weighed untrimmed)	111	24.7
Canned, solids & liq:			
(Comstock)	½ cup	60	13.0
(Greenwood)	½ cup	60	13.0
Savory (USDA) raw, whole	1 lb. (weighed untrimmed)	86	16.5
(Stouffer's) *Lean Cuisine*	10¾ oz. pkg.	220	19.0
CABERNET SAUVIGNON:			
(Louis M. Martini) 12½% alcohol	3 fl. oz.	62	.2
(Paul Masson) 11.9% alcohol	3 fl. oz.	70	.2
CAFE COMFORT, 55 proof	1 fl. oz.	79	8.8

Food and Description	Measure or Quantity	Calories	Carbo-hydrates (grams)
CAKE:			
Non-frozen:			
Plain:			
Home recipe, with butter & boiled white icing	1/9 of 9″ square	401	70.5
Home recipe, with butter & chocolate icing	1/9 of 9″ square	453	73.1
Angel food:			
Home recipe	1/12 of 8″ cake	108	24.1
(Dolly Madison)	1/6 of 10½-oz. cake	120	17.0
Apple (Dolly Madison) Dutch, *Buttercrumb*	1½-oz. piece	170	28.0
Apple spice (Entenmann's) fat & cholesterol free	1-oz. slice	80	17.0
Banana crunch (Entenmann's) fat & cholesterol free	1-oz. slice	80	18.0
Blueberry crunch (Entenmann's) fat & cholesterol free	1-oz. slice	70	16.0
Butter streusel (Dolly Madison) *Buttercrumb*	1½-oz. piece	150	23.0
Caramel, home recipe:			
Without icing	1/9 of 9″ square	322	46.2
With caramel icing	1/9 of 9″ square	331	50.2
Carrot (Dolly Madison) *Lunch Cake*	3¼-oz. serving	350	64.0
Chocolate, home recipe, with chocolate icing, 2-layer	1/12 of 9″ cake	365	55.2
Chocolate (Dolly Madison) German, *Lunch Cake*	3¼-oz. serving	440	54.0
Cinnamon (Dolly Madison) *Buttercrumb*	1½-oz. piece	170	27.0
Coffee (Entenmann's) fat & cholesterol free, cherry or cinnamon apple	1.3-oz. piece	90	20.0
Creme (Dolly Madison) *Lunch Cake*	7/8-oz. piece	90	17.0

(USDA) = United States Department of Agriculture
(HHS/FAO) = Health and Human Services/Food and Agriculture Organization
* = prepared as package directs

Food and Description	Measure or Quantity	Calories	Carbo-hydrates (grams)
Crumb (Hostess)	1¼-oz. piece	131	21.7
Devil's food, home recipe:			
Without icing	3″ × 2″ × 1½″ piece	201	28.6
With chocolate icing, 2-layer	1/16 of 9″ cake	277	41.8
Fruit, home recipe:			
Dark	1/30 of 8″ loaf	57	9.0
Light, made with butter	1/30 of 8″ loaf	58	8.6
Hawaiian spice (Dolly Madison) *Lunch Cake*	3¼-oz. piece	350	58.0
Honey (Holland Honey Cake) low sodium:			
Fruit and raisin	½″ slice (.9 oz.)	80	19.0
Orange and premium unsalted	½″ slice (.9 oz.)	70	17.0
Honey 'n spice (Dolly Madison) *Lunch Cake*	3¼-oz. piece	330	57.0
Pineapple crunch (Entenmann's) fat & cholesterol free	1-oz. slice	70	16.0
Pound, home recipe:			
Equal weights flour, sugar, butter and eggs	3½″ × 3½″ slice (1.1 oz.)	142	14.1
Pound (Dolly Madison)	1/6 of 14-oz. cake	220	33.0
Traditional, made with butter	3½″ × 3½″ slice (1.1 oz.)	123	16.4
Sponge, home recipe	1/12 of 10″ cake	196	35.7
White, home recipe:			
Made with butter, without icing, 2-layer	1/9 of 9″ wide, 3″ high cake	353	50.8
Made with butter, with coconut icing, 2-layer	1/12 of 9″ wide, 3″ high cake	386	63.1
White & coconut (Dolly Madison), layer	1/12 of 30-oz. cake	220	37.0
Yellow, home recipe, made with butter, without icing, 2-layer	1/9 of cake	351	56.3
Frozen:			
Black Forest (Weight Watchers)	3-oz. serving	180	32.0
Boston cream:	¼ of 11¾-oz.		
(Pepperidge Farm)	cake	290	39.0
(Weight Watchers)	3-oz. serving	190	35.0

Food and Description	Measure or Quantity	Calories	Carbo-hydrates (grams)
Carrot:			
(Pepperidge Farm)	⅛ of 11¾-oz. cake	150	19.0
(Weight Watchers)	3-oz. serving	170	27.0
Cheesecake:			
(Pepperidge Farm)			
Manhattan strawberry	4¼-oz. serving	300	49.0
(Weight Watchers):			
Regular	4-oz. serving	220	30.0
Brownie	3½-oz. serving	200	30.0
Strawberry	4-oz. serving	180	28.0
Chocolate:			
(Pepperidge Farm):			
Classic	2¼-oz. serving	250	29.0
Layer:			
Fudge	1⅝-oz. serving	180	23.0
Fudge stripe	1⅝-oz. serving	170	20.0
German	1⅝-oz. serving	180	22.0
Light, mousse cake	2½-oz. serving	190	25.0
Supreme	2⅞-oz. serving	300	37.0
(Weight Watchers):			
Regular	2½-oz. serving	190	31.0
German	2½-oz. serving	200	31.0
Coconut (Pepperidge Farm):			
Classic	2¼-oz. serving	230	31.0
Layer	1⅝-oz. serving	180	24.0
Devil's food (Pepperidge Farm) layer	¹⁄₁₀ of 17-oz. cake	180	24.0
Golden (Pepperidge Farm) layer	¹⁄₁₀ of 17-oz. cake	180	24.0
Lemon (Pepperidge Farm) *Supreme*	2¾-oz. serving	170	26.0
Lemon cream (Pepperidge Farm)	1⅝-oz. serving	170	21.0
Pineapple cream (Pepperidge Farm)	¹⁄₁₂ of 24-oz. cake	190	28.0
Pound (Pepperidge Farm) cholesterol free	1 oz.	110	13.0
Strawberry cream (Pepperidge Farm)	¹⁄₁₂ of 12-oz. cake	190	30.0

(USDA) = United States Department of Agriculture
(HHS/FAO) = Health and Human Services/Food and Agriculture Organization
* = prepared as package directs

Food and Description	Measure or Quantity	Calories	Carbo-hydrates (grams)
Strawberry shortcake (Pepperidge Farm) dessert lights	3-oz. serving	170	30.0
Vanilla (Pepperidge Farm) layer	1/10 of 17-oz. cake	190	25.0
Vanilla fudge swirl (Pepperidge Farm)	2¼-oz. serving	250	33.0

CAKE OR COOKIE ICING (Pillsbury):

All flavors except chocolate	1 T.	70	12.0
Chocolate	1 T.	60	11.0

CAKE ICING:

Amaretto almond (Betty Crocker) *Creamy Deluxe*	1/12 of can	160	27.0
Butter pecan (Betty Crocker) *Creamy Deluxe*	1/12 of can	170	26.0
Caramel, home recipe (USDA)	4 oz.	408	86.8
Caramel pecan (Pillsbury) *Frosting Supreme*	1/12 of can	160	21.0
Cherry (Betty Crocker) *Creamy Deluxe*	1/12 of can	160	27.0
Chocolate:			
(USDA) home recipe	½ cup (4.9 oz.)	519	93.0
(Betty Crocker) *Creamy Deluxe:*			
Regular	1/12 of can	160	24.0
With candy-coated chocolate chips	1/12 of can	160	24.0
Chip	1/12 of can	170	27.0
With dinosaurs	1/12 of can	160	24.0
Fudge, dark Dutch	1/12 of can	160	22.0
Milk	1/12 of can	160	25.0
Sour cream	1/12 of can	160	23.0
(Duncan Hines):			
Regular	1/12 of can	152	23.3
Fudge, dark Dutch	1/12 of can	149	22.5
Milk	1/12 of can	151	22.9
(Mrs. Wright's) fudge, creamy	1/12 of can	170	25.0
(Pillsbury):			
Regular, fudge	1/8 of can	110	17.0

Food and Description	Measure or Quantity	Calories	Carbohydrates (grams)
Frosting Supreme:			
Chip	1/12 of can	150	27.0
Fudge	1/12 of can	150	24.0
Milk	1/12 of can	150	23.0
Mint	1/12 of can	150	24.0
Coconut almond (Pillsbury)			
Frosting Supreme	1/12 of can	150	17.0
Coconut pecan (Pillsbury)			
Frosting Supreme	1/12 of can	160	17.0
Cream cheese:			
(Betty Crocker)			
Creamy Deluxe	1/12 of can	160	27.0
(Duncan Hines)	1/12 of can	152	23.6
(Pillsbury) *Frosting Supreme*	1/12 of can	160	26.0
Double Dutch (Pillsbury)			
Frosting Supreme	1/12 of can	140	22.0
Lemon:			
(Betty Crocker) *Creamy Deluxe*	1/12 of can	170	28.0
(Pillsbury) *Frosting Supreme*	1/12 of can	160	26.0
Polka dot (Duncan Hines):			
Milk chocolate	1/12 of can	168	24.7
Pink vanilla	1/12 of can	154	23.3
Rainbow chip (Betty Crocker *Creamy Deluxe*	1/12 of can	170	27.0
Rocky road minimorsels (Betty Crocker) *Creamy Deluxe*	1/12 of can	150	20.0
Strawberry (Pillsbury) *Frosting Supreme*	1/12 of can	160	26.0
Vanilla:			
(Betty Crocker) *Creamy Deluxe*	1/12 of can	160	27.0
(Duncan Hines)	1/12 of can	151	23.6
(Pillsbury) *Frosting Supreme*, regular or sour cream	1/12 of can	160	27.0
White:			
Home recipe, boiled (USDA)	4 oz.	358	91.1
Home recipe, uncooked (USDA)	4 oz.	426	92.5

(USDA) = United States Department of Agriculture
(HHS/FAO) = Health and Human Services/Food and Agriculture Organization
* = prepared as package directs

Food and Description	Measure or Quantity	Calories	Carbo-hydrates (grams)
(Betty Crocker) *Creamy Deluxe*, sour cream	1/12 of can	160	27.0
(Mrs. Wright's)	1/12 of can	160	25.0

*CAKE ICING MIX:
  Regular:
    Chocolate:
      (Betty Crocker) creamy:

Fudge	1/12 of pkg.	180	30.0
Milk	1/12 of pkg.	170	29.0
(Pillsbury)	1/8 of pkg.	50	12.0
Coconut almond (Pillsbury)	1/12 of pkg.	160	16.0

Coconut pecan:

(Betty Crocker) creamy	1/12 of pkg.	150	19.0
(Pillsbury)	1/12 of pkg.	150	20.0
Lemon (Betty Crocker) creamy	1/12 of pkg.	170	31.0

Vanilla:

(Betty Crocker) creamy	1/12 of pkg.	170	32.0
(Pillsbury) *Rich 'n Easy*	1/12 of pkg.	150	25.0

White:

(Betty Crocker) Fluffy	1/12 of pkg.	70	16.0
(Pillsbury) fluffy	1/12 of pkg.	60	15.0
Dietetic (Estee)	1½ tsp.	50	10.0

CAKE MEAL (Manischewitz)	½ cup (2.6 oz.)	286	NA

CAKE MIX:
  Regular:
    Angel food:
      (Betty Crocker):

Confetti, lemon custard or white	1/12 of pkg.	150	34.0
Traditional	1/12 of pkg.	130	30.0
(Duncan Hines)	1/12 of pkg.	124	28.9
*(Mrs. Wright's) deluxe	1/12 of cake	130	31.0

  *Apple cinnamon (Betty Crocker) *Supermoist:*

Regular	1/12 of cake	250	36.0
No cholesterol recipe	1/12 of cake	210	36.0

  *Apple streusel (Betty Crocker) *MicroRave:*

Regular	1/6 of cake	240	33.0
No cholesterol recipe	1/6 of cake	210	33.0

Food and Description	Measure or Quantity	Calories	Carbo-hydrates (grams)
*Banana (Pillsbury) *Pillsbury Plus*	1/12 of cake	250	36.0
*Black Forest cherry (Pillsbury) *Bundt*	1/16 of cake	240	38.0
*Boston cream (Pillsbury) *Bundt*	1/16 of cake	270	43.0
*Butter (Pillsbury) *Pillsbury Plus*	1/12 of cake	260	34.0
Butter Brickle (Betty Crocker) *Supermoist*:			
Regular	1/12 of cake	250	38.0
No cholesterol recipe	1/12 of cake	220	38.0
Butter pecan (Betty Crocker) *Supermoist*:			
Regular	1/12 of cake	250	35.0
No cholesterol recipe	1/12 of cake	220	35.0
*Carrot (Betty Crocker) *Supermoist*:			
Regular	1/12 of cake	250	35.0
No cholesterol recipe	1/12 of cake	220	35.0
*Carrot'n spice (Pillsbury) *Pillsbury Plus*	1/12 of cake	260	36.0
*Cheesecake:			
(Jello-O)	1/8 of cake	283	36.5
(Royal) No Bake:			
Lite	1/8 of cake	210	23.0
Real	1/8 of cake	280	31.0
*Cherry chip (Betty Crocker) *Supermoist*	1/12 of cake	190	37.0
Chocolate:			
*(Betty Crocker):			
MicroRave:			
Fudge, with vanilla frosting	1/6 of cake	310	40.0
German, with coconut pecan frosting	1/6 of cake	320	37.0
Pudding	1/6 of cake	230	44.0
Supermoist:			
Butter recipe	1/12 of cake	270	35.0

(USDA) = United States Department of Agriculture
(HHS/FAO) = Health and Human Services/Food and Agriculture Organization
* = prepared as package directs

Food and Description	Measure or Quantity	Calories	Carbohydrates (grams)
Chip:			
Regular	1/12 of cake	280	36.0
No cholesterol			
recipe	1/12 of cake	220	36.0
Chocolate chip	1/12 of cake	260	34.0
Fudge	1/12 of cake	260	34.0
German:			
Regular	1/12 of cake	260	35.0
No cholesterol			
recipe	1/12 of cake	210	35.0
Sour cream:			
Regular	1/12 of cake	260	33.0
No cholesterol			
recipe	1/12 of cake	220	35.0
(Duncan Hines) fudge	1/12 of pkg.	187	34.8
*(Pillsbury):			
Bundt:			
Macaroon	1/16 of cake	240	36.0
Tunnel of Fudge	1/16 of cake	260	37.0
Microwave:			
Plain	1/8 of cake	210	23.0
Frosted:			
With chocolate			
frosting	1/8 of cake	300	35.0
With vanilla frosting	1/8 of cake	300	36.0
Supreme, double	1/8 of cake	330	39.0
Tunnel of Fudge	1/8 of cake	290	36.0
Pillsbury Plus:			
Chocolate chip	1/12 of cake	270	33.0
Fudge, dark	1/12 of cake	250	32.0
Fudge, marble	1/12 of cake	270	36.0
German	1/12 of cake	250	36.0
*Cinnamon (Pillsbury)			
Streusel Swirl,			
microwave	1/8 of cake	240	33.0
*Cinnamon pecan streusel			
(Betty Crocker)			
MicroRave:			
Regular	1/6 of cake	290	39.0
No cholesterol recipe	1/6 of cake	240	39.0
Coffee cake:			
*(Aunt Jemima)	1/8 of cake	170	29.0
*(Pillsbury) apple			
cinnamon	1/8 of cake	240	40.0

Food and Description	Measure or Quantity	Calories	Carbo- hydrates (grams)
Devil's food:			
*(Betty Crocker):			
MicroRave, with chocolate frosting:			
Regular	⅙ of cake	310	37.0
No cholesterol recipe	⅙ of cake	240	37.0
Supermoist:			
Regular	¹⁄₁₂ of cake	260	35.0
No cholesterol recipe	¹⁄₁₂ of cake	220	35.0
(Duncan Hines) deluxe	¹⁄₁₂ of pkg.	189	35.6
(Mrs. Wright's) deluxe	¹⁄₁₂ of cake	190	32.0
*(Pillsbury) *Pillsbury Plus*	¹⁄₁₂ of cake	270	32.0
Fudge (see Chocolate)			
Gingerbread (See **GINGERBREAD**)			
Golden (Duncan Hines) butter recipe	¹⁄₁₂ of pkg.	188	36.5
Lemon:			
(Betty Crocker):			
MicroRave, with lemon frosting	⅙ of cake	300	37.0
Pudding	⅙ of cake	230	45.0
Supermoist:			
Regular	¹⁄₁₂ of cake	290	36.0
No cholesterol recipe	¹⁄₁₂ of cake	220	36.0
*(Pillsbury):			
Bundt, Tunnel of Lemon	¹⁄₁₆ of cake	270	45.0
Microwave:			
Plain	⅛ of cake	220	23.0
With lemon frosting	⅛ of cake	300	37.0
Supreme, double	⅛ of cake	300	40.0
Pillsbury Plus	¹⁄₁₂ of cake	250	34.0
Streusel Swirl	¹⁄₁₆ of cake	270	39.0
*Marble (Betty Crocker)			
Supermoist:			
Regular	¹⁄₁₂ of cake	250	35.0
No cholesterol recipe	¹⁄₁₂ of cake	210	35.0
*Pineapple creme (Pillsbury) *Bundt*	¹⁄₁₆ of cake	260	41.0
Pound:			
*(Betty Crocker) golden	¹⁄₁₂ of cake	200	28.0

(USDA) = United States Department of Agriculture
(HHS/FAO) = Health and Human Services/Food and Agriculture Organization
* = prepared as package directs

Food and Description	Measure or Quantity	Calories	Carbo-hydrates (grams)
*(Dromedary)	½" slice (¹⁄₁₂ of pkg.)	150	21.0
*((Mrs. Wright's) deluxe	¹⁄₁₂ of cake	200	32.0
*Spice (Betty Crocker) *Supermoist*:			
Regular	¹⁄₁₂ of cake	260	36.0
No cholesterol recipe	¹⁄₁₂ of cake	220	36.0
Strawberry*(Pillsbury) *Pillsbury Plus*	¹⁄₁₂ of cake	260	37.0
*Upside down (Betty Crocker) pineapple:			
Regular	¹⁄₉ of cake	250	39.0
No cholesterol recipe	¹⁄₉ of cake	240	39.0
*Vanilla (Betty Crocker) golden, *Supermoist*	¹⁄₁₂ of cake	280	34.0
White:			
*(Betty Crocker):			
MicroRave, golden, with rainbow chip frosting	⅙ of cake	320	40.0
Supermoist:			
Regular	¹⁄₁₂ of cake	280	36.0
No cholesterol recipe	¹⁄₁₂ of cake	220	36.0
(Duncan Hines) deluxe	¹⁄₁₂ of pkg.	188	36.1
(Mrs. Wright's)	¹⁄₁₂ of pkg.	180	34.0
*(Pillsbury) *Pillsbury Plus*	¹⁄₁₂ of cake	240	35.0
Yellow:			
(Betty Crocker):			
MicroRave, with chocolate frosting:			
Regular	⅙ of cake	300	36.0
No cholesterol recipe	⅙ of cake	230	36.0
Supermoist:			
Plain:			
Regular	¹⁄₁₂ of cake	260	36.0
No cholesterol recipe	¹⁄₁₂ of cake	220	36.0
Butter recipe	¹⁄₁₂ of cake	260	37.0
(Duncan Hines) deluxe	¹⁄₁₂ of pkg.	188	37.0
(Mrs. Wright's)	¹⁄₁₂ of pkg.	190	33.0
*(Pillsbury):			
Microwave:			
Plain	⅛ of cake	220	23.0
With chocolate frosting	⅛ of cake	300	36.0
Pillsbury Plus	¹⁄₁₂ of cake	260	36.0

Food and Description	Measure or Quantity	Calories	Carbo-hydrates (grams)
*Dietetic (Estee)	1/10 of cake	100	18.0
CAMPARI, 45 proof	1 fl. oz.	66	7.1

CANDY, GENERIC. The follow
ing values of candies from the
U.S. Department of Agriculture
are representative of the types
sold commercially. These values
may be useful when individual
brands or sizes are not known:

Food and Description	Measure or Quantity	Calories	Carbo-hydrates (grams)
Almond:			
Chocolate-coated	1 cup (6.3 oz.)	1024	71.3
Chocolate-coated	1 oz.	161	11.2
Sugar-coated or Jordan	1 oz.	129	19.9
Butterscotch	1 oz.	113	26.9
Candy corn	1 oz.	103	25.4
Caramel:			
Plain	1 oz.	113	21.7
Plain with nuts	1 oz.	121	20.0
Chocolate	1 oz.	113	21.7
Chocolate with nuts	1 oz.	121	20.0
Chocolate-flavored roll	1 oz.	112	23.4
Chocolate:			
Bittersweet	1 oz.	135	13.3
Milk:			
Plain	1 oz.	147	16.1
With almonds	1 oz.	151	14.5
With peanuts	1 oz.	154	12.6
Semisweet	1 oz.	144	16.2
Sweet	1 oz.	150	16.4
Chocolate discs, sugar coated	1 oz.	132	20.6
Coconut center, chocolate-coated	1 oz.	124	20.4
Fondant, plain	1 oz.	103	25.4
Fondant, chocolate-covered	1 oz.	116	23.0
Fudge:			
Chocolate fudge	1 oz.	113	21.3

(USDA) = United States Department of Agriculture
(HHS/FAO) = Health and Human Services/Food and Agriculture
                 Organization
* = prepared as package directs

Food and Description	Measure or Quantity	Calories	Carbohydrates (grams)
Chocolate fudge, chocolate-coated	1 oz.	122	20.7
Chocolate fudge with nuts	1 oz.	121	19.6
Chocolate fudge with nuts, chocolate-coated	1 oz.	128	19.1
Vanilla fudge	1 oz.	113	21.2
Vanilla fudge with nuts	1 oz.	120	19.5
With peanuts & caramel, chocolate-coated	1 oz.	130	16.6
Gum drops	1 oz.	98	24.8
Hard	1 oz.	109	27.6
Honeycombed hard candy, with peanut butter, chocolate-covered	1 oz.	131	20.0
Jelly beans	1 oz.	104	26.4
Marshmallow	1 oz.	90	22.8
Mints, uncoated	1 oz.	103	25.4
Nougat & caramel, chocolate-covered,	1 oz.	118	20.6
Peanut bar	1 oz.	146	13.4
Peanut brittle	1 oz.	119	23.0
Peanuts, chocolate-covered	1 oz.	159	11.1
Raisins, chocolate-covered	1 oz.	120	20.0
Vanilla creams, chocolate-covered	1 oz.	123	19.9

CANDY, COMMERCIAL:

Food and Description	Measure or Quantity	Calories	Carbohydrates (grams)
Almond, Jordan (Banner)	1¼-oz. box	154	27.9
Almond Joy (Hershey's)	1.76-oz. bar	250	28.0
Apricot Delight (Sahadi)	1 oz.	100	25.0
Baby Ruth	2-oz. piece	260	36.0
Bar None (Hershey's)	1½-oz. serving	240	23.0
Bit-O-Honey (Nestlé)	1.7-oz. serving	200	41.0
Bonkers! (Nabisco)	1 piece	20	5.0
Breath Saver, any flavor	1 piece	8	2.0
Bridge Mix (Nabisco)	1 piece	10	2.0
Butterfinger	2-oz. bar	260	38.0
Butternut (Hollywood Brands)	2¼-oz. bar	310	36.0
Caramello (Hershey's)	1.6-oz. serving	220	28.0
Caramel Nip (Pearson)	1 piece	30	5.7
Charleston Chew	2-oz. bar	240	44.0

Food and Description	Measure or Quantity	Calories	Carbo- hydrates (grams)
Cherry, chocolate-covered (Welch's):			
Dark	1 piece	90	16.0
Milk	1 piece	85	16.0
Chocolate bar:			
Alpine white (Nestlé)	1 oz.	170	13.0
Brazil Nut (Cadbury's)	2-oz. serving	310	32.0
Caramello (Cadbury's)	2-oz. serving	280	37.0
Crunch (Nestlé)	1⅙-oz. bar	160	19.0
Fruit & nut (Cadbury's)	2-oz. serving	300	33.0
Hazelnut (Cadbury's)	2-oz. serving	310	32.0
Milk:			
(Cadbury's)	2-oz. serving	300	34.0
(Hershey's)	1.55-oz. bar	240	25.0
(Nestlé)	.35-oz. bar	53	6.0
(Nestlé)	1¹/₁₆-oz. bar	159	18.1
Special Dark (Hershey's)	1.45-oz. bar	220	25.0
Chocolate bar with almonds:			
(Cadbury's)	2-oz. serving	310	31.0
(Hershey's):			
Milk	1.45-oz. bar	230	20.0
Golden Almond	3.2-oz. bar	520	40.0
(Nestlé)	1-oz.	160	15.0
Chocolate Parfait (Pearson)	1 piece (6.5 grams)	30	5.7
Chocolate, Petite (Andes)	1 piece	26	2.6
Chuckles	1 oz.	100	23.0
Clark Bar	1.5-oz. bar	201	30.4
Coffee Nip (Pearson)	1 piece (6.5 grams)	30	5.7
Coffioca (Pearson)	1 piece (6.5 grams)	30	5.7
Creme De Menthe (Andes)	1 piece	25	2.6
Dutch Treat Bar (Clark)	1¹/₁₆-oz. bar	160	20.3
Eggs:			
(Nabisco) *Chuckles*	½ oz.	55	13.5
(Hershey's):			
Creme	1 oz.	136	19.2
Mini	1 oz.	140	20.0
5th Avenue (Hershey's)	2.1-oz. serving	290	39.0

(USDA) = United States Department of Agriculture
(HHS/FAO) = Health and Human Services/Food and Agriculture Organization
* = prepared as package directs

Food and Description	Measure or Quantity	Calories	Carbohydrates (grams)
Fruit bears (Flavor Tree) assorted	½ of 2.1-oz. pkg.	117	25.4
Fruit circus (Flavor Tree) assorted	½ of 2.1-oz. pkg.	117	25.4
Fruit roll (Flavor Tree):			
Apple, cherry, grape or raspberry	¾-oz. piece	75	18.5
Apricot	¾-oz. piece	76	17.7
Fruit punch or strawberry	¾-oz. piece	74	18.0
Fudge bar (Nabisco)	1 piece (.7 oz.)	85	14.5
Fun Fruit (Sunkist) any type	.9-oz. piece	100	21.8
Goobers (Nestlé)	1 oz.	160	13.0
Good & Plenty	1 oz.	100	24.8
Good Stuff (Nabisco)	1.8-oz. piece	250	29.0
Halvah (Sahadi) original and marble	1 oz.	150	13.0
Hard (Jolly Rancher):			
All flavors except butterscotch	1 piece	23	5.7
Butterscotch	1 piece	25	5.6
Holidays (M&M/Mars):			
Plain	1 oz.	140	19.0
Peanut	1 oz.	140	16.0
Jelly bar, Chuckles	1 oz.	100	25.0
Jelly bean, Chuckles	½ oz.	55	13.0
Jelly rings, Chuckles	½ oz.	50	11.0
JuJubes, Chuckles	½ oz.	55	12.5
Kisses (Hershey's)	1 piece (.2 oz.)	24	2.5
Kit Kat (Hershey's)	1.65-oz. bar	250	29.0
Krackle Bar	1.55-oz. bar	230	27.0
Licorice:			
Licorice Nips (Pearson)	1 piece (6.5 grams)	30	5.7
(Switzer) bars, bites or stix:			
Black	1 oz.	94	22.1
Cherry or strawberry	1 oz.	98	23.2
Chocolate	1 oz.	97	22.7
Life Savers	1 piece	7	3.0
Lollipops (Life Savers)	.1-oz. pop	45	11.0
Mallo Cup (Boyer)	.6-oz. piece	54	11.2
Mars Bar (M&M/Mars)	1.7-oz. bar	240	30.0
Marshmallow (Campfire)	1 oz.	111	24.9
Marshmallow eggs, Chuckles	1 oz.	110	27.0
Mary Jane (Miller):			
Small size	¼-oz. piece	19	3.5

Food and Description	Measure or Quantity	Calories	Carbo-hydrates (grams)
Large size	1½-oz. bar	110	20.3
Milk Duds (Clark)	¾-oz. bar	89	17.8
Milk Shake (Hollywood Brands)	2.4-oz. bar	300	51.0
Milky Way (M&M/Mars)	2.24-oz. bar	290	44.0
Mint Parfait:			
(Andes)	.2-oz. piece	27	2.7
(Pearson)	.2-oz. piece	30	5.7
Mint or peppermint:			
Canada Mint (Necco)	.1-oz. piece	12	3.1
Junior mint pattie (Nabisco)	1 piece (.1 oz.)	10	2.0
Peppermint pattie:			
(Nabisco)	1 piece (.5 oz.)	55	12.5
York (Hershey's)	1¼-oz. serving	160	28.0
M&M's:			
Peanut	1.83-oz. pkg.	270	30.0
Plain	1.69-oz. pkg.	240	33.0
Mounds (Hershey's)	1.9-oz. bar	260	31.0
Mr. Goodbar (Hershey's)	1.85-oz. bar	300	24.0
Munch bar (M&M/Mars)	1.42-oz. bar	220	19.0
My Buddy (Tom's)	1.8-oz. piece	250	30.0
Naturally Nut & Fruit Bar (Planters):			
Almond/apricot; almond/ pineapple; peanut/raisin	1 oz.	140	17.0
Walnut/apple	1 oz.	150	16.0
Necco Wafers:			
Assorted	2.02-oz. roll	227	56.5
Chocolate	2.02-oz. roll	228	56.3
Nougat centers, *Chuckles*	1 oz.	110	26.0
Oh Henry! (Nestlé)	1 oz.	140	16.0
$100,000 Bar (Nestlé)	1¼-oz. bar	175	23.8
Orange slices, *Chuckles*	1 oz.	110	24.0
Park Avenue (Tom's)	1.8-oz. piece	230	34.0
Payday (Hollywood Brands):			
Regular	1.9-oz. piece	250	28.0
Chocolate coated	2-oz. piece	290	30.0
Peanut bar (Planters)	1.6-oz. piece	240	21.0
Peanut, chocolate-covered:			
(Curtiss)	1 piece	5	1.0

(USDA) = United States Department of Agriculture
(HHS/FAO) = Health and Human Services/Food and Agriculture Organization
* = prepared as package directs

Food and Description	Measure or Quantity	Calories	Carbo-hydrates (grams)
(Nabisco)	1 piece (4.1 grams)	11	1.0
Peanut butter cup:			
(Boyer)	1.5-oz. pkg.	148	17.4
(Reese's)	.9-oz. cup	140	13.0
Peanut Butter Pals (Tom's)	1.3-oz. serving	200	19.0
Peanut crunch (Sahadi)	¾-oz. bar	110	9.0
Peanut Parfait:			
(Andes)	1 piece	28	2.5
(Pearson)	1 piece	30	5.7
Peanut Plank (Tom's)	1.7-oz. piece	230	28.0
Peanut Roll (Tom's)	1.7-oz. piece	230	29.0
Pom Poms (Nabisco)	1 oz.	100	15.0
Powerhouse (Hershey's)	2-oz. serving	260	38.0
Raisin, chocolate-covered (Nabisco)	1 piece	5	.7
Raisinets (Nestlé)	1 oz.	120	20.0
Reese's Pieces (Hershey's)	1.95-oz. pkg.	270	31.0
Reggie Bar	2-oz. bar	290	29.0
Rolo (Hershey's)	1 piece (6 grams)	34	4.6
Royals, mint chocolate (M&M/Mars)	1.52-oz. pkg.	212	29.5
Sesame Crunch (Sahadi)	¾-oz. bar	110	7.0
Sesame Tahini (Sahadi)	1 oz.	190	4.0
Skittles (M&M/Mars)	1 oz.	113	26.3
Skor (Hershey's)	1.4-oz. bar	220	22.0
Sky Bar (Necco)	1.5-oz. bar	198	31.5
Snickers (M&M/Mars)	2.16-oz. bar	290	36.0
Solitaires (Hershey's)	½ of 3.2-oz. pkg.	260	20.0
Spearmint leaves, *Chuckles*	1 oz.	110	15.0
Starburst (M&M/Mars)	1-oz. serving	120	24.0
Sugar Babies (Nabisco):	1⅝-oz. pkg.	180	40.0
Sugar Daddy (Nabisco) caramel sucker	1⅜-oz.	150	33.0
Sugar Mama (Nabisco)	1 piece (.8 oz.)	90	17.0
Symphony (Hershey's):			
Almond	1.4-oz. serving	220	20.0
Milk	1.4-oz. serving	220	22.0
3 Musketeers	2.13-oz. bar	260	46.0
Ting-A-Ling (Andes)	1 piece	24	2.8
Tootsie Roll:			
Chocolate	.23-oz. midgee	26	5.3
Chocolate	1/16-oz. bar	72	14.3

Food and Description	Measure or Quantity	Calories	Carbo-hydrates (grams)
Chocolate	1-oz. bar	115	22.9
Flavored	.6-oz. square	19	3.8
Pop, all flavors	.49-oz. pop	55	12.5
Pop drop, all flavors	4.7-gram piece	19	4.2
Twizzler (Y & S) strawberry	1-oz. serving	100	23.0
Whatchamacallit (Hershey's)	1.8-oz. bar	260	30.0
Wispa (Hershey's)	1 oz.	150	17.0
Y & S Bites	1 oz.	100	23.0
Zagnut Bar (Clark)	.7-oz. bar	85	12.5
Zero (Hollywood Brands)	2-oz. bar	210	34.0
CANDY, DIETETIC:			
Caramel (Estee)	1 piece	30	5.0
Chocolate or chocolate-flavored:			
(Estee):			
Coconut	.2-oz. square	30	2.0
Crunch	.2-oz. square	22	2.0
Fruit & nut	.2-oz. square	30	2.5
Milk	.2-oz. square	30	2.5
(Louis Sherry):			
Bittersweet	.2-oz. piece	30	3.0
Coffee-flavored	.2-oz. piece	22	2.0
Estee-ets, with peanuts (Estee)	1 piece (1.4 grams)	7	.8
Gum drops (Estee) any flavor	1 piece (1.8 grams)	6	1.5
Gummy Bears (Estee)	1 piece	7	1.3
Hard candy:			
(Estee) assorted fruit	1 piece (.1 oz.)	12	3.0
(Louis Sherry)	1 piece (.1 oz.)	12	3.0
Lollipop (Estee)	1 piece (.2 oz.)	25	6.0
Peanut brittle (Estee)	¼ oz.	35	5.0
Peanut butter cup (Estee)	1 cup (.3 oz.)	40	3.0
Raisins, chocolate-covered (Estee)	1 piece (1.2 grams)	3	.5
CANDY APPLE COOLER DRINK, canned (Hi-C)	6 fl. oz.	94	23.1

(USDA) = United States Department of Agriculture
(HHS/FAO) = Health and Human Services/Food and Agriculture Organization
* = prepared as package directs

Food and Description	Measure or Quantity	Calories	Carbohydrates (grams)
CANNELONI, frozen:			
(Armour) *Dining Lite*, cheese	9-oz. meal	310	38.0
(Celentano) florentine	12-oz. pkg.	350	48.0
(Stouffer's) *Lean Cuisine:*			
Beef & pork with mornay sauce	9⅝-oz. pkg.	260	25.0
Cheese with tomato sauce	9⅛-oz. pkg.	260	22.0
CANTALOUPE, fresh (USDA):			
Whole, medium	1 lb. (weighed with skin & cavity contents)	68	17.0
Cubed or diced	½ cup (2.9 oz.)	24	6.1
CAP'N CRUNCH, cereal (Quaker):			
Regular	¾ cup (1 oz.)	121	22.9
Crunchberry	¾ cup (1 oz.)	120	22.9
Peanut butter	¾ cup (1 oz.)	127	20.9
CARAWAY SEED (French's)	1 tsp (1.8 grams)	8	.8
***CARL'S JR.* RESTAURANT:**			
Bacon	2 strips (10 grams)	50	0.
Cake, chocolate	3.2-oz. serving	380	43.0
California Roast Beef'n Swiss Sandwich	7.3-oz. serving	360	43.0
Cheese:			
American	.6-oz. serving	63	1.0
Swiss	.6-oz. serving	57	1.0
Chicken sandwich:			
Charbroiler BBQ	6.3-oz. serving	320	40.0
Charbroiler Club	8.2-oz. serving	510	53.0
Cookie, chocolate chip	2¼-oz. serving	330	44.0
Danish	3½-oz. piece	300	49.0
Eggs, scrambled	2.4-oz. serving	120	2.0
Fish sandwich, filet	7.9-oz. serving	550	58.0
French toast dips, excluding syrup	4.7-oz. serving	480	54.0

Food and Description	Measure or Quantity	Calories	Carbo-hydrates (grams)
Hamburger:			
Plain:			
Famous Star	8.1-oz. serving	590	42.0
Happy Star	3.0-oz. serving	220	26.0
Old Time Star	6.9-oz. serving	400	38.0
Super Star	10.6-oz. serving	770	44.0
Cheeseburger, *Western*			
Bacon:			
Regular	7½-oz. serving	630	49.0
Double	10.4-oz. serving	890	61.0
Hot cakes, with margarine, excluding syrup	5½-oz. serving	360	59.0
Milk, 2% lowfat	10 fl. oz.	175	16.0
Muffins:			
Blueberry	3½-oz. muffin	256	40.0
Bran	4-oz. nuffin	220	34.0
English, with margarine	2-oz. muffin	180	28.0
Onion rings	3.2-oz. serving	310	38.0
Orange juice, small	8 fl. oz.	94	21.0
Potato:			
Baked:			
Bacon & cheese	14.1-oz. serving	650	63.0
Broccoli & cheese	14-oz. serving	470	61.0
Cheese	14.2-oz. serving	550	72.0
Fiesta	15.2-oz. serving	550	60.0
Lite	9.8-oz. serving	250	54.0
Sour cream & chive	10.4-oz. serving	350	49.0
French fries, regular	6-oz. serving	360	43.0
Hash brown nuggets	3-oz. serving	170	20.0
Salad dressing:			
Regular:			
Blue cheese	2-oz. serving	150	3.0
House	2-oz. serving	186	6.0
1000 Island	2-oz. serving	231	7.0
Dietetic, Italian	2-oz. serving	80	0.
Sausage	1½-oz. patty	190	1.0
Shakes	1 regular size shake	353	61.0
Soft drink:			

(USDA) = United States Department of Agriculture
(HHS/FAO) = Health and Human Services/Food and Agriculture Organization
* = prepared as package directs

Food and Description	Measure or Quantity	Calories	Carbohydrates (grams)
Regular	1 regular size soft drink	243	62.0
Dietetic	1 regular size soft drink	2	0.
Soup:			
Broccoli, cream of	6 fl. oz.	140	14.0
Chicken & noodle	6 fl. oz.	80	11.0
Chowder, clam, Boston	6 fl. oz.	140	12.0
Vegetable, Lumber Jack mix	6 fl. oz.	70	10.0
Steak sandwich, *Country Fried*	7.2-oz. serving	610	54.0
Sunrise Sandwich:			
Bacon	4½-oz. serving	370	32.0
Sausage	6.1-oz. serving	500	31.0
Tea, iced	1 regular size drink	2	0.
Zucchini	4.3-oz. serving	300	33.0

CARNATION DO-IT-YOURSELF DIET PLAN:

Chocolate	2 scoops (1.1 oz.)	110	21.0
Vanilla	2 scoops (1.1 oz.)	110	22.0

CARNATION INSTANT BREAKFAST:

Bar:			
Chocolate chip	1 bar (1.44 oz.)	200	20.0
Chocolate crunch	1 bar (1.34 oz.)	190	20.0
Honey nut	1 bar (1.35 oz.)	190	18.0
Peanut butter with chocolate chips	1 bar (1.4 oz.)	200	20.0
Peanut butter crunch	1 bar (1.35 oz.)	200	20.0
Drink packets:			
Chocolate or egg nog	1 packet	130	23.0
Chocolate malt	1 packet	130	22.0
Coffee, strawberry or vanilla	1 packet	130	24.0

CARROT:

Raw (USDA):			
Whole	1 lb. (weighed with full tops)	112	26.0

Food and Description	Measure or Quantity	Calories	Carbo-hydrates (grams)
Partially trimmed	1 lb. (weighed without tops, with skins)	156	36.1
Trimmed	5½" × 1" carrot (1.8 oz.)	21	4.8
Trimmed	25 thin strips (1.8 oz.)	21	4.8
Chunks	½ cup (2.4 oz.)	29	6.7
Diced	½ cup (1½ oz.)	30	7.0
Grated or shredded	½ cup (1.9 oz.)	23	5.3
Slices	½ cup (2.2 oz.)	27	6.2
Strips	½ cup (2 oz.)	24	5.6
Boiled, drained (USDA):			
Chunks	½ cup (2.9 oz.)	25	5.8
Diced	½ cup (2½ oz.)	24	5.2
Slices	½ cup (2.7 oz.)	24	5.4
Canned, regular pack, solids & liq.:			
(Comstock)	½ cup (4.2 oz.)	35	6.0
(Larsen) *Freshlike*, solids & liq.	½ cup	30	6.0
Canned, dietetic pack, solids & liq.:			
(Featherweight) sliced	½ cup	30	6.0
(Larsen) *Fresh-Lite*, sliced, low sodium	½ cup (4.4 oz.)	25	6.0
(S&W) *Nutradiet*, green label	½ cup	30	7.0
Frozen:			
(Bel-Air) whole, baby	3.3 oz.	40	9.0
(Birds Eye) whole, baby deluxe	⅓ of pkg. (3.3 oz.)	32	7.0
(Frosty Acres) cut or whole	3.3-oz. serving	40	9.0
(Green Giant) cuts, in butter sauce	½ cup	80	16.0
CASABA MELON (USDA):			
Whole	1 lb. (weighed whole)	61	14.7
Flesh only, cubed or diced	4 oz.	31	7.4

(USDA) = United States Department of Agriculture
(HHS/FAO) = Health and Human Services/Food and Agriculture Organization
* = prepared as package directs

Food and Description	Measure or Quantity	Calories	Carbo-hydrates (grams)
CASHEW NUT:			
(USDA)	1 oz.	159	8.3
(USDA)	½ cup (2.5 oz.)	393	20.5
(USDA)	5 large or 8 med.	60	3.1
(Beer Nuts)	1 oz.	170	8.0
(Eagle Snacks):			
Honey Roast:			
Regular	1 oz.	170	9.0
With peanuts	1 oz.	170	8.0
Lightly salted	1 oz.	170	7.0
(Fisher):			
Dry roasted	¼ cup (1.2 oz.)	160	8.0
Honey roasted	1 oz.	150	7.0
Oil roasted	¼ cup (1.2 oz.)	170	8.0
(Party Pride) dry roasted	1 oz.	170	9.0
(Planters):			
Dry roasted, salted or unsalted	1 oz.	160	9.0
Honey roasted:			
Plain	1 oz.	170	11.0
With peanuts	1 oz.	170	9.0
Oil roasted	1 oz.	170	8.0
(Tom's)	1 oz.	178	7.8
CASHEW BUTTER			
(Hain) raw or toasted	1 T.	95	4.0
CATFISH, freshwater (USDA)			
raw fillet	4 oz.	117	0.
CATSUP:			
Regular:			
(Heinz)	1 T.	18	4.0
(Hunt's)	1 T. (.5 oz.)	15	4.0
(Smucker's)	1 T.	24	6.0
(Town House)	1 T.	15	4.0
Dietetic or low calorie:			
(Estee)	1 T. (.5 oz.)	6	1.0
(Heinz) lite	1 T.	8	2.0
(Hunt's) no salt added	1 T.	20	5.0
(Weight Watchers)	1 T.	12	3.0

Food and Description	Measure or Quantity	Calories	Carbo-hydrates (grams)
CAULIFLOWER:			
Raw (USDA):			
Whole	1 lb. (weighed untrimmed)	49	9.2
Flowerbuds	½ cup (1.8 oz.)	14	2.6
Slices	½ cup (1.5 oz.)	11	2.2
Boiled (USDA) flowerbuds, drained	½ cup (2.2 oz.)	14	2.5
Frozen:			
(Birds Eye):			
Regular or florets, deluxe	⅓ of 10-oz. pkg.	23	5.0
With cheese sauce	½ of 10-oz. pkg.	130	12.0
(Frosty Acres)	3.3-oz. serving	25	5.0
(Green Giant):			
In cheese sauce, regular	3.3 oz.	50	7.5
Cuts, polybag	½ cup	12	3.0
(Larsen)	3.3 oz. serving	25	5.0
CAULIFLOWER, PICKLED			
(Vlasic) hot & spicy	1 oz.	4	1.0
CAVATELLI, frozen			
(Celentano)	⅕ of 16-oz. pkg.	250	52.0
CAVIAR, STURGEON			
(USDA):			
Pressed	1 oz.	90	1.4
Whole eggs	1 T. (.6 oz.)	42	.5
CELERIAC ROOT, raw			
(USDA):			
Whole	1 lb. (weighed unpared)	156	39.2
Pared	4 oz.	45	9.6
CELERY, all varieties (USDA):			
Fresh:			
Whole	1 lb. (weighed untrimmed)	58	13.3

(USDA) = United States Department of Agriculture
(HHS/FAO) = Health and Human Services/Food and Agriculture Organization
* = prepared as package directs

Food and Description	Measure or Quantity	Calories	Carbo-hydrates (grams)
1 large outer stalk	8″ × 1½″ at root end (1.4 oz.)	7	1.6
Diced, chopped or cut in chunks	½ cup (2.1 oz.)	10	2.3
Slices	½ cup (1.9 oz.)	9	2.1
Boiled, drained solids:			
Diced or cut in chunks	½ cup (2.7 oz.)	10	2.4
Slices	½ cup (3 oz.)	12	2.6
Frozen (Larsen)	3½ oz. serving	14	3.0
CELERY SALT (French's)	1 tsp.	2	Tr.
CELERY SEED (French's)	1 tsp.	11	1.1
CEREAL BAR			
(Kellogg's) *Smart Start:*			
Common Sense, oat bran, with raspberry filling	1.5-oz. bar	170	28.0
Cornflakes with mixed berry filling	1.5-oz. bar	170	27.0
Nutri-Grain, blueberry or strawberry	1.5-oz. bar	180	26.0
Raisin bran	1.5-oz. bar	160	28.0
Rice Krispies, with almonds	1-oz. bar	130	18.0
CERTS	1 piece	6	1.5
CERVELAT:			
(USDA):			
Dry	1 oz.	128	.5
Soft	1 oz.	87	.5
(Hormel) Viking	1-oz. serving	90	0.
CEREAL (See individual listings such as **BRAN BREAKFAST CEREAL;** *COCOA PUFFS;* **CORN FLAKES; NATURAL CEREAL;** *NUTRI-GRAIN;* **OATMEAL;** etc.)			
CHABLIS WINE:			
(Almaden) light	3 fl. oz.	42	DNA
(Carlo Rossi)	3 fl. oz.	66	1.5

Food and Description	Measure or Quantity	Calories	Carbo-hydrates (grams)
(Gallo):			
White	3 fl. oz.	60	.5
Pink	3 fl. oz.	60	3.0
(Louis M. Martini) 12½% alcohol	3 fl. oz.	59	.2
(Paul Masson):			
Regular, 11.8% alcohol	3 fl. oz.	71	2.7
Light, 7.1% alcohol	3 fl. oz.	45	2.7
CHAMPAGNE:			
(Great Western):			
Regular, 12% alcohol	3 fl. oz.	71	2.5
Brut, 12% alcohol	3 fl. oz.	74	3.4
Pink, 12% alcohol	3 fl. oz.	81	4.9
(Taylor) dry, 12½% alcohol	3 fl. oz.	78	3.9
CHARD, Swiss (USDA):			
Raw, whole	1 lb. (weighed untrimmed)	104	19.2
Raw, trimmed	4 oz.	29	5.2
Boiled, drained solids	½ cup (3.4 oz.)	17	3.2
CHARDONNAY WINE (Louis M. Martini) 12½% alcohol	3 fl. oz.	60	.2
CHARLOTTE RUSSE, homemade recipe (USDA)	4 oz.	324	38.0
CHEERIOS, cereal (General Mills):			
Regular	1¼ cups (1 oz.)	110	20.0
Apple cinnamon	¾ cup (1 oz.)	110	22.0
Honey & nut	¾ cup (1 oz.)	110	23.0
CHEERIOS-TO-GO (General Mills):			
Plain	¾-oz. pkg.	80	15.0
Apple cinnamon	1-oz. pkg.	110	22.0
Honeynut	1-oz. pkg.	110	23.0

(USDA) = United States Department of Agriculture
(HHS/FAO) = Health and Human Services/Food and Agriculture Organization
* = prepared as package directs

Food and Description	Measure or Quantity	Calories	Carbo-hydrates (grams)
CHEESE:			
American or cheddar:			
(USDA):			
Regular	1 oz.	105	.5
Cube, natural	1″ cube (.6 oz.)	68	.3
(Borden) *Lite-Line*	1 oz.	70	1.0
(Churny) cheddar, lite, mild or sharp	1 oz.	80	1.0
(Dorman's):			
American:			
Lo-chol	1 oz.	90	1.0
Low sodium	1 oz.	110	1.0
Cheddar:			
Light, regular or *Cheddar-Jack*	1 oz.	80	1.0
Lo-chol	1 oz.	100	1.0
(Kraft):			
American singles	1 oz.	90	2.0
Cheddar, regular or *Old English*	1 oz.	110	1.0
Laughing Cow, natural	1 oz.	100	Tr.
(Land O' Lakes):			
American, process:			
Regular	1 oz.	110	1.0
Sharp	1 oz.	100	1.0
Cheddar, natural:			
Regular	1 oz.	110	<1.0
& bacon	1 oz.	110	1.0
Extra sharp	1 oz.	100	1.0
(Lucerne):			
American slices	1 oz.	110	1.0
Cheddar	1 oz.	110	0.
(Polly-O) cheddar, shredded	1 oz.	110	1.0
(Safeway) American	1 oz.	110	1.0
Wispride	1 oz.	115	1.0
Blue:			
(USDA) natural	1 oz.	104	.6
Laughing Cow	¾-oz. wedge	55	.5
(Safeway)	1 oz.	100	1.0
(Sargento) cold pack or crumbled	1 oz.	100	1.0
Bonbino, *Laughing Cow*, natural	1 oz.	103	Tr.
Brick:			
(USDA) natural	1 oz.	105	.5

Food and Description	Measure or Quantity	Calories	Carbo-hydrates (grams)
(Land O' Lakes)	1 oz.	110	1.0
(Safeway) mild	1 oz.	100	1.0
Brie (Sargento) *Danish Danko*	1 oz.	80	.1
Burgercheese (Sargento) *Danish Danko*	1 oz.	106	1.0
Camembert (USDA) domestic	1 oz.	85	.5
Colby:			
(Churny) lite	1 oz.	80	1.0
(Dorman's) *Lo-chol*	1 oz.	100	1.0
(Kraft)	1 oz.	110	1.0
(Land O' Lakes)	1 oz.	110	1.0
(Lucerne) loaf or shredded	1 oz.	110	0.
(Safeway)	1 oz.	110	0.
Cottage:			
Unflavored:			
(USDA) creamed	½ cup (4.3 oz.)	130	3.5
(Breakstone):			
Low fat	4 oz.	90	4.0
Smooth & creamy or tangy	4 oz.	110	4.0
(Friendship) California style	1 oz	30	1.0
(Johanna):			
Large or small curd	½ cup	120	4.0
Low fat or no salt	½ cup	90	4.0
(Land O' Lakes)	1 oz.	30	1.0
(Lucerne):			
Dry curd	½ cup	80	3.0
Farmers or farmer curd, large or small curd	½ cup	120	4.0
Low fat, regular or unsalted	½ cup	100	4.0
(Weight Watchers):			
1%	½ cup	90	4.0
2%	½ cup	100	4.0
Flavored (Friendship) pineapple, regular	1 oz.	35	3.8
Cream:			
(USDA)	1 oz.	106	.6
(Friendship)	1 oz.	103	.8

(USDA) = United States Department of Agriculture
(HHS/FAO) = Health and Human Services/Food and Agriculture
            Organization
* = prepared as package directs

Food and Description	Measure or Quantity	Calories	Carbo- hydrates (grams)
(Kraft) Philadelphia Brand:			
Regular	1 oz.	100	1.0
With chive & onion	1 oz.	100	2.0
Light	1 oz.	60	2.0
Olive & pimento	1 oz.	90	2.0
(Lucerne) plain, regular or soft	1 oz.	100	1.0
Edam:			
(Churny) May-Bud	1 oz.	100	0.0
(Kaukauna)	1 oz.	100	<1.0
(Land O' Lakes)	1 oz.	100	<1.0
Laughing Cow	1 oz.	100	Tr.
Farmer:			
(Churny) May-Bud	1 oz.	90	1.0
(Friendship) regular or no salt added	1 oz.	40	1.0
(Kaukauna)	1 oz.	100	<1.0
Wispride	1 oz.	100	1.0
Feta:			
(Churny)	1 oz.	75	1.2
(Safeway)	1 oz.	75	1.0
Gjetost *(Sargento)* Norwegian	1 oz.	118	13.0
Gouda:			
(Churny) May-Bud:			
Regular	1 oz.	100	1.0
Lite	1 oz.	81	1.0
(Kaukauna)	1 oz.	100	<1.0
(Land O' Lakes)	1 oz.	100	1.0
Laughing Cow:			
Regular	1 oz.	110	Tr.
Mini, waxed	¾ oz.	80	Tr.
(Lucerne)	1 oz.	100	1.0
Gruyère, *Swiss Knight*	1 oz.	100	Tr.
Havarti *(Sargento):*			
Creamy	1 oz.	90	.2
Creamy, 60% mild	1 oz.	177	.2
Hoop *(Friendship)* natural	1 oz.	21	.5
Hot pepper *(Sargento)* sliced	1 oz.	112	1.0
Jalapeño Jack *(Land O' Lakes)*	1 oz.	90	1.0
Jarlsberg *(Safeway)* Norwegian	1 oz.	100	0.
Kettle Moraine *(Sargento)*	1 oz.	100	1.0
Limburger *(Sargento)* natural	1 oz.	93	14.0
Longhorn:			
(Lucerne)	1 oz.	110	0.

Food and Description	Measure or Quantity	Calories	Carbo-hydrates (grams)
(Safeway)	1 oz.	110	0.
Monterey Jack:			
(Churny) lite	1 oz.	80	0.
(Kaukauna)	1 oz.	110	<1.0
(Kraft)	1 oz.	110	0.
(Land O' Lakes)	1 oz.	110	<1.0
(Lucerne)	1 oz.	105	0.
(Safeway)	1 oz.	105	0.
Mozzarella:			
(Dorman's) light	1 oz.	80	1.0
(Kraft)	1 oz.	80	0.
(Land O' Lakes) part skim milk	1 oz.	80	1.0
(Lucerne) shredded, sliced or whole	1 oz.	80	0.
(Polly-O):			
Fior di Latte	1 oz.	80	1.0
Lite	1 oz.	70	1.0
Part skim milk, regular or shredded	1 oz.	80	1.0
Smoked	1 oz.	85	1.0
Whole milk:			
Regular	1 oz.	90	1.0
Old fashioned, regular	1 oz.	70	1.0
(Sargento):			
Bar, rounds, shredded regular or with spices, sliced for pizza or square	1 oz.	79	1.0
Whole milk	1 oz.	100	1.0
Muenster:			
(Dorman's):			
Light	1 oz.	80	0.
Lo-chol	1 oz.	100	1.0
Low sodium	1 oz.	110	0.
(Kaukauna)	1 oz.	110	<1.0
(Land O' Lakes)	1 oz.	100	<1.0
(Safeway)	1 oz.	105	0.
Wispride	1 oz.	100	Tr.

(USDA) = United States Department of Agriculture
(HHS/FAO) = Health and Human Services/Food and Agriculture Organization
* = prepared as package directs

Food and Description	Measure or Quantity	Calories	Carbo-hydrates (grams)
Parmesan:			
(USDA):			
Regular	1 oz.	111	.8
Grated	½ cup (not packed)	169	1.2
(Lucerne) grated	1 oz.	110	1.0
(Polly-O) grated	1 oz.	130	1.0
(Progresso) grated	1 T.	23	*1.0
Pot (Sargento) regular, French onion or garlic	1 oz.	30	1.0
Provolone:			
(Frigo)	1 oz.	90	1.0
Laughing Cow:			
Cube	⅙ oz.	12	.1
Wedge	¾ oz.	55	.5
Ricotto:			
(Frigo) part skim milk	1 oz.	43	.9
(Polly-O):			
Lite	1 oz.	40	1.5
Old-fashioned	1 oz.	50	1.0
Part skim milk	1 oz.	45	1.0
Whole milk	1 oz.	50	1.0
(Sargento):			
Part skim milk	1 oz.	39	1.0
Whole milk	1 oz.	49	1.0
Romano (Polly-O) wedge	1 oz.	130	1.0
Roquefort, natural (USDA)	1 oz.	104	.6
Samsoe (Sargento) Danish	1 oz.	101	.2
Scamorze (Frigo)	1 oz.	79	.3
Semisoft:			
Bel Paese	1 oz.	90	.3
Laughing Cow:			
Babybel:			
Regular	1 oz.	91	Tr.
Mini	¾ oz.	74	Tr.
Bonbel:			
Regular	1 oz.	100	Tr.
Mini	¾ oz.	74	Tr.
Reduced calorie	1 oz.	45	Tr.
Slim Jack (Dorman's)	1 oz.	80	1.0
Stirred curd (Frigo)	1 oz.	110	1.0
Swiss:			
(USDA) domestic, natural or process	1 oz.	105	.5

Food and Description	Measure or Quantity	Calories	Carbo-hydrates (grams)
(Churny) lite	1 oz.	90	1.0
(Dorman's) light	1 oz.	90	0.
(Lucerne)	1 oz.	100	0.
(Safeway)	1 oz.	100	0.
Taco (Sargento) shredded	1 oz.	105	1.0
Washed curd (Frigo)	1 oz.	110	1.0

CHEESE ENTREE (See MACARONI & CHEESE; SOUFFLE, Cheese; WELSH RAREBIT)

CHEESE FONDUE,
  Swiss Knight | 1 oz. | 60 | 1.0 |

CHEESE FOOD:
  American or cheddar:

Food and Description	Measure or Quantity	Calories	Carbo-hydrates (grams)
(USDA) process	1 oz.	92	2.0
(Borden) *Lite-Line*	1 oz.	50	1.0
(Fisher) *Ched-O-Mate* or *Sandwich-Mate*	1 oz.	90	1.0
(Land O' Lakes)	¾-oz. slice	70	2.0
(Lucerne)	1 oz.	90	2.0
(Shedd's) *Country Crock*	1 oz.	70	3.0
Cheez-ola (Fisher)	1 oz.	90	1.0
Chef's Delight (Fisher)	1 oz.	70	4.0
Garlic & Herb, *Wispride*	1 oz.	90	4.0
Hot pepper (Lucerne)	1 oz.	90	2.0
Italian herb (Land O' Lakes)	1 oz.	90	2.0
Jalapeño (Borden) *Lite-Line*	1 oz.	50	1.0
Low sodium (Borden) *Lite-Line*	1 oz.	70	2.0
Muenster (Borden) *Lite-Line*	1 oz.	50	1.0
Mun-chee (Pauly)	1 oz.	100	2.0
Neufchatel (Shedd's) *Country Crock*	1 oz.	70	1.0
Onion (Land O' Lakes)	1 oz.	90	2.0
Pepperoni (Land O' Lakes)	1 oz.	90	1.0
Pimiento (Lucerne)	1 oz.	80	2.0
Salami (Land O' Lakes)	1 oz.	90	2.0

(USDA) = United States Department of Agriculture
(HHS/FAO) = Health and Human Services/Food and Agriculture Organization
* = prepared as package directs

Food and Description	Measure or Quantity	Calories	Carbo-hydrates (grams)
Swiss:			
(Borden) *Lite-Line*	1 oz.	50	1.0
(Kraft) reduced fat	1 oz.	90	1.0
(Pauly)	.8-oz. slice	74	1.6
CHEESE SPREAD:			
American or cheddar:			
(USDA)	1 T. (.5 oz.)	40	1.1
(Fisher)	1 oz.	80	2.0
Laughing Cow	1 oz.	72	.7
(Nabisco) *Easy Cheese*	1 tsp.	16	.4
Blue, *Laughing Cow*	1 oz.	72	.7
Cheese 'n Bacon (Nabisco) *Easy Cheese*	1 tsp.	16	.4
Golden velvet (Land O' Lakes)	1 oz.	80	2.0
Gruyère, *Laughing Cow,* *La Vache Que Rit*:			
Regular	1 oz.	72	.7
Reduced calorie	1 oz.	46	1.3
Nacho (Nabisco) *Easy Cheese*	1 tsp.	16	.4
Pimiento:			
(Nabisco) *Snack Mate*	1 tsp.	15	.3
(Price)	1 oz.	80	2.0
Provolone, *Laughing Cow*	1 oz.	72	.7
Velveeta (Kraft)	1 oz.	80	2.0
CHENIN BLANC WINE (Louis M. Martini) 12½% alcohol	3 fl. oz.	56	.9
CHERRY:			
Sour:			
Fresh (USDA):			
Whole	1 lb. (weighed with stems)	213	52.5
Whole	1 lb. (weighed without stems)	242	59.7
Pitted	½ cup (2.7 oz.)	45	11.1
Canned, syrup pack, pitted:			
(USDA):			
Light syrup	4 oz. (with liq.)	84	21.2
Heavy syrup	½ cup (with liq.)	116	29.5
Extra heavy syrup	4 oz. (with liq.)	127	32.4
(Thank You Brand)	½ cup (4.5 oz.)	123	29.4
Canned, water pack, pitted, solid & liq.	½ cup (4.3 oz.)	52	13.1

Food and Description	Measure or Quantity	Calories	Carbo-hydrates (grams)
Frozen, pitted:			
Sweetened	½ cup (4.6 oz.)	146	36.1
Unsweetened	4 oz.	62	15.2
Sweet:			
Fresh (USDA):			
Whole	1 lb. (weighed with stems)	286	71.0
Whole, with stems	½ cup (2.3 oz.)	41	10.2
Pitted	½ cup (2.9 oz.)	57	14.3
Canned, syrup pack: (USDA):			
Light syrup, pitted	4 oz. (with liq.)	74	18.7
Heavy syrup, pitted	½ cup (with liq., 4.2 oz.)	96	24.2
Extra heavy syrup, pitted	4 oz. (with liq.)	113	29.0
(Del Monte) solids & liq.:			
Dark	½ cup (4.3 oz.)	90	23.0
Light	½ cup (4.3 oz.)	100	26.0
(Stokely-Van Camp) pitted, solids & liq.	½ cup (4.2 oz.)	50	11.0
(Thank You Brand) heavy syrup	½ cup (4.5 oz.)	98	23.0
Canned, dietetic or water pack, solids & liq.:			
(Diet Delight)	½ cup (4.4 oz.)	70	17.0
(Featherweight):			
Dark	½ cup	60	13.0
Light	½ cup	50	11.0
(Thank You Brand) water pack	½ cup (4.5 oz.)	61	14.1
CHERRY, CANDIED (USDA)	1 oz.	96	24.6
CHERRY, MARASCHINO (USDA)	1 oz. (with liq.)	33	8.3
CHERRY DRINK:			
Canned:			
(Hi-C)	6 fl. oz.	100	24.7

(USDA) = United States Department of Agriculture
(HHS/FAO) = Health and Human Services/Food and Agriculture
                        Organization
* = prepared as package directs

Food and Description	Measure or Quantity	Calories	Carbo-hydrates (grams)
(Johanna Farms) *Ssips*	8.45-fl.-oz. container	130	32.0
(Lincoln) cherry berry	6 fl. oz.	100	25.0
(Smucker's)	8 fl. oz.	130	31.0
Squeezit (General Mills)	6¾-fl.-oz. container	110	27.0
*Mix (Funny Face)	8 fl. oz.	88	22.0
CHERRY HEERING			
(Hiram Walker)	1 fl. oz.	80	10.0
CHERRY JELLY:			
Sweetened (Smucker's)	1 T. (.5 oz.)	54	12.0
Dietetic (Featherweight)	1 T.	16	4.0
CHERRY LIQUEUR			
(DeKuyper) 50 proof	1 fl. oz.	75	8.5
CHERRY PRESERVES OR JAM:			
Sweetened (Smucker's)	1 T. (.7 oz.)	54	12.0
Dietetic:			
(Estee)	1 T. (.6 oz.)	6	0.
(Louis Sherry)	1 T. (.6 oz.)	6	0.
(S&W) *Nutradiet*, red label	1 T. (.6 oz.)	12	3.0
CHESTNUT (USDA):			
Fresh:			
In shell	1 lb. (weighed in shell)	713	154.7
Shelled	4 oz.	220	47.7
Dried:			
In shell	1 lb. (weighed in shell)	1402	292.4
Shelled	4 oz.	428	89.1
CHEWING GUM:			
Sweetened:			
Bazooka, bubble	1 slice	18	4.5
Beechies	1 piece	6	2.0

Food and Description	Measure or Quantity	Calories	Carbo-hydrates (grams)
Beech Nut; Beeman's, Big Red; Black Jack; Clove; Doublemint; Freedent; Fruit Punch; Juicy Fruit, Spearmint (Wrigley's); *Teaberry*	1 stick	10	2.3
Bubble Yum	1 piece	25	7.0
Dentyne	1 piece	4	1.2
Extra (Wrigley's)	1 piece	8	Tr.
Hubba Bubba (Wrigley's)	1 piece (8 grams)	23	5.8
Dietetic:			
Bubble Yum	1 piece	20	5.0
(*Care*Free*)	1 piece	8	2.0
(Estee) bubble or regular	1 piece	5	1.4
Orbit (Wrigley's)	1 piece	8	Tr.
CHEX, cereal (Ralston Purina):			
Bran (See **BRAN BREAKFAST CEREAL**)			
Corn	1 cup (1 oz.)	110	25.0
Double	⅔ cup (1 oz.)	100	24.0
Honey graham	⅔ cup (1 oz.)	110	25.0
Oat, honey nut	½ cup (1 oz.)	100	22.0
Rice	1⅛ cups (1 oz.)	110	25.0
Wheat	⅔ cup (1 oz.)	110	23.0
CHIANTI WINE (Italian Swiss Colony) 13% alcohol	3 fl. oz.	64	1.5
CHICKEN (USDA):			
Broiler, cooked, meat only	4 oz.	154	0.
Capon, raw, with bone	1 lb. (weighed ready-to-cook)	937	0.
Fryer:			
Raw:			
Ready-to-cook	1 lb. (weighed ready-to-cook)	382	0.
Breast	1 lb. (weighed with bone)	394	0.

(USDA) = United States Department of Agriculture
(HHS/FAO) = Health and Human Services/Food and Agriculture Organization
* = prepared as package directs

Food and Description	Measure or Quantity	Calories	Carbo-hydrates (grams)
Leg or drumstick	1 lb. (weighed with bone)	313	0.
Thigh	1 lb. (weighed with bone)	435	0.
Fried. A 2½-lb. chicken (weighed before cooking with bone) will give you:			
Back	1 back (2.2 oz.)	139	2.7
Breast	½ breast (3⅓ oz.)	154	1.1
Leg or drumstrick	1 leg (2 oz.)	87	.4
Neck	1 neck (2.1 oz.)	121	1.9
Rib	1 rib (.7 oz.)	42	.8
Thigh	1 thigh (2¼ oz.)	118	1.2
Wing	1 wing (1¾ oz.)	78	.8
Fried, frozen (See **CHICKEN, FRIED**, frozen)			
Fried skin	1 oz.	199	2.6
Hen and cock:			
Raw	1 lb. (weighed ready-to-cook)	987	0.
Stewed:			
Meat only	4 oz.	236	0.
Chopped	½ cup (2.5 oz.)	150	0.
Diced	½ cup (2.4 oz.)	139	0.
Ground	½ cup (2 oz.)	116	0.
Roaster:			
Raw:	1 lb. (weighed ready-to-cook)	791	0.
Roasted:			
Dark meat without skin	4 oz.	209	0.
Light meat without skin	4 oz.	206	0.
CHICKEN À LA KING:			
Home recipe (USDA)	1 cup (8.6 oz.)	468	12.3
Canned (Swanson)	½ of 10½-oz. can	190	9.0
Frozen:			
(Armour) *Classics Lite*	11¼-oz. meal	290	38.0
(Banquet)	4-oz. pkg.	110	9.0
(Le Menu):	10¼-oz. dinner	320	29.0
Regular	10¼-oz. dinner	330	29.0
Healthy entree	8¼-oz. entree	240	29.0
(Stouffer's) with rice	9½-oz. pkg.	290	34.0
(Weight Watchers)	9-oz. pkg.	220	15.0

Food and Description	Measure or Quantity	Calories	Carbo-hydrates (grams)
CHICKEN BOUILLON:			
Regular:			
(Herb-Ox):			
Cube	1 cube	6	.6
Packet	1 packet	12	1.9
(Knorr)	1 packet	16	.6
(Maggi) cube	1 cube	7	1.0
(Wyler's)	1 cube	8	1.0
Low sodium:			
(Borden) *Lite-Line,*	1 tsp.	12	2.0
(Featherweight)	1 tsp.	18	2.0
CHICKEN, BONED, canned:			
Regular:			
(USDA)	1 cup (7.2 oz.)	406	0.
(Hormel) chunk:			
Breast	6¾-oz. serving	350	0.
Dark	6¾-oz. serving	327	0.
White & dark:			
Regular	6¾-oz. serving	340	0.
Low salt	6¾-oz. serving	330	0.
(Swanson) chunk:			
Mixin' chicken	2½ oz.	130	1.0
White	2½ oz.	90	0.
Low sodium (Featherweight)	2½ oz.	154	0.
CHICKEN CHUNKS, frozen (Country Pride):			
Regular	3 oz.	240	15.0
Southern fried	3 oz.	280	14.0
CHICKEN, CREAMED, frozen (Stouffer's)	6½ oz. pkg.	300	5.9
CHICKEN DINNER OR ENTREE:			
Canned:			
(Hunt's) Minute Gourmet, microwave entree maker:			
Barbecued	6.8-oz. serving	320	37.0

(USDA) = United States Department of Agriculture
(HHS/FAO) = Health and Human Services/Food and Agriculture
                    Organization
* = prepared as package directs

Food and Description	Measure or Quantity	Calories	Carbo-hydrates (grams)
Cacciatore	8.3-oz. serving	280	20.0
Sweet & sour	7.8-oz. serving	300	32.0
(Swanson) & dumplings	7½-oz. serving	220	19.0
Frozen:			
(Armour):			
Classics Lite:			
Breast medallion marsala	10½-oz. meal	250	27.0
Burgundy	10½-oz. meal	210	25.0
Oriental	10-oz. meal	180	24.0
Sweet & sour	11-oz. meal	240	39.0
Dining Lite, glazed	9-oz. meal	220	30.0
Dinner Classics:			
Glazed	10¾-oz. dinner	300	24.0
Mesquite	9½-oz. dinner	370	42.0
Parmigiana	11½-oz. dinner	370	27.0
With wine and mush-room sauce	10¾-oz. dinner	280	24.0
(Banquet):			
Cookin' Bag & vegetable primavera	4-oz. serving	100	14.0
Dinner:			
Regular:			
& dumplings	10-oz. dinner	430	34.0
Fried	10-oz. dinner	400	45.0
Extra Helping:			
Fried	16-oz. dinner	570	70.0
Fried, all white meat	16-oz. dinner	570	70.0
Nuggets:			
BBQ sauce	10-oz. dinner	640	56.0
Sweet & Sour Sauce	10-oz. dinner	650	54.0
Family Entree:			
& dumplings	¼ of 28-oz. pkg.	280	28.0
& vegetable primavera	¼ of 28-oz. pkg.	140	18.0
Platter:			
Boneless:			
Drumsnacker	7-oz. meal	430	49.0
Nuggets	6.4-oz. meal	430	46.0
Pattie	7½-oz. meal	380	34.0
Fried, all white meat, any type	9-oz. meal	430	21.0
(Celentano):			
Parmigiana, cutlets	9-oz. pkg.	400	21.0
Primavera	11½-oz. pkg.	260	26.0

Food and Description	Measure or Quantity	Calories	Carbo-hydrates (grams)
(Chun King):			
Imperial	13-oz. entree	300	54.0
Walnut, crunchy	13-oz. entree	310	49.0
(Healthy Choice):			
À l'orange	9½-oz. meal	260	39.0
Glazed	8½-oz. meal	230	28.0
Herb roasted	11-oz. meal	260	38.0
Mesquite	10½-oz. meal	310	52.0
Oriental	11¼-oz. meal	220	31.0
Parmigiana	11½-oz. meal	280	38.0
& pasta divan	11½ oz. meal	310	45.0
Sweet & sour	11½-oz. meal	280	44.0
(Kid Cuisine):			
Fried	7¼-oz. meal	420	41.0
Nuggets	6¼-oz. meal	400	46.0
(La Choy) *Fresh & Lite:*			
Almond, with rice			
& vegetables	9¾-oz. meal	270	40.1
Imperial	11-oz. meal	260	45.0
Oriental, spicy	9¾-oz. meal	270	52.0
Sweet & sour	10-oz. meal	260	50.1
(Le Menu):			
Regular, dinner:			
Cordon bleu	11-oz. dinner	460	47.0
Parmigiana	11¾-oz. dinner	410	31.0
Sweet & sour	11¼-oz. dinner	400	41.0
In wine sauce	10-oz. dinner	280	27.0
Healthy style dinner:			
Glazed breast	10-oz. dinner	230	25.0
Herb roasted	10-oz. dinner	240	18.0
Sweet & sour	10-oz. dinner	250	29.0
Healthy style entree:			
Dijon	8-oz. entree	240	21.0
Empress	8¼-oz. entree		
(Morton):			
Regular:			
Boneless	11-oz. dinner	329	44.7
Boneless	17-oz. dinner	627	84.0
Fried	11-oz. dinner	431	64.1
Light, boneless	11-oz. dinner	250	30.0

(USDA) = United States Department of Agriculture
(HHS/FAO) = Health and Human Services/Food and Agriculture
            Organization
* = prepared as package directs

Food and Description	Measure or Quantity	Calories	Carbo-hydrates (grams)
(Stouffer's):			
Regular:			
Cashew, in sauce with rice	9½-oz. meal	380	29.0
Creamed	6½-oz. meal	300	8.0
Divan	8½-oz. meal	320	11.0
Escalloped, & noodles	10-oz. meal	420	27.0
Lean Cuisine:			
À l'orange, with almond rice	8-oz. meal	260	30.0
Breast, in herbed cream sauce	9½-oz. meal	260	11.0
Breast, marsala, with vegetables	8⅛-oz. meal	190	11.0
Breast, Parmesan	10-oz. meal	260	19.0
Cacciatore, with vermicelli	10⅞-oz. meal	250	26.0
Fiesta	8½-oz. meal	250	29.0
Glazed, with vegetable rice	8½-oz. meal	270	23.0
Oriental	9⅜-oz. meal	230	23.0
& vegetables with vermicelli	11¾-oz. meal	270	29.0
Right Course:			
Italiano, with fettucini & vegetables	9⅝-oz. meal	280	29.0
Sesame	10-oz. meal	320	34.0
Tenderloins in barbecue sauce with rice pilaf	8¾-oz. meal	270	38.0
Tenderloins in peanut sauce with linguini & vegetables	9¼-oz. meal	330	32.0
(Swanson):			
Regular, 4-compartment dinner:			
Fried:			
BBQ flavor	10-oz. dinner	540	61.0
Dark meat	9¾-oz. dinner	560	55.0
White meat	10¼-oz. dinner	550	60.0
Nuggets	8¾-oz. dinner	470	47.0
Homestyle Recipe, entrees:			
Cacciatore	10.95 oz. meal	260	33.0
Fried	7-oz. meal	390	33.0
Nibbles	4¼-oz. meal	340	29.0
Hungry Man, dinner:			
Boneless	17¾-oz. dinner	700	65.0

Food and Description	Measure or Quantity	Calories	Carbo-hydrates (grams)
Fried:			
Dark meat	14½-oz. dinner	860	77.0
White meat	14½-oz. dinner	870	80.0
(Tyson):			
À l'orange	9½-oz. meal	300	36.0
Dijon	8½-oz. meal	310	17.0
Francais	9½-oz. meal	280	20.0
Kiev	9¼-oz. meal	520	40.0
Marsala	10½-oz. meal	300	26.0
Mesquite	9½-oz. meal	320	35.0
Oriental	10¼-oz. meal	270	32.0
Parmigiana	11¼-oz. meal	380	37.0
Sweet & sour	11-oz. meal	420	50.0
(Weight Watchers):			
Cordon bleu, breaded	8-oz. meal	230	15.0
Fettucini	8¼-oz. meal	290	26.0
Imperial	9¼-oz. meal	220	26.0
Nuggets	5.9-oz. meal	270	24.0
Patty, southern fried	6½-oz. meal	340	31.0
Sweet & sour tenders	10.2-oz. meal	240	43.0
Mix (Lipton) *Microeasy*:			
Barbecue	¼ pkg.	108	24.1
Country	¼ pkg.	78	14.9
CHICKEN FRICASEE (USDA)			
home recipe	1 cup (8.5 oz.)	386	7.7
CHICKEN, FRIED, frozen:			
(Banquet):			
Assorted	2-lb. pkg.	1650	145.0
Breast portion	11½-oz. pkg.	440	26.0
Hot & spicy	32-oz. pkg.	1650	145.0
Thigh & drumstick	25-oz. pkg.	1000	56.0
(Country Pride) southern fried:			
Chunks	3 oz.	276	14.0

(USDA) = United States Department of Agriculture
(HHS/FAO) = Health and Human Services/Food and Agriculture Organization
* = prepared as package directs

Food and Description	Measure or Quantity	Calories	Carbo-hydrates (grams)
(Swanson):			
Assorted	3¼-oz. serving	270	16.0
Breast portion	4½-oz. serving	360	21.0
Nibbles	3¼-oz. serving	300	19.0
Thighs & drumsticks	3¼-oz. serving	290	17.0
CHICKEN GIZZARD (USDA):			
Raw	4 oz.	128	.8
Simmered	4 oz.	168	.8
CHICKEN HELPER			
(General Mills):			
& biscuits, crispy	⅕ of pkg.	710	45.0
& dumplings	⅕ of pkg.	530	41.0
& mushrooms	⅕ of pkg.	470	29.0
Potato & gravy	⅕ of pkg.	600	45.0
& seasoned rice, crispy	⅕ of pkg.	689	47.0
Stuffing	⅕ of pkg.	570	34.0
Teriyaki	⅕ of pkg.	480	35.0
Tetrazzini	⅕ of pkg.	340	38.0
CHICKEN & NOODLES,			
frozen:			
(Armour):			
Dining Lite	9-oz. meal	240	28.0
Dinner Classics	11-oz. meal	230	23.0
(Stouffer's) homestyle	10-oz. meal	310	21.0
CHICKEN NUGGETS, frozen:			
(Country Pride)	3-oz. serving	250	14.0
(Empire Kosher)	12-oz. pkg.	708	56.0
(Swanson)	3-oz. serving	230	14.0
CHICKEN, PACKAGED:			
(Carl Buddig) smoked, sliced	1 oz.	60	1.0
(Eckrich) breast	1 slice	20	.5
(Louis Rich) breast, oven roasted	1-oz. slice	40	Tr.
(Oscar Mayer) breast:			
Oven roasted	1-oz. slice	30	.6
Smoked	1-oz. slice	26	.5
(Weaver):			
Bologna	1 slice	44	.5
Breast	1 slice	25	.5
Roll	1 slice	46	.5

Food and Description	Measure or Quantity	Calories	Carbo-hydrates (grams)
CHICKEN PATTIES, frozen:			
(County Pride) regular	12-oz. pkg.	1000	56.0
(Empire Kosher)	12-oz. pkg.	792	52.0
CHICKEN PIE, frozen:			
(Banquet)	7-oz pie	550	39.0
(Empire Kosher)	8-oz. pie	463	49.0
(Morton)	7-oz. pie	420	27.0
(Stouffer's)	10-oz. pie	530	35.0
(Swanson):			
Regular	7-oz. pie	380	35.0
Hungry Man	16-oz. pie	630	57.0
CHICKEN, POTTED (USDA)	1 oz.	70	0.
CHICKEN SALAD (Carnation)	¼ of 7½-oz. can	120	3.8
CHICKEN SOUP (See **SOUP**, Chicken)			
CHICKEN STEW, canned, regular	7³⁄₈-oz.	160	15.0
CHICKEN STICKS, frozen (County Pride)	12-oz. pkg.	960	64.0
CHICK-FIL-A:			
Brownie, fudge, with nuts	2.8 oz.	369	45.0
Chicken, without bun	3.6 oz.	219	1.5
Chicken nuggets, 8 pack	4 oz.	287	12.5
Chicken salad:			
Regular, plate	11.8 oz.	475	60.2
Sandwich, regular wheat bread	5.7 oz.	449	35.2
Sandwich, deluxe, regular	7.45 oz.	368	29.8
Cole slaw	3.7 oz. cup	175	11.2
Icedream	4½ oz.	134	18.9
Pie, lemon	4.1-oz. slice	329	63.8
Potato, *Waffle Potato Fries*	3 oz.	270	33.0
Potato salad	3.8-oz. cup	198	13.9

(USDA) = United States Department of Agriculture
(HHS/FAO) = Health and Human Services/Food and Agriculture Organization
* = prepared as package directs

Food and Description	Measure or Quantity	Calories	Carbo-hydrates (grams)
Salad, tossed:			
Plain	4½ oz.	21	4.2
With dressing:			
Honey french	6 oz.	246	6.9
Italian, lite	6 oz.	46	6.3
1000 Island	6 oz.	231	8.7
Soup, hearty, small	8½ oz.	152	11.1
CHICK-PEAS OR			
GARBANZOS:			
Dry (USDA)	1 cup (7.1 oz.)	720	122.0
Canned, regular pack, solids & liq.:			
(Allen's)	½ cup	110	18.0
(Furman's)	⅓ cup (2.6 oz.)	237	13.5
(Goya)	½ cup (4 oz.)	110	17.0
(Old El Paso)	½ cup	190	16.0
(Progresso)	½ cup	120	22.0
Canned, dietetic pack, solids & liq.			
(S&W) *Nutradiet*	½ cup	105	19.0
CHILI, OR CHILI CON			
CARNE:			
Canned, regular pack:			
Beans only:			
(Comstock)	½ cup (4.4 oz.)	140	23.0
(Hormel) in sauce	5 oz.	130	19.0
(Hunt's)	½ cup (3.5 oz.)	100	18.0
(Town House)	½ cup	110	20.0
With beans:			
(Gebhardt) hot	½ of 15-oz. can	470	46.0
(Hormel):			
Regular	7½-oz. serving	310	23.0
Hot	½-oz. serving	310	24.0
Short Orders	7½-oz. can	300	23.0
(Hunt's) *Just Rite:*			
Regular	4 oz.	200	16.0
Hot	4 oz.	195	16.0
(Old El Paso)	1 cup	349	12.3
Without beans:			
(Gebhardt)	½ of 15-oz. can	410	13.0
(Hunt's) *Just Rite*	4 oz.	180	9.0

Food and Description	Measure or Quantity	Calories	Carbo-hydrates (grams)
Canned, dietetic pack:			
(Estee) with beans	7½-oz. serving	370	27.0
(Featherweight) with beans	7½-oz.	270	25.0
Frozen:			
(Stouffer's):			
Regular, with beans	8⅓-oz. meal	260	24.0
Right Choice, vegetarian	9¾-oz. meal	280	45.0
(Swanson) *Homestyle Recipe*	8¼-oz. meal	270	26.0
Mix, *Manwich, Chili Fixins*:			
Sauce only	5.3 oz.	110	20.0
*Prepared	8-oz. serving	290	20.0
CHILI SAUCE:			
(USDA)	½ cup (4.8 oz.)	142	33.8
(El Molino) green, mild	1 T.	5	1.0
(Heinz)	1 T.	17	3.0
(LaVictoria) green	1 T.	3	1.0
(Ortega) green:			
Hot	1 oz.	9	1.9
Medium or mild	1 oz.	7	1.7
CHILI SEASONING MIX:			
(French's) *Chili-O*:			
Plain	⅙ of pkg.	25	5.0
Onion	⅙ of pkg.	35	7.0
(Lawry's)	1.6-oz. pkg.	143	26.6
CHIMICHANGA, frozen:			
(Fred's) *Marquez*:			
Beef, shredded	5-oz. serving	351	35.0
Chicken	5-oz. serving	350	42.0
(Old El Paso):			
Regular:			
Beef	1 piece	370	34.0
Chicken	1 piece	360	33.0
Dinner, festive:			
Beef	11-oz. dinner	540	65.0
Beef & cheese	11-oz. dinner	510	53.0

(USDA) = United States Department of Agriculture
(HHS/FAO) = Health and Human Services/Food and Agriculture Organization
* = prepared as package directs

Food and Description	Measure or Quantity	Calories	Carbo-hydrates (grams)
Entree:			
Bean & cheese	1 piece	350	36.0
Beef	1 piece	380	35.0
Beef & pork	1 piece	340	35.0
Chicken	1 piece	370	35.0
CHIPS (See **CRACKERS, PUFFS & CHIPS**)			
CHIVES (USDA) raw	1 T. (3 grams)	1	.2
CHOCOLATE, BAKING:			
(Baker's):			
Bitter or unsweetened	1-oz. square	180	8.6
Semi-sweet:			
Regular	1-oz. square	156	16.8
Chips	¼ cup (1½ oz.)	207	31.7
Sweetened, *German's*	1 oz. square	158	17.3
(Hershey's):			
Bitter or unsweetened	1 oz.	190	7.0
Sweetened:			
Dark chips, regular or mini	1 oz.	151	17.8
Milk, chips	1 oz.	150	18.0
Semi-sweet, chips	1 oz.	147	17.3
(Nestlé):			
Bitter or unsweetened, *Choco-bake*	1-oz. packet	180	8.0
Sweet or semi-sweet, morsels	1 oz.	150	17.0
***CHOCOLATE DRINK;**			
Canned (Yoo-hoo)	8 fl. oz	130	28.0
Mix (Lucerne)	8 fl. oz	240	32.0
CHOCOLATE ICE CREAM (See **ICE CREAM**, Chocolate)			
CHOCOLATE SYRUP (See **SYRUP**, Chocolate)			
CHOP SUEY:			
Home recipe (USDA) with meat	1 cup (8.8 oz.)	300	12.8
Frozen (Stouffer's) beef, with rice	12-oz. pkg.	340	43.0

Food and Description	Measure or Quantity	Calories	Carbo-hydrates (grams)
CHOWDER (See **SOUP,** Chowder)			
CHOW CHOW (USDA):			
Sour	1 cup (8.5 oz.)	70	9.8
Sweet	1 cup (8.6 oz.)	284	66.2
CHOW MEIN:			
Canned:			
(Chun King) Divider-pak:			
Beef	¼ of pkg.	91	11.6
Chicken	½ of 24-oz. pkg.	110	12.7
Pork	¼ of pkg.	116	11.2
Shrimp	¼ of pkg.	91	13.0
(La Choy):			
Regular:			
Beef	7 oz.	60	6.0
Chicken	7 oz.	70	6.0
Meatless	¾ cup	35	6.0
Shrimp	¾ cup	45	4.0
*Bi-pack:			
Beef	¾ cup	70	8.0
Beef pepper oriental or shrimp	¾ cup	80	10.0
Chicken	¾ cup	80	8.0
Pork	¾ cup	80	7.0
Vegetable	¾ cup	50	8.0
Frozen:			
(Armour) *Dining Lite,* chicken, & rice	9-oz. meal	180	31.0
*(Chun King) chicken	13-oz. entree	370	53.0
(Empire Kosher)	7½-oz. serving	97	12.0
(Healthy Choice) chicken	8½-oz. meal	220	31.0
(La Choy):			
Chicken:			
Dinner	12-oz. dinner	260	44.0
Entree	⅔ cup	90	11.0
Shrimp:			
Dinner	12-oz. dinner	220	47.0
Entree	¾ cup	70	11.0

(USDA) = United States Department of Agriculture
(HHS/FAO) = Health and Human Services/Food and Agriculture Organization
* = prepared as package directs

Food and Description	Measure or Quantity	Calories	Carbo-hydrates (grams)
(Morton) chicken, light:			
Dinner	11-oz. meal	260	43.0
Entree	8-oz. meal	210	35.0
(Stouffer's)			
Regular, chicken	8-oz. pkg.	130	11.0
Lean Cuisine, chicken,			
with rice	11¼-oz. serving	250	36.0
*Mix (Betty Crocker)	¼ pkg.	260	43.0
CHOW MEIN SEASONING			
MIX (Kikkoman)	1⅛-oz. pkg.	98	13.8
CHURCH'S FRIED CHICKEN:			
Chicken:			
Breast	4.3-oz serving	278	9.4
Leg	2.9-oz. serving	147	4.5
Thigh	4.2-oz. servng	306	9.2
Wing-breast	4.8-oz. serving	303	8.9
Corn, with butter oil	1 ear	237	32.9
French fries	1 regular order	138	20.1
CINNAMON, GROUND	1 tsp.		
(French's)	(1.7 grams)	6	1.4
CINNAMON SUGAR (French's)	1 tsp.		
	(4.3 grams)	16	4.0
CINNAMON TOAST CRUNCH,			
cereal (General Mills)	¾ cup (1 oz.)	120	22.0
CITRUS COOLER DRINK,			
canned (Hi-C)	6 fl. oz.	95	23.3
CITRUS DRINK, chilled or *frozen (Five Alive)	6 fl. oz.	87	21.8
CLAM:			
Raw (USDA):			
Hard or round:			
Meat & liq.	1 lb. (weighed in shell)	71	6.1
Meat only	1 cup (8 oz.)	182	13.4
Soft:			
Meat & liq.	1 lb. (weighed in shell)	142	5.3

Food and Description	Measure or Quantity	Calories	Carbo-hydrates (grams)
Meat only	1 cup (8 oz.)	186	3.0
Canned:			
(Doxsee):			
Chopped or minced:			
Drained solids	½ cup	97	1.9
Solids & liq.	½ cup	59	3.2
Whole:			
Drained solids	½ cup	97	1.9
Solids & liq.	½ cup	58	3.1
(Gorton's) minced, drained solids	1 can	140	8.0
(Progresso) minced	½ cup	70	2.0
Frozen:			
(Gorton's) fried strips, crunchy	3½ oz.	330	24.0
(Mrs. Paul's) fried, light	2½-oz. serving	200	21.0
CLAMATO COCKTAIL			
(Mott's)	6 fl. oz.	96	23.0
CLAM JUICE (USDA)	½ cup	23	2.5
CLARET WINE:			
(Gold Seal) 12% alcohol	3 fl. oz.	82	.4
(Taylor) 12.5% alcohol	3 fl. oz.	72	2.4
CLUSTERS, cereal			
(General Mills)	½ cup (1 oz.)	110	20.0
COBBLER, frozen			
(Pet-Ritz):			
Apple or strawberry	⅙ of 26-oz. pkg.	290	50.0
Blackberry	⅙ of 26-oz. pkg.	270	39.0
Blueberry	⅙ of 26-oz. pkg.	270	50.0
Cherry	⅙ of 26-oz. pkg.	280	46.0
Peach	⅙ of 26-oz. pkg.	260	46.0
COCKTAIL (See individual listings)			

(USDA) = United States Department of Agriculture
(HHS/FAO) = Health and Human Services/Food and Agriculture Organization
* = prepared as package directs

Food and Description	Measure or Quantity	Calories	Carbo-hydrates (grams)
COCKTAIL MIX (See individual listings such as **PIÑA COLADA COCKTAIL** or **WHISKEY SOUR COCKTAIL**)			
COCOA:			
Dry, unsweetened:			
(USDA):			
Low fat	1 T. (5 grams)	10	3.1
High fat	1 T. (5 grams)	14	2.8
(Hershey's) American process	1 T. (5 grams)	22	2.3
Mix, regular:			
(Carnation) all flavors	1-oz. pkg.	110	23.0
(Hershey's)	1 T.	27	5.7
(Nestlé)	1¼ oz.	150	26.0
(Ovaltine) hot'n rich	1 oz.	120	22.0
Swiss Miss:			
Regular:			
Double rich	1 envelope	110	19.1
Milk chocolate or with mini marshmallows	1 envelope or 3-4 heaping tsps.	110	20.0
European creme:			
Amaretto or chocolate	1 envelope	150	29.0
Creme de menthe	1¼-oz. envelope	145	25.0
Mocha	1¼-oz. envelope	140	24.0
Mix, dietetic:			
(Carnation):			
70 Calorie	¾-oz. packet	70	15.0
Sugar free	.5-oz. envelope	50	8.0
*(Estee)	6 fl. oz.	50	9.0
(Lucerne)	1 envelope	50	8.0
(Ovaltine) reduced calorie	.45-oz. envelope	50	8.0
Swiss Miss:			
Lite	1 envelope	70	17.0
Milk chocolate	.5-oz. envelope	50	10.0
With sugar-free mini marshmallows	.5-oz. envelope	50	9.0
(Weight Watchers)	1 envelope	60	10.0
COCOA KRISPIES, cereal			
(Kellogg's)	¾ cup (1 oz.)	110	25.0
COCOA PUFFS, cereal			
(General Mills)	1 cup (1 oz.)	110	25.0

Food and Description	Measure or Quantity	Calories	Carbo-hydrates (grams)
COCONUT:			
Fresh (USDA):			
Whole	1 lb. (weighed in shell)	816	22.2
Meat only	4 oz.	392	10.7
Grated or shredded, loosely packed	½ cup (1.4 oz.)	225	6.1
Dried, canned or packaged:			
(Baker's):			
Angel Flake:			
Packaged in bag	⅓ cup (.9 oz.)	118	10.6
Canned	⅓ cup (.9 oz.)	120	10.4
Cookie cut	⅓ cup (1.3 oz.)	186	17.1
Premium shred	⅓ cup (1 oz.)	138	12.4
Southern style	⅓ cup (.9 oz.)	118	10.3
(Town House) flakes or shredded	1 oz.	150	12.0
COCONUT, CREAM OF, canned:			
(Coco Lopez)	1 T.	60	10.0
(Holland House)	1 oz.	81	18.0
COCO WHEATS, cereal (Little Crow):			
Regular	1 T. (.42 oz.)	43	9.3
Instant	1¼-oz. serving	130	29.0
COD:			
(USDA):			
Raw, meat only	4 oz.	88	0.
Broiled	4 oz.	193	0.
Dehydrated, lightly salted	4 oz.	425	0.
Frozen:			
(Captain's Choice) fillet	3-oz. fillet	89	0.
(Frionor) Norway Gourmet	4-oz. fillet	70	0.
(Gorton's) Fishmarket Fresh	5 oz.	110	0.
(National Sea Products):			
Plain	5 oz. raw	110	0.

(USDA) = United States Department of Agriculture
(HHS/FAO) = Health and Human Services/Food and Agriculture Organization
* = prepared as package directs

Food and Description	Measure or Quantity	Calories	Carbo-hydrates (grams)
Butter crumb, center cut or loin	5 oz. raw	160	4.0
Lemon pepper crumb, center cut or loin	5 oz. raw	170	6.0
Marinara crumb, center cut or loin	5 oz. raw	160	5.0
(Van de Kamp's) *Today's Catch*	4 oz.	80	0.

COD DINNER OR ENTREE,
frozen:

(Armour) *Dinner Classics,* almondine	12-oz. meal	360	33.0
(Mrs. Paul's) fillet, light	1 piece	240	22.0
(Frionor) *Norway Gourmet:*			
With dill sauce	4½-oz. fillet	80	1.0
With toasted bread crumbs	4½-oz. fillet	160	3.0

COD LIVER OIL

(Hain) regular, cherry or mint	1 T.	120	0.

COFFEE:
Regular:

Max-Pax; Maxwell House Electra Perk; Yuban, Yuban Electra Matic	6 fl. oz.	2	0.
Mellow Roast	6 fl. oz.	8	2.0
Decaffeinated:			
Brim, regular or electric perk	6 fl. oz.	2	0.
Brim, freeze-dried; *Decaf; Nescafe*	6 fl. oz.	4	1.0
Sanka, regular or electric perk	6 fl. oz.	2	0.
Instant:			
(Maxwell House)	6 fl. oz.	4	1.0
Mellow Roast	6 fl. oz.	8	2.0
Sunrise	6 fl. oz.	6	1.0
Mix (General Foods) International Coffee:			
Café Amaretto	6 fl. oz.	59	7.0
Café Français	6 fl. oz.	59	6.6

Food and Description	Measure or Quantity	Calories	Carbo-hydrates (grams)
Café Vienna, Orange Capuccino	6 fl. oz.	65	10.3
Irish Mocha Mint	6 fl. oz.	55	7.4
Suisse Mocha	6 fl. oz.	58	7.6
COFFEE CAKE (See CAKE, Coffee)			
COFFEE LIQUEUR (DeKuyper)	1 fl. oz.	93	12.4
COFFEE SOUTHERN	1 fl. oz.	79	8.8
COGNAC (See DISTILLED LIQUOR)			
COLA SOFT DRINK (See SOFT DRINK, Cola)			
COLD DUCK WINE (Great Western) pink, 12% alcohol	3 fl. oz.	92	7.7
COLESLAW, solids & liq. (USDA):			
Prepared with commercial French dressing	4-oz. serving	108	8.6
Prepared with homemade French dressing	4-oz. serving	146	5.8
Prepared with mayonnaise	4-oz. serving	163	5.4
Prepared with mayonnaise type salad dressing	1 cup (4.2 oz.)	119	8.5
***COLESLAW MIX** (Libby's) *Super Slaw*	½ cup	240	11.0
COLLARDS:			
Raw (USDA):			
Leaves, including stems	1 lb.	181	32.7
Leaves only	½ lb.	70	11.6
Boiled (USDA) drained:			

(USDA) = United States Department of Agriculture
(HHS/FAO) = Health and Human Services/Food and Agriculture Organization
* = prepared as package directs

Food and Description	Measure or Quantity	Calories	Carbo-hydrates (grams)
Leaves, cooked in large amount of water	½ cup (3.4 oz.)	29	4.6
Leaves & stems, cooked in small amount of water	½ cup (3.4 oz.)	31	4.8
Canned (Allen's) chopped, solids & liq.	½ cup (4.1 oz.)	25	2.0
Frozen, chopped:			
(Bel-Air)	3.3 oz.	25	4.0
(Birds Eye)	⅓ pkg. (3.3 oz.)	31	4.4
(Frosty Acres)	3.3-oz. serving	25	4.0
(McKenzie)	⅓ pkg. (3.3 oz.)	25	4.0
CONCORD WINE (Gold Seal) 13—14% alcohol	3 fl. oz.	125	9.8
COOKIE:			
Home recipe (USDA):			
Brownie with nuts	1¾″ × 1¾″ × ⅞″	97	10.2
Chocolate chip	1 oz.	146	17.0
Sugar, soft, thick	1 oz.	126	19.3
Packaged:			
Almond toast (Stella D'oro)	1 piece	60	10.0
Angel bar (Stella D'oro)	1 piece	80	7.0
Angelic Goodies (Stella D'oro)	1 piece	110	16.0
Angel wings (Stella D'oro)	1 piece	70	7.0
Anginetti (Stella D'oro)	1 piece	30	5.0
Animal:			
(USDA)	1 piece (3 grams)	11	2.1
(FFV)	1 piece (.1 oz.)	14	3.0
(Gerber)	.2-oz. piece	30	5.0
(Nabisco) *Barnum's Animals*	1 piece	12	1.9
(Ralston)	1 piece (2 grams)	8	1.5
(Sunshine)	1 piece	8	1.4
(Tom's)	1.7 oz.	210	37.0
Anisette sponge (Stella D'oro)	1 piece	50	10.0
Anisette toast (Stella D'oro):			
Regular	1 piece	50	9.0
Jumbo	1 piece	110	23.0
Apple Newtons (Nabisco)	1 piece	73	14.0
Apple N'Raisin (Archway)	1 cookie	120	20.0

Food and Description	Measure or Quantity	Calories	Carbohydrates (grams)
Apricot Raspberry (Pepperidge Farm)	1 piece (.4 oz.)	50	7.5
Assortment:			
(Nabisco) Famous:			
Baronet	1 piece	47	6.7
Butter flavor	1 piece	22	3.3
Biscos sugar wafer	1 piece	19	2.5
Cameo creme sandwich	1 piece	47	7.0
Kettle cookie	1 piece	32	5.0
Lorna Doone	1 piece	35	4.5
Oreo, chocolate	1 piece	47	6.7
(Stella D'oro) Hostess or *Lady Stella*	1 piece	40	6.0
Blueberry Newtons (Nabisco)	1 piece	73	14.0
Bordeaux (Pepperidge Farm)	1 piece (7.1 grams)	35	5.5
Breakfast Treats (Stella D'oro)	1 piece	100	15.0
Brown edge wafer (Nabisco)	1 piece (.2 oz.)	28	4.0
Brownie:			
(Nabisco) *Almost Home*, fudge & nut	1 piece	160	23.0
(Pepperidge Farm):			
Chocolate nut	.4-oz. piece	55	5.5
Nut, large	.9-oz. piece	140	15.0
Brussels (Pepperidge Farm):			
Regular	1 piece	55	6.5
Mint	1 piece	65	8.5
Butter flavored:			
(Nabisco)	1 piece (.2 oz.)	22	3.3
(Sunshine)	1 piece (.2 oz.)	30	4.5
Cappucino (Pepperidge Farm)	9 grams	50	6.0
Capri (Pepperidge Farm)	1 piece (.5 oz.)	80	10.0
Caramel Patties (FFV)	1 piece	75	10.0
Cherry Newtons (Nabisco)	1 piece	73	13.3
Chessman (Pepperidge Farm)	1 piece (.3 oz.)	45	6.0
Chinese dessert (Stella D'oro)	1 piece	170	20.0

(USDA) = United States Department of Agriculture
(HHS/FAO) = Health and Human Services/Food and Agriculture Organization
* = prepared as package directs

Food and Description	Measure or Quantity	Calories	Carbo-hydrates (grams)
Chocolate & chocolate-covered:			
(Keebler)			
fudge strips	1 piece (.4 oz.)	50	7.0
(Nabisco):			
Famous wafer	1 piece (.2 oz.)	22	5.2
Pinwheel, cake	1 piece (1.1 oz.)	130	20.0
Snap	1 piece (.14 oz.)	19	3.0
(Sunshine) nuggets	1 piece	23	3.3
Chocolate chip or chunk:			
(Archway) & toffee	.1-oz. piece	150	21.0
(Keebler):			
Chips deluxe	1 piece (.5 oz.)	90	10.0
Rich 'n chips	1 piece (.5 oz.)	80	10.0
(Nabisco):			
Almost Home, fudge or real	1 piece (.5 oz.)	65	10.0
Chips Ahoy!:			
Regular	1 piece (.3 oz.)	47	6.0
Chewy	1 piece (.5 oz.)	65	9.0
Chips 'n More:			
Coconut	1 piece (.5 oz.)	75	9.0
Fudge	1 piece (.3 oz.)	47	6.3
Original	1 piece (.5 oz.)	75	9.0
Snaps	1 piece (.2 oz.)	22	3.5
(Pepperidge Farm):			
Regular	1 piece (.3 oz.)	50	6.0
Chesapeake, with pecans	1 piece	120	14.0
Nantucket	1 piece	120	15.0
Pecan	1 piece	70	8.0
Mocha	1 piece	40	5.3
(Sunshine):			
Chip-A-Roos:			
Regular	1 piece (.5 oz.)	60	8.0
Chocolate	1 piece (.5 oz.)	60	7.0
Chippy Chews	1 piece	50	8.0
(Tom's)	1.7-oz. serving	230	34.0
Chocolate peanut bar (Nabisco) Ideal	1 piece (.6 oz.)	75	8.5
Cinnamon raisin (Nabisco) *Almost Home*	1 piece (.5 oz.)	70	8.0
Coconut fudge (FFV)	1 piece	80	10.0
Como Delights (Stella D'oro)	1 piece	150	18.0
Danish (Nabisco) imported	1 piece (.2 oz.)	30	3.6

Food and Description	Measure or Quantity	Calories	Carbo-hydrates (grams)
Date pecan (Pepperidge Farm)	1 piece (.4 oz.)	55	7.5
Devil's food cake (Nabisco)	1 piece	140	30.0
Dinosaurs (FFV)	1 oz.	130	20.0
Dutch apple bar (Stella D'oro)	1 piece	110	19.0
Dutch cocoa (Archway)	1 piece	110	19.0
Egg biscuit (Stella D'oro):			
Regular	1 piece	80	14.0
Roman	1 piece	140	20.0
Fig bar:			
(FFV)	1 piece	70	12.0
(Nabisco): *Fig Newtons*	1 piece (.5 oz.)	50	10.0
(Sunshine) Chewies	1 piece (.5 oz.)	50	11.0
(Tom's) bar	1 oz.	100	21.0
Fruit stick (Nabisco) *Almost Home*	1 piece (.7 oz.)	70	14.0
Fudge (Stella D'oro):			
Deep night	1 piece	65	8.0
Swiss	1 piece	70	9.0
Geneva (Pepperidge Farm)	1 piece (.4 oz.)	65	7.0
Gingerboys (FFV)	1 oz.	120	20.0
Gingerman (Pepperidge Farm)	1 piece	35	5.0
Gingersnap:			
(Archway)	1 piece (.5oz.)	25	4.0
(FFV)	1 oz.	130	22.0
(Nabisco)	1 piece	30	5.5
(Sunshine)	1 piece (.2 oz.)	20	3.0
Golden bars (Stella D'oro)	1 piece	110	16.0
Golden fruit raisin (Sunshine)	1 piece (smallest portion after breaking on scoreline) (.6 oz.)	70	14.0
Hazelnut (Pepperidge Farm)	1 piece (.4 oz.)	55	7.5
Heyday (Nabisco)	1 piece	140	15.0
Jelly tart (FFV)	1 piece	60	11.0
Ladyfinger (USDA)	3¼″ × 1⅜″ × 1⅛″ (.4 oz.)	40	7.1

(USDA) = United States Department of Agriculture
(HHS/FAO) = Health and Human Services/Food and Agriculture Organization
* = prepared as package directs

Food and Description	Measure or Quantity	Calories	Carbo-hydrates (grams)
Lemon (Archway)	1 piece	155	23.0
Lemon Cooler (Sunshine)	1 piece (.2 oz.)	30	4.3
Lemon nut crunch (Pepperidge Farm)	1 piece (.4 oz.)	55	6.5
Lido (Pepperidge Farm)	1 piece (.6 oz.)	90	10.0
Linzer (Pepperidge Farm)	1 piece	120	20.0
Macaroon (Nabisco) soft	1 piece	190	23.0
Mallo Puffs (Sunshine)	1 piece (.6 oz.)	70	12.0
Margherite (Stella D'oro)	1 piece	70	10.0
Marshmallow: (Nabisco):			
Mallomars	1 piece (.5 oz.)	65	9.0
Puffs, cocoa covered	1 piece (.1 oz.)	120	20.0
Sandwich	1 piece (.3 oz.)	30	5.5
Twirls cakes	1 piece (1 oz.)	130	19.0
(Planters) banana pie	1 oz.	127	22.0
Milano (Pepperidge Farm)	1 piece (.4 oz.)	75	8.5
Mint fudge (FFV)	1 piece	80	11.0
Molasses (Nabisco) Pantry	1 piece (.5 oz.)	65	10.5
Molasses crisp (Pepperidge Farm)	1 piece (.2 oz.)	35	4.0
Nassau (Pepperidge Farm)	1 piece (.5 oz.)	80	9.0
Nilla wafer (Nabisco)	1 piece (.1 oz.)	19	3.0
Oatmeal: (Archway):			
Regular	1 piece	110	19.0
Apple bran	1 piece	107	18.0
Apple filled	1 piece	90	18.0
Date filled, raisin or raisin bran	1 piece	100	18.0
Golden, Ruth's	1 piece	120	20.0
Iced	1 piece	140	22.0
(FFV):			
Regular	1 piece	26	4.0
Bar	1 piece	70	11.0
(Keebler) old fashioned	1 piece (18 grams)	80	12.0
(Nabisco) Bakers Bonus	1 piece (.5 oz.)	65	10.0
Cookie Little	1 piece (.1 oz.)	6	1.0
(Pepperidge Farm):			
Irish	1 piece	45	6.5
Milk chocolate, Dakota	1 piece	110	15.0
Raisin:			
Regular	1 piece	55	7.5
Santa Fe	1 piece	100	16.0

Food and Description	Measure or Quantity	Calories	Carbo-hydrates (grams)
(Sunshine):			
Country style	1 piece	60	8.0
Peanut sandwich	1 piece	70	9.0
Orbits (Sunshine):			
Butter flavored	1 piece	15	2.5
Chocolate	1 piece	15	2.3
Orleans (Pepperidge Farm) regular	1 piece (.2 oz.)	30	3.6
Peanut & peanut butter:			
(Nabisco):			
Almost Home	1 piece	70	8.0
Nutter Butter:			
Creme pattie	1 piece (.3 oz.)	37	4.3
Sandwich	1 piece (.5 oz.)	70	9.0
(Sunshine) wafer	1 piece	40	5.0
Pecan Sandies (Keebler)	1 piece (16 grams)	80	9.0
Pfeffernusse (Stella D'oro)	1 piece	40	7.0
Pirouettes (Pepperidge Farm)	1 piece	35	4.5
Praline Pecan (FFV)	1 piece	40	10.0
Raisin (USDA)	1 oz.	107	22.9
Raisin bran (Pepperidge Farm)	1 piece (.4 oz.)	53	6.5
Rocky road (Archway)	1 piece	130	20.0
Royal Dainty (FFV)	1 piece	60	7.0
Royal Nuggets (Stella D'oro)	1 piece	2	.1
Sandwich:			
(Keebler):			
Fudge creme	1 piece (12 grams)	60	8.0
Oatmeal cream	(.5 oz.)	80	11.0
Pitter Patter	1 piece (17 grams)	90	11.0
(Nabisco):			
Almost Home	1 piece	140	20.0
Baronet	1 piece (.3 oz.)	47	6.7
Cameo	1 piece (.3 oz.)	47	7.0
Gaity, fudge chocolate	1 piece (.3 oz.)	50	6.3
Giggles	1 piece (.3 oz.)	70	8.5
I Screams	1 piece (.5 oz.)	75	10.0

(USDA) = United States Department of Agriculture
(HHS/FAO) = Health and Human Services/Food and Agriculture Organization
* = prepared as package directs

Food and Description	Measure or Quantity	Calories	Carbo-hydrates (grams)
Mystic Mint	1 piece (.5 oz.)	75	9.5
Oreo:			
Regular	1 piece (.3 oz.)	47	6.7
Double Stuf	1 piece (.5 oz.)	70	9.5
Mint	1 piece (.5 oz.)	70	10.0
Vanilla, *Cookie Break* (Sunshine):	1 piece (.3 oz.)	47	6.7
Regular:			
Chocolate fudge or cup custard	1 piece (.5 oz.)	70	9.0
Hydrox	1 piece (.4 oz.)	50	7.0
Vienna Fingers	1 piece	70	11.0
Chips 'n Middles:			
Fudge	1 piece (.5 oz.)	70	10.0
Peanut butter	1 piece (.5 oz.)	70	9.0
Tru Blue, any flavor	1 piece (.6 oz.)	80	11.0
Sesame (Stella D'oro)			
Regina	1 piece	50	6.0
Shortbread or shortcake:			
(FFV) country	1 piece	70	9.0
(Nabisco):			
Fudge striped	1 piece	50	6.3
Lorna Doone	1 piece (.3 oz.)	35	4.5
Pecan	1 piece (.5 oz.)	75	8.0
(Pepperidge Farm):			
Regular	1 piece	75	8.5
Pecan	1 piece	70	7.0
Social Tea, biscuit (Nabisco)	1 piece	22	3.5
Sprinkles (Sunshine)	1 piece (.6 oz.)	70	12.0
Strawberry (Pepperidge Farm)	1 piece (.4 oz.)	50	7.5
Sugar:			
(Nabisco) rings, *Bakers Bonus*	1 piece (.5 oz.)	65	10.0
(Pepperidge Farm)	1 piece (.4 oz.)	50	6.5
Sugar wafer:			
(Dutch Twin) any flavor	1 piece (.3 oz.)	36	4.7
(Nabisco) *Biscos*	1 piece (.1 oz.)	19	2.5
(Sunshine)	1 piece (.3 oz.)	45	6.0
Super Heroes (Nabisco)	1 piece (.1 oz.)	12	1.8
Tahiti (Pepperidge Farm)	1 piece (.5 oz.)	90	9.0
Tango (FFV)	1 piece	80	13.0
Toy (Sunshine)	1 piece (.1 oz.)	12	2.0
Trolley Cakes (FFV)	1 piece	60	12.5
Vanilla wafer (Keebler)	1 piece (4 grams)	20	2.7

Food and Description	Measure or Quantity	Calories	Carbo-hydrates (grams)
Waffle creme:			
(Dutch Twin)	1 piece (.3 oz.)	45	5.7
(Nabisco)	1 piece (.3 oz.)	50	6.7
Zanzibar (Pepperidge Farm)	1 piece (.3 oz.)	40	4.3
COOKIE, DIETETIC:			
Apple pastry (Stella D'oro)	1 piece	90	14.0
Chocoalte chip (Estee)	1 piece (.2 oz.)	30	4.0
Coconut:			
(Estee)	1 piece	30	4.0
(Stella D'oro)	1 piece	50	6.0
Egg biscuit (Stella D'oro)	1 piece	40	7.0
Fruit & honey (Entenmann's) fat & cholesterol free	1 piece	40	9.0
Fudge (Estee)	1 piece	30	4.0
Kichel (Stella D'oro)	1 piece	8	.7
Lemon (Estee) thin	1 piece (.2 oz.)	30	4.0
Oatmeal raisin:			
(Entenmann's) fat & choles-terol free	1 piece (.4 oz.)	40	8.5
(Estee)	1 piece (.2 oz.)	30	4.0
Peach apricot pastry (Stella D'oro)	1 piece	90	13.0
Prune pastry (Stella D'oro)	1 piece	90	13.0
Sandwich (Estee)	1 piece	45	6.0
Sesame (Stella D'oro) Regina	1 piece	40	6.0
Wafer, chocolate-covered (Estee)	1 piece (.85 oz.)	130	14.0
Wafer, creme filled (Estee):			
Assorted	1 piece	20	3.0
Chocolate or vanilla	1 piece	20	3.0
COOKIE CRISP, cereal			
(Ralston Purina) any flavor	1 cup (1 oz.)	110	25.0

(USDA) = United States Department of Agriculture
(HHS/FAO) = Health and Human Services/Food and Agriculture
  Organization
* = prepared as package directs

Food and Description	Measure or Quantity	Calories	Carbo-hydrates (grams)
*COOKIE DOUGH:			
Refrigerated (Pillsbury):			
Brownie, fudge			
microwave	⅑ of pkg.	70	9.0
Chocolate chip or sugar	1 cookie	70	9.0
Peanut butter	1 cookie	70	8.0
Frozen (Rich's):			
Chocolate chip	1 cookie	138	20.3
Oatmeal	1 cookie	125	18.3
Oatmeal & raisins	1 cookie	122	19.1
Peanut butter	1 cookie	128	14.6
Sugar	1 cookie	118	17.4
COOKIE MIX:			
Regular:			
Brownie:			
*(Betty Crocker):			
Regular:			
Chocolate chip	¹⁄₂₄ of pan	140	20.0
Frosted	¹⁄₂₄ of pan	160	26.0
Fudge:			
Regular size	¹⁄₁₆ of pan	150	23.0
Family size	¹⁄₂₄ of pan	140	22.0
Supreme	¹⁄₂₄ of pan	120	21.0
German chocolate	¹⁄₂₄ of pan	160	24.0
Walnut	¹⁄₁₆ of pan	140	18.0
MicroRave:			
Frosted	1 piece	180	27.0
Fudge	1 piece	150	22.0
Walnut	1 piece	160	21.0
(Duncan Hines)	¹⁄₂₄ of pkg.	119	22.0
Chewey recipe	¹⁄₂₄ of pkg.	98	17.9
Fudge, original	¹⁄₂₄ of pkg.	122	22.4
Milk chocolate	¹⁄₂₄ of pkg.	128	22.1
Peanut butter	¹⁄₂₄ of pkg.	120	16.6
Truffle	¹⁄₁₆ of pkg.	200	32.4
Turtle	¹⁄₁₆ of pkg.	166	32.4
*(Pillsbury) fudge:			
Deluxe:			
Plain	¹⁄₁₆ of pkg.	150	21.0
Family size	¹⁄₂₄ of pkg.	150	20.0
With walnuts	¹⁄₁₆ of pkg.	150	19.0
Microwave	⅑ of pkg.	190	25.0

Food and Description	Measure or Quantity	Calories	Carbo-hydrates (grams)
Ultimate:			
Caramel chunk or chunky triple	1/16 of pkg.	170	25.0
Double	1/16 of pkg.	160	24.0
Rocky road	1/16 of pkg.	170	24.0
*Robin Hood (General Mills) fudge	1/16 of pkg.	100	16.0
Chocolate (Duncan Hines) double	1/36 of pkg.	67	9.2
Chocolate chip:			
*(Betty Crocker)			
Big Batch	1 cookie	60	8.0
(Duncan Hines)	1/36 of pkg.	73	9.2
Date bar (Betty Crocker)	1/24 of pkg.	60	9.0
Oatmeal (Duncan Hines) raisin	1/36 of pkg.	68	9.1
Peanut butter (Duncan Hines)	1/36 pkg.	68	7.5
Sugar (Duncan Hines) golden	1/36 of pkg.	59	8.4
*Dietetic (Estee) brownie	2" × 2"-sq. cookie	50	8.0
COOKING SPRAY:			
Mazola No Stick	2½-second spray	6	0.
(Weight Watchers)	1-second spray	2	0.
Wesson Lite	2-second spray	<1	0.
CORIANDER SEED (French's)	1 tsp. (1.4 grams)	6	.8
CORN:			
Fresh, white or yellow (USDA):			
Raw:			
Untrimmed, on the cob	1 lb. (weighed in husk)	167	36.1
Trimmed, on cob	1 lb. (husk removed)	240	55.1
Boiled:			
Kernels, cut from cob, drained	1 cup (5.8 oz.)	137	31.0

(USDA) = United States Department of Agriculture
(HHS/FAO) = Health and Human Services/Food and Agriculture Organization
* = prepared as package directs

Food and Description	Measure or Quantity	Calories	Carbo-hydrates (grams)
Whole	4.9-oz. ear (5" × 1¾")	70	16.2
Trimmed, on the cob	5" × 1¾" ear	70	16.2
Canned, regular pack: (USDA):			
Golden or yellow, whole kernel, solids & liq., vacuum pack	½ cup (3.7 oz.)	87	21.6
Golden or yellow, whole kernel, wet pack	½ cup (4.5 oz.)	84	20.1
Golden or yellow, whole kernel, drained solids, wet pack	½ cup (3 oz.)	72	16.4
White kernel, drained solids	½ cup (2.8 oz.)	70	16.4
White, whole kernel, drained liq., wet pack	4 oz.	29	7.8
Cream style	½ cup (4.4 oz.)	105	25.6
(Allen's) whole kernel, golden	½ cup (4.2 oz.)	80	3.0
(Green Giant) solids & liq.:			
Cream style	½ cup	100	24.0
Whole kernel or shoe peg, golden	4¼ oz.	90	18.0
Whole kernel, vacuum pack	½ cup	80	16.0
Whole kernel, Mexicorn	3½ oz.	80	19.0
Whole kernel, white, vacuum pack	½ cup	80	20.0
(Larsen) Freshlike:			
Whole kernel, vacuum pack	½ cup (3.9 oz.)	100	22.0
Whole kernel, vacuum pack, with pepper	½ cup (4 oz.)	90	23.0
(Stokely-Van Camp) solids & liq.:			
Cream style, golden	½ cup (4.5 oz.)	105	23.5
Cream style, white	½ cup (4.6 oz.)	110	24.5
Whole kernel, golden	½ cup	90	19.5
(Town House):			
Cream style	½ cup	80	18.0
Whole kernel	½ cup	70	17.0
Canned, dietetic pack, solids & liq.:			
(Diet Delight) whole kernel	½ cup	60	15.0
(Green Giant)	½ cup	80	18.0

Food and Description	Measure or Quantity	Calories	Carbo-hydrates (grams)
(Larsén) *Fresh-Lite*, whole kernel, no salt added	½ cup (4.5 oz.)	80	19.0
Frozen:			
(Bel-Air)):			
On the cob:			
Regular	1 ear	120	29.0
Short ears	1 ear	65	15.0
Whole kernel	3.3 oz.	80	20.0
(Birds Eye):			
On the cob:			
Regular	4.4-oz. ear	120	28.7
Big Ears	5.7-oz. ear	156	37.0
Little Ears	4.6-oz. ear	126	30.0
Whole kernel:			
Cob corn, deluxe baby	⅓ of 8-oz. pkg.	23	4.0
Deluxe, petite	⅓ of 8-oz. pkg.	66	1.6
Sweet:			
Regular	¼ of 12-oz. pkg.	74	18.0
Butter sauce	⅓ of 10-oz. pkg.	85	17.0
Deluxe, tender	⅓ of 10-oz. pkg.	82	20.0
(Frosty Acres):			
On the cob	1 ear	120	29.0
Whole kernel	3.3-oz. serving	80	20.0
(Green Giant):			
On the cob:			
Nibbler, regular	1 ear	60	13.0
Niblet Ear, regular	1 ear	120	26.0
Cream style	½ cup	110	25.0
Whole kernel, *Niblets:*			
In butter sauce, golden	½ cup	100	19.0
Harvest Fresh, golden	3 oz.	80	17.0
Polybag, white	½ cup	70	15.0
(Larsen):			
On the cob:			
3-inch piece	2.2-oz. piece	60	15.0
5-inch piece	4.4-oz. piece	120	29.0
Cut	3.3 oz.	80	20.0

CORNBREAD:
  Home recipe (USDA):

(USDA) = United States Department of Agriculture
(HHS/FAO) = Health and Human Services/Food and Agriculture Organization
* = prepared as package directs

Food and Description	Measure or Quantity	Calories	Carbo-hydrates (grams)
Corn pone, prepared with white, whole-ground cornmeal	4 oz.	231	41.1
Johnnycake, prepared with yellow, degermed cornmeal	4 oz.	303	51.6
Southern style, prepared with degermed cornmeal	2½″ × 2½″ × 1⅝″ piece	186	28.8
Southern style, prepared with whole-ground cornmeal	4 oz.	235	33.0
Spoon bread, prepared with white, whole-ground cornmeal	4 oz.	221	19.2
*Mix:			
(Aunt Jemima)	⅙ of pkg.	220	34.0
(Dromedary)	2″ × 2″ piece (¹⁄₁₆ of pkg.)	130	20.0
Gold Medal	⅙ of pkg.	150	22.0
(Pillsbury) Ballard	⅛ of recipe	140	25.0
*CORN DOG, frozen:			
(Fred's) Little Juan	2¾-oz. serving	231	24.6
(Hormel)	1 piece	220	21.0
CORNED BEEF:			
Cooked (USDA), boneless, medium fat	4-oz. serving	422	0.
Canned, regular pack:			
Dinty Moore (Hormel)	2-oz. serving	130	0.
(Libby's)	⅓ of 7-oz. can	160	2.0
Packaged:			
(Eckrich) sliced	1-oz. slice	40	1.0
(Carl Buddig) smoked, sliced	1 oz.	40	Tr.
(Oscar Mayer)	.6-oz. slice	16	.1
CORNED BEEF HASH, canned:			
(Libby's)	⅓ of 24-oz. can	420	21.0
Mary Kitchen (Hormel):			
Regular	½ of 15-oz. can	360	19.0
Short Orders	7½-oz. can	360	17.0
CORNED BEEF SPREAD, canned:			
(Hormel)	1 oz.	70	0.
(Underwood)	½ of 4½-oz. can	120	Tr.

Food and Description	Measure or Quantity	Calories	Carbo-hydrates (grams)
CORN FLAKE CRUMBS			
(Kellogg's)	¼ cup (1 oz.)	100	24.0
CORN FLAKES, cereal:			
(General Mills) *Country*	1 cup (1 oz.)	110	25.0
(Kellogg's):			
Regular	1 cup (1 oz.)	100	24.0
Sugar Frosted Flakes	¾ cup (1 oz.)	110	26.0
(Malt-O-Meal):			
Plain	1 cup (1 oz.)	106	24.8
Sugar coated	¾ cup (1 oz.)	109	26.0
(Post) *Post Toasties*	1¼ cups (1 oz.)	111	24.0
(Safeway) plain	1 cup (1 oz.)	110	25.0
CORNMEAL, WHITE OR YELLOW:			
Dry:			
Bolted:			
(USDA)	1 cup (4.3 oz.)	442	90.9
(Aunt Jemima/Quaker)	1 cup (4 oz.)	408	84.8
Degermed:			
(USDA)	1 cup (4.9 oz.)	502	108.2
(Aunt Jemima/Quaker)	1 cup (4 oz.)	404	88.8
Self-rising degermed:			
(USDA)	1 cup (5 oz.)	491	105.9
(Aunt Jemima)	1 cup (6 oz.)	582	126.0
Self-rising, whole ground			
(USDA)	1 cup (5 oz.)	489	101.4
Whole ground, unbolted			
(USDA)	1 cup (4.3 oz.)	433	90.0
Cooked:			
(USDA)	1 cup (8.5 oz.)	120	25.7
(Albers) degermed	1 cup	119	25.5
Mix (Aunt Jemima/Quaker) bolted	1 cup (4 oz.)	392	80.4
CORN POPS, cereal (Kellogg's)	1 cup (1 oz.)	110	26.0
CORN PUDDING, home recipe			
(USDA)	1 cup (8.6 oz.)	255	31.9

(USDA) = United States Department of Agriculture
(HHS/FAO) = Health and Human Services/Food and Agriculture Organization
* = prepared as package directs

Food and Description	Measure or Quantity	Calories	Carbo-hydrates (grams)
CORN PUREE, canned (Larsen) no salt added	½ cup	100	22.5
CORNSTARCH (Argo; Kingsford's)	1 tsp. (8 grams)	10	8.3
CORN SYRUP (See **SYRUP,** Corn)			
COTTAGE PUDDING, home recipe (USDA):			
Without sauce	2 oz.	180	30.8
With chocolate sauce	2 oz.	195	32.1
With strawberry sauce	2 oz.	166	27.4
COUGH DROP:			
(Beech-Nut)	1 drop	10	2.5
(Pine Bros.)	1 drop	10	2.4
COUNT CHOCULA, cereal (General Mills)	1 oz. (1 cup)	110	24.0
COWPEA (USDA):			
Immature seeds:			
Raw, whole	1 lb. (weighed in pods)	317	54.4
Raw, shelled	½ cup (2.5 oz.)	92	15.8
Boiled, drained solids	½ cup (2.9 oz.)	89	15.0
Canned, solids & liq.	4 oz.	79	14.1
Frozen (See **BLACK-EYED PEAS,** frozen)			
Young pods with seeds:			
Raw, whole	1 lb. (weighed untrimmed)	182	39.2
Boiled, drained solids	4 oz.	39	7.9
Mature seeds, dry:			
Raw	1 lb.	1556	279.9
Raw	½ cup (3 oz.)	292	52.4
Boiled	½ cup (4.4 oz.)	95	17.2
CRAB:			
Fresh, steamed (USDA):			
Whole	½ lb. (weighed in shell)	202	1.1

Food and Description	Measure or Quantity	Calories	Carbo-hydrates (grams)
Meat only	4 oz.	105	.6
Canned, drained (USDA)	4 oz.	115	1.2
Frozen (Wakefield's)	4 oz.	86	.7
CRAB APPLE, flesh only (USDA)	¼ lb.	71	20.2
CRAB APPLE JELLY (Smucker's)	1 T. (.7 oz.)	53	13.5
CRAB, DEVILED:			
Home recipe (USDA)	4 oz.	213	15.1
Frozen (Mrs. Paul's):			
Regular	1 cake	180	18.0
Miniature	3½ oz.	240	25.0
CRAB, IMITATION:			
(Louis Kemp) *Crab Delights*, chunks, flakes or legs	2-oz. serving	60	7.0
CRAB IMPERIAL:			
Home recipe (USDA)	1 cup (7.8 oz.)	323	8.6
Frozen (Gorton's) Light Recipe, stuffed	1 pkg.	340	36.0
CRACKERS, PUFFS & CHIPS:			
Animal (FFV)	1 oz.	130	21.0
Arrowroot biscuit (Nabisco)	1 piece (.2 oz.)	22	3.5
Bacon-flavored thins (Nabisco)	1 piece (.1 oz.)	10	1.3
Bravos (Wise)	1 oz.	150	18.0
Bugles (Tom's)	1 oz.	150	18.0
Butter (Pepperidge Farm) thin	1 piece	17	2.5
Cafe Cracker (Sunshine)	1 piece (smallest portion after breaking on scoreline)	20	2.3

(USDA) = United States Department of Agriculture
(HHS/FAO) = Health and Human Services/Food and Agriculture Organization
* = prepared as package directs

Food and Description	Measure or Quantity	Calories	Carbohydrates (grams)
Cheese flavored:			
American Heritage (Sunshine):			
Cheddar	1 piece	16	1.6
Parmesan	1 piece	18	1.8
Better Blue Cheese (Nabisco)	1 piece	7	.8
Better Cheddar (Nabisco)	1 piece	6	.7
Better Nacho (Nabisco)	1 piece	8	.9
Better Swiss (Nabisco)	1 piece	7	.8
Cheddar Sticks (Flavor Tree)	1 oz.	160	12.0
Cheese Bites (Tom's)	1½ oz.	200	26.0
Cheese 'n Crunch (Nabisco)	1 piece	4	.4
Cheese Doodles (Wise):			
Crunchy	1 oz.	160	16.0
Fried	1 oz.	150	16.0
Chee-Tos, crunchy or puffy	1 oz.	160	15.0
Cheez Balls (Planters)	1 oz.	160	14.0
Cheez Curls (Planters)	1 oz.	160	14.0
Cheez-It (Sunshine)	1 piece	6	.6
Corn cheese (Tom's):			
Crunchy	⅝ oz.	280	25.0
Puffed, baked	1⅛ oz.	180	18.0
Curls (Old Dutch)	1 oz.	160	14.0
Dip In A Chip (Nabisco)	1 piece (.1 oz.)	9	1.0
(Dixie Belle)	1 piece	6	.7
(Eagle)	1 oz.	130	18.0
Nacho cheese cracker (Old El Paso)	1 oz.	76	15.3
Nips (Nabisco)	1 piece (.04 oz.)	5	.7
(Planters) squares	1 oz.	140	15.0
(Ralston Purina)	1 piece (1.1 grams)	6	.7
Sandwich (Nabisco)	1 piece	35	4.0
Tid-Bit (Nabisco)	1 piece	4	.5
Chicken in a Biskit (Nabisco)	1 piece (.1 oz.)	11	1.1
Chipsters (Nabisco)	1 piece	2	.3
Cinnamon Treats (Nabisco)	1 piece	30	5.5
Club cracker (Keebler)	1 piece (3.2 grams)	15	2.0
Corn chips:			
Dippy Doodle (Wise)	1 oz.	160	12.0
(Flavor Tree)	1 oz.	150	17.0
Fritos:			
Regular	1 oz.	160	16.0
Barbecue flavor	1 oz.	150	15.5

Food and Description	Measure or Quantity	Calories	Carbo-hydrates (grams)
Happy Heart (TKI Foods)	⅜-oz. pkg.	40	8.0
Heart Lovers (TKI Foods)	⅜-oz. pkg.	40	8.0
(Laura Scudder's)	1 oz.	160	15.0
(Old Dutch)	1 oz.	160	15.0
(Tom's) regular	1 oz.	105	17.0
Corn Smackers (Weight Watchers)	.5-oz. pkg.	60	10.0
Corn Stick (Flavor Tree)	1 oz.	160	15.0
Country Cracker (Nabisco)	1 piece	16	1.8
Crown Pilot (Nabisco)	1 piece (.6 oz.)	70	11.0
Diggers (Nabisco)	1 piece	4	.5
Dip In A Chip (Nabisco)	1 piece	9	1.0
Doo Dads (Nabisco)	1 oz.	140	18.0
English Water Biscuit (Pepperidge Farm)	1 piece (.1 oz.)	27	3.2
Escort (Nabisco)	1 piece (.1 oz.)	23	3.0
Flutters (Pepperidge Farm):			
Garden herb	¾ oz.	100	14.0
Golden sesame or toasted wheat	¾ oz.	110	13.0
Original butter	¾ oz.	100	15.0
Goldfish (Pepperidge Farm):			
Thins, cheese	1 piece	12	2.0
Tiny:			
Cheddar cheese or parmesan	1 oz.	120	19.0
Original	1 oz.	130	18.0
Pizza flavored	1 oz.	130	19.0
Pretzel	1 oz.	110	20.0
Graham:			
(Dixie Belle) sugar-honey coated	1 piece	15	2.6
FlavorKist (Schulze and Burch) sugar-honey coated	1 double cracker	57	10.0
Honey Maid (Nabisco)	1 piece (.25 oz.)	30	5.5
(Keebler):			
Cinnamon Crisp	1 piece	17	2.7
Honey coated	1 piece	17	3.0
Party Graham (Nabisco)	1 piece	47	6.0

(USDA) = United States Department of Agriculture
(HHS/FAO) = Health and Human Services/Food and Agriculture Organization
* = prepared as package directs

Food and Description	Measure or Quantity	Calories	Carbohydrates (grams)
(Ralston Purina) sugar-honey coated	1 piece	15	2.6
(Rokeach)	8 pieces	120	21.0
(Sunshine):			
Cinnamon	1 piece (.1 oz.)	17	2.8
Honey	1 piece	15	2.5
Graham, chocolate or cocoa-covered (Keebler) deluxe	1 piece (.3 oz.)	40	5.5
Great Crisps (Nabisco):			
Cheese & chive, real bacon, sesame or tomato & celery	1 piece	8	.9
French onion	1 piece	10	1.1
Nacho	1 piece	9	1.0
Savory garlic	1 piece	9	1.1
Great Snackers (Weight Watchers)	.5-oz. pkg.	60	8.0
Hi Ho Crackers (Sunshine)	1 piece	20	2.0
Meal Mates (Nabisco)	1 piece	23	3.0
Melba Toast (See **MELBA TOAST**)			
Nachips (Old El Paso)	1 piece	17	1.7
Nacho Rings (Tom's)	1 oz.	160	15.0
Oat thins (Nabisco)	1 piece (.1 oz.)	9	1.2
Ocean Crisp (FFV)	1 piece	60	10.0
Onion rings (Wise)	1 oz.	130	21.0
Oyster:			
(Dixie Belle)	1 piece (.03 oz.)	4	.6
(Keebler) *Zesta*	1 piece	2	.3
(Nabisco) *Dandy* or *Oysterettes*	1 piece (.03 oz.)	3	.5
(Ralston Purina)	1 piece	4	.6
(Sunshine)	1 piece	4	.6
Party Mix (Flavor Tree)	1 oz.	160	11.0
Peanut butter & cheese (Eagle)	1.8-oz. serving	280	26.0
Pizza Crunchies (Planters)	1 oz.	160	15.0
Potato chips (see **POTATO CHIPS**)			
Ritz (Nabisco)	1 piece (.1 oz.)	17	2.3
Ritz Bits (Nabisco):			
Regular, low salt or cheese	1 piece	3	.4

Food and Description	Measure or Quantity	Calories	Carbo- hydrates (grams)
Cheese or peanut butter sandwich	1 piece	13	1.2
Rich & Crisp (Dixie Bell; Ralston Purina)	1 piece	14	1.9
Roman Meal Wafer, boxed	1 piece	11	1.3
Royal Lunch (Nabisco)	1 piece	60	10.0
Rye toast (Keebler)	1 piece	16	2.0
RyKrisp (Ralston Purina):			
Natural	1 triple cracker	20	5.5
Seasoned	1 triple cracker	22	5.5
Saltine:			
(Dixie Belle) regular or unsalted	1 piece (.1 oz.)	12	2.0
Flavor Kist (Schulze and Burch)	1 piece	12	2.0
Krispy (Sunshine)	1 piece	12	2.2
Premium (Nabisco):			
Regular, low salt, unsalted top or whole wheat	1 piece	12	2.0
Bits	1 piece	4	.6
(Ralston Purina) regular or unsalted	1 piece	12	2.0
(Rokeach)	1 piece	12	2.0
Zesta (Keebler)	1 piece	13	2.1
Schooners (FFV):			
Regular	½ oz.	60	10.0
Whole wheat	½ oz.	70	8.0
Sea Rounds (Nabisco)	1 piece (.5 oz.)	50	10.0
Sesame:			
(Estee)	½ oz.	70	9.0
(Flavor Tree):			
Chip	1 oz.	150	13.0
Crunch	1 oz.	150	10.0
Sticks:			
Plain	1 oz.	150	13.0
With bran	1 oz.	160	11.0
No salt added	1 oz.	160	12.0
(Keebler) toasted	1 piece	16	2.0

(USDA) = United States Department of Agriculture
(HHS/FAO) = Health and Human Services/Food and Agriculture Organization
* = prepared as package directs

Food and Description	Measure or Quantity	Calories	Carbo-hydrates (grams)
(Sunshine) *American Heritage*	1 piece	17	2.0
Sesame wheat (Natures Cupboard)	1 piece	11	1.4
Snack Cracker (Rokeach)	1 piece (.1 oz.)	14	2.1
Snackers (Dixie Bell; Ralston Purina)	1 piece	17	2.2
Snacks Sticks (Pepperidge Farm):			
Cheese, three	1 piece	16	2.4
Pretzel	1 piece	15	2.9
Pumpernickel or sesame	1 piece	17	2.5
Sociables (Nabisco)	1 piece	12	1.5
Sour cream & onion stick (Flavor Tree)	1 oz.	150	13.0
Spirals (Wise)	1 oz.	160	15.0
Taco chips (Laura Scudder) mini	1 oz.	150	17.0
Tortilla chips:			
Doritos, nacho or taco:	1 oz.	140	18.0
Regular or *Salsa Rio*	1 oz.	140	19.0
Cool Ranch:			
Regular	1 oz.	140	18.0
Light	1 oz.	120	21.0
Nacho cheese:			
Regular	1 oz.	140	18.0
Light	1 oz.	120	21.0
Taco	1 oz.	140	18.0
(Eagle)	1 oz.	150	17.0
(Nabisco):			
Nacho	1 piece	12	1.3
Toasted corn	1 piece	11	1.4
(Old Dutch):			
Nacho	1 oz.	156	15.0
Taco	1 oz.	152	15.0
(Old El Paso)	1 oz.	150	17.0
(Planters)	1 oz.	150	18.0
(Tom's) nacho	1 oz.	140	18.0
Tostitos:			
Jalapeño & cheese or sharp nacho	1 oz.	150	17.0
Traditional	1 oz.	140	18.0

Food and Description	Measure or Quantity	Calories	Carbo-hydrates (grams)
Town House Cracker (Keebler)	1 piece (3.1 grams)	16	1.8
Triscuit (Nabisco):			
Regular, low salt or wheat & bran	1 piece	20	3.3
Bits	1 piece	7	1.2
Tuc (Keebler)	1 piece (.2 oz.)	23	2.7
Twiddle Sticks (Nabisco)	1 piece	53	7.0
Twigs (Nabisco)	1 piece (.1 oz.)	14	1.6
Uneeda Biscuit (Nabisco)	1 piece	30	5.0
Unsalted (Estee)	1 piece (.1 oz.)	15	2.5
Vegetable thins (Nabisco)	1 piece	10	1.1
Waverly (Nabisco)	1 piece	17	2.5
Wheat:			
(Dixie Belle) snack	1 piece	9	1.2
(Estee) *6 calorie*	1 piece	6	2.0
(Featherweight) wafer, unsalted	1 piece	13	2.3
(Flavor Tree) nuts	1 oz.	200	5.0
(Nabisco):			
Wheat Thins:			
Regular or low salt	1 piece (.1 oz.)	9	1.1
Cheese	1 piece (.1 oz.)	8	1.0
Nutty	1 piece (.1 oz.)	11	1.1
Wheatsworth	1 piece	14	1.9
(Pepperidge Farm):			
Cracked	1 piece	33	4.7
Hearty	1 piece	25	3.2
Toasted, with onion	1 piece	20	3.0
(Sunshine):			
American Heritage	1 piece	15	2.0
Wafer	1 piece	10	1.2
CRACKER CRUMBS, graham:			
(Nabisco)	⅛ of 9″ pie shell (2 T.)	60	11.0
(Sunshine)	½ cup	275	47.5

(USDA) = United States Department of Agriculture
(HHS/FAO) = Health and Human Services/Food and Agriculture Organization
* = prepared as package directs

Food and Description	Measure or Quantity	Calories	Carbo-hydrates (grams)
CRACKER MEAL (Nabisco)	2 T.	50	12.0
***CRANAPPLE* JUICE DRINK** (Ocean Spray) canned:			
Regular	6 fl. oz.	127	31.1
Dietetic	6 fl. oz.	41	10.0
CRANBERRY, fresh (Ocean Spray)	½ cup (2 oz.)	25	6.0
CRANBERRY-APPLE DRINK, canned (Town House)	6 fl. oz.	130	32.0
CRANBERRY JUICE COCKTAIL: Canned:			
Regular pack:			
(Ardmore Farms)	6 fl. oz.	77	19.1
(Ocean Spray)	6 fl. oz.	103	25.4
(Town House)	6 fl. oz.	110	26.0
Dietetic (Ocean Spray)	6 fl. oz.	41	9.8
*Frozen (Sunkist)	6 fl. oz.	110	28.2
CRANBERRY SAUCE: Home recipe (USDA) sweetened, unstrained	4 oz.	202	51.6
Canned: (Ocean Spray):			
Regular:			
Jellied	2 oz.	87	21.7
Whole berry	2 oz.	93	23.1
Cran-Fruit:			
& apple	2 oz.	100	24.0
& orange, raspberry or strawberry	2 oz.	100	23.0
(Town House) jellied	2 oz.	100	25.0
CRANICOT (Ocean Spray)	6 fl. oz.	110	26.0
***CRAN-BLUEBERRY* JUICE DRINK,** canned (Ocean Spray)	6 fl. oz.	120	30.0

Food and Description	Measure or Quantity	Calories	Carbo-hydrates (grams)
CRAN-RASPBERRY JUICE DRINK, canned (Ocean Spray):			
Regular	6 fl. oz.	110	27.0
Dietetic	6 fl. oz.	40	10.0
CRANTASTIC JUICE DRINK, canned (Ocean Spray)	6 fl. oz.	110	27.0
CREAM:			
Half & half (Dairylea)	1 fl. oz.	40	1.0
Light, table or coffee (Sealtest) 16% fat	1 T.	26	.6
Light, whipping, 30% fat (Sealtest)	1 T. (.5 oz.)	45	1.0
Heavy, whipping:			
(Johanna Farms) 36% butterfat	1 T. (.5 oz.)	52	1.0
(Land O' Lakes)	1 T. (.5 oz.)	50	*1.0
Sour:			
(Friendship):			
Regular	1 T. (.5 oz.)	27	.5
Light	1 T. (.5 oz.)	17	.1
(Johanna Farms)	¼ cup	123	1.4
(Land O' Lakes):			
Regular	1 T. (.5 oz.)	30	1.0
Light, plain or with chives	1 T.	20	2.0
(Lucerne) light	1 T.	22	1.0
(Weight Watchers)	1 T. (.5 oz.)	17	1.0
Substitute (See **CREAM SUBSTITUTE)**			
CREAM PUFF, home recipe (USDA) custard filling	3½" × 2" piece	303	26.7
CREAM SUBSTITUTE:			
Coffee Mate (Carnation)	1 tsp.	11	1.1
Coffee Rich (Rich's)	½ oz.	22	2.2

(USDA) = United States Department of Agriculture
(HHS/FAO) = Health and Human Services/Food and Agriculture Organization
* = prepared as package directs

Food and Description	Measure or Quantity	Calories	Carbo-hydrates (grams)
Coffee Tone (Lucerne):			
Regular	1 tsp.	10	1.0
Frozen	1 T.	24	2.0
Non-dairy	½ fl. oz.	16	1.0
Cremora (Borden)	1 tsp.	12	1.0
Dairy Light (Alba)	2.8-oz. envelope	10	1.0
Mocha Mix (Presto Food Products)	1 T. (.5 oz.)	19	1.2
N-Rich	1 tsp.	10	2.0
CREAM OF WHEAT, cereal (Nabisco):			
Regular	1 T.	40	8.8
Instant	1 T.	40	8.8
*Mix'n Eat:			
Regular	1-oz. packet	100	21.0
Baked apple & cinnamon	1.25-oz. packet	130	30.0
Brown sugar	1.25-oz. packet	130	30.0
Maple & brown sugar	1.25-oz. packet	130	30.0
Strawberry	1.25-oz. packet	140	29.0
Quick	1 T.	40	8.8
CREME DE BANANA LIQUEUR (Mr. Boston):			
Regular, 27% alcohol	1 fl. oz.	93	12.1
Connoisseur, 21% alcohol	1 fl. oz.	82	11.4
CREME DE CACAO:			
(Hiram Walker) (27% alcohol)	1 fl. oz.	104	15.0
(Mr. Boston) 27% alcohol:			
Brown	1 fl. oz.	102	14.3
White	1 fl. oz.	93	12.0
CREME DE CASSIS			
(Mr. Boston) 17½% alcohol	1 fl. oz.	85	14.1
CREME DE MENTHE:			
(De Kuyper)	1 fl. oz.	94	11.3
(Mr. Boston) 27% alcohol:			
Green	1 fl. oz.	109	16.0
White	1 fl. oz.	97	13.0

Food and Description	Measure or Quantity	Calories	Carbo-hydrates (grams)
CREME DE NOYAUX			
(Mr. Boston) 27% alcohol	1 fl. oz.	99	13.5
CREPE, frozen:			
(Mrs. Paul's):			
Crab	5½-oz. pkg.	248	24.6
Shrimp	5½-oz. pkg.	252	23.8
(Stouffer's):			
Chicken with mushroom sauce	8¼-oz. pkg.	390	19.0
Ham & asparagus	6¼-oz. pkg.	325	21.0
Ham & swiss cheese with cheddar cheese sauce	7½-oz. pkg.	410	23.0
Spinach with cheddar cheese sauce	9½-oz. pkg.	415	30.0
CRISPIX, cereal (Kellogg's)	¾ cup (1 oz.)	110	25.0
CRISP RICE CEREAL:			
(Malt-O-Meal) *Crisp 'N Crackling Rice*	1 cup (1 oz.)	108	24.8
(Safeway)	1 cup	110	25.0
CRISPY CRITTERS, cereal (Post)	1 cup (1 oz.)	110	24.0
CRISPY WHEATS 'N RAISINS, cereal (General Mills)	¾ cup (1 oz.)	110	23.0
CROAKER (USDA):			
Atlantic:			
Raw, whole	1 lb. (weighed whole)	148	0.
Raw, meat only	4 oz.	109	0.
Baked	4 oz.	151	0.
White, raw meat only	4 oz.	95	0.
Yellowfin, raw, meat only	4 oz.	101	0.

(USDA) = United States Department of Agriculture
(HHS/FAO) = Health and Human Services/Food and Agriculture Organization
* = prepared as package directs

Food and Description	Measure or Quantity	Calories	Carbohydrates (grams)
CROUTON:			
(Kellogg's) *Croutettes*	⅔ cup (.7 oz.)	70	14.0
(Mrs. Cubbison's):			
Cheese & garlic or seasoned	½ oz.	60	9.0
Onion & garlic	½ oz.	70	10.0
(Pepperidge Farm)	½ oz	70	9.0
CUCUMBER (USDA):			
Eaten with skin	8-oz. cucumber (weighed whole)	32	7.4
Pared	7½" × 2" pared (7.3 oz.)	29	6.6
Pared	3 slices (.9 oz.)	4	.5
CUMIN SEED (French's)	1 tsp.	7	.7
CUPCAKE:			
Home recipe (USDA):			
Without icing	1.4-oz. cupcake	146	22.4
With chocolate icing	1.8-oz. cupcake	184	29.7
With boiled white icing	1.8-oz. cupcake	176	30.9
With uncooked white icing	1.8-oz. cupcake	184	31.6
Regular:			
(Dolly Madison) chocolate	1.6-oz. piece	170	29.0
(Hostess):			
Chocolate	1⅜-oz. piece	166	29.8
Orange	1½-oz. piece	151	26.8
CURACAO LIQUEUR:			
(Bols)	1 fl. oz.	105	10.3
(Hiram Walker)	1 fl. oz.	96	11.8
CURRANT:			
Fresh (USDA):			
Black European:			
Whole	1 lb. (weighed with stems)	240	58.2
Stems removed	4 oz.	61	14.9
Red and white:			
Whole	1 lb. (weighed with stems)	220	53.2
Stems removed	1 cup (3.9 oz.)	55	13.3

Food and Description	Measure or Quantity	Calories	Carbo- hydrates (grams)
Dried:			
(Del Monte) Zante	½ cup (2.4 oz.)	200	53.0
(Sun-Maid)	½ cup	220	53.0
CUSTARD:			
Home recipe (USDA)	½ cup (4.7 oz.)	152	14.7
Canned (Thank You Brand) egg	½ cup (4.6 oz.)	135	18.2
C.W. POST, cereal	¼ cup (1 oz.)	128	21.4

(USDA) = United States Department of Agriculture
(HHS/FAO) = Health and Human Services/Food and Agriculture Organization
* = prepared as package directs

Food and Description	Measure or Quantity	Calories	Carbo-hydrates (grams)

D

DAIQUIRI MIX:

Food and Description	Measure or Quantity	Calories	Carbo-hydrates (grams)
Dry (Holland House)	.56-oz. pkg.	65	16.0
Liquid:			
(Bar-Tender's)	3½ fl. oz.	177	18.0
(Holland House):			
Regular	1 fl. oz.	36	9.0
Raspberry	1 fl. oz.	30	7.0
Strawberry	1 fl. oz.	31	7.0
*Frozen (Bacardi):			
Peach	4 fl. oz.	98	16.3
Raspberry	4 fl. oz.	97	15.9
Strawberry	4 fl. oz.	102	17.1
DAIRY QUEEN/BRAZIER:			
Banana split	13.5-oz. serving	540	103.0
Brownie Delight, hot fudge	9.4-oz. serving	600	85.0
Buster Bar	5¼-oz. piece	460	41.0
Chicken sandwich	7.8-oz. sandwich	670	46.0
Cone:			
Plain, any flavor:			
Small	3-oz. cone	140	22.0
Regular	5-oz. cone	240	38.0
Large	7½-oz. cone	340	57.0
Dipped, chocolate:			
Small	3¼-oz. cone	190	25.0
Regular	5½-oz. cone	340	42.0
Large	8¼-oz. cone	510	64.0
Dilly Bar	3-oz. piece	210	21.0
Double Delight	9-oz. serving	490	69.0
DQ Sandwich	2.1-oz. sandwich	140	24.0
Fish sandwich:			
Plain	6-oz. sandwich	400	41.0
With cheese	6¼-oz. sandwich	440	39.0
Float	14-oz. serving	410	82.0
Freeze, vanilla	12-oz. serving	500	89.0

Food and Description	Measure or Quantity	Calories	Carbohydrates (grams)
French fries:			
Regular	2½-oz. serving	200	25.0
Large	4-oz. serving	320	40.0
Hamburger:			
Plain:			
Single	5.2-oz. burger	360	33.0
Double	7.4-oz. burger	530	33.0
Triple	9.6-oz. burger	710	33.0
With cheese:			
Single	5.7-oz. burger	410	33.0
Double	8.4-oz. burger	650	34.0
Triple	10.63-oz. burger	820	34.0
Hot dog:			
Regular:			
Plain	3.5-oz. serving	280	21.0
With cheese	4-oz. serving	330	21.0
With chili	4½-oz. serving	320	23.0
Super:			
Plain	6.2-oz. serving	520	44.0
With cheese	6.9-oz. serving	580	45.0
With chili	7.7-oz. serving	570	47.0
Malt, chocolate:			
Small	10¼-oz. serving	520	91.0
Regular	14¾-oz. serving	760	134.0
Large	20¾-oz. serving	1060	187.0
Mr. Misty:			
Plain:			
Small	8¼-oz. serving	190	48.0
Regular	11.64-oz. serving	250	63.0
Large	15½-oz. serving	340	84.0
Kiss	3.14-oz. serving	70	17.0
Float	14.5-oz. serving	390	74.0
Freeze	14.5-oz. serving	500	94.0
Onion rings	3-oz. serving	280	31.0
Parfait	10-oz. serving	430	76.0
Peanut Butter Parfait	10¾-oz. serving	750	94.0
Shake, chocolate:			
Small	10¼-oz. serving	490	82.0
Regular	14¾-oz. serving	710	120.0
Large	20¾-oz. serving	990	168.0

(USDA) = United States Department of Agriculture
(HHS/FAO) = Health and Human Services/Food and Agriculture
            Organization
* = prepared as package directs

Food and Description	Measure or Quantity	Calories	Carbo-hydrates (grams)
Strawberry shortcake	11-oz. serving	540	100.0
Sundae, chocolate:			
Small	3¾-oz. serving	190	33.0
Regular	6¼-oz. serving	310	56.0
Large	8¾-oz. serving	440	78.0
Tomato	½ oz.	4	1.0

DAMSON PLUM (See **PLUM**)

DANDELION GREENS, raw (USDA):

Trimmed	1 lb.	204	41.7
Boiled, drained	½ cup (3.2 oz.)	30	5.8

DANISH (See **ROLL OR BUN**)

DATE, dry:
Domestic:
(USDA):

With pits	1 lb. (weighed with pits)	1081	287.7
Without pits	4 oz.	311	82.7
Without pits chopped	1 cup (6.1 oz.)	477	126.8
(Dromedary):			
Without pits	1 date	20	4.6
Without pits, chopped	¼ cup (1¼ oz.)	130	31.0

DESSERT (See individual listings such as **APPLE BROWN BETTY; CAKE; FROZEN DESSERT; ICE CREAM; PRUNE WHIP; PUDDING** etc.)

DILL SEED (French's)	1 tsp. (2.1 grams)	9	1.2
DINERSAURS, cereal (Ralston Purina)	1 cup (1 oz.)	110	25.0

DINNER, FROZEN (See individual listings such as **BEAN & FRANKFURTER DINNER; BEEF DINNER** or

Food and Description	Measure or Quantity	Calories	Carbo-hydrates (grams)
ENTREE; LASAGNA, frozen; etc.)			
DIP:			
Acapulco (Ortega):			
Plain	1 oz.	8	1.8
American cheese	1 oz.	60	1.1
Cheddar cheese	1 oz.	64	1.2
Monterey Jack cheese	1 oz.	59	1.4
Bean (Eagle)	1 oz.	35	4.0
Blue cheese:			
(Dean) tang	1 oz.	61	2.3
(Nalley's)	1 oz.	110	.9
Chili (La Victoria)	1 T.	6	1.0
Enchilada, *Fritos*	1 oz.	37	3.9
Guacamole (Calavo)	1 oz.	55	3.5
Hot bean (Hain)	1 T.	17	2.5
Jalapeño (Wise)	1 T.	12	2.5
Onion (Hain) natural	1 T.	17	2.5
Picante sauce (Wise)	1 T.	6	1.5
Taco (Thank You Brand)	1 T. (.8 oz.)	44	2.0
DIP 'UM SAUCE, canned (French's):			
BBQ	1 T.	22	5.0
Creamy mustard	1 T.	40	6.0
Hot mustard	1 T.	35	7.0
Sweet 'n Sour	1 T.	40	10.0

DISTILLED LIQUOR. The values below would apply to unflavored bourbon whiskey, brandy, Canadian whiskey, gin, Irish whiskey, rum, rye whiskey, Scotch whisky, tequila and vodka. The caloric content of distilled liquors depends on the percentage of alcohol. The proof is twice the alcohol

(USDA) = United States Department of Agriculture
(HHS/FAO) = Health and Human Services/Food and Agriculture
                Organization
* = prepared as package directs

Food and Description	Measure or Quantity	Calories	Carbo-hydrates (grams)
percent and the following values apply to all brands (USDA):			
80 proof	1 fl. oz.	65	Tr.
86 proof	1 fl. oz.	70	Tr.
90 proof	1 fl. oz.	74	Tr.
94 proof	1 fl. oz.	77	Tr.
100 proof	1 fl. oz.	83	Tr.
DOUGHNUT:			
(USDA):			
Cake type	1.1-oz. piece	125	16.4
Yeast leavened	2-oz. piece	235	21.4
(Dolly Madison):			
Regular:			
Plain	1¼-oz. piece	140	17.0
Chocolate coated	1¼-oz. piece	150	18.0
Coconut crunch	1¼-oz. piece	140	20.0
Powdered sugar	1¼-oz. piece	140	19.0
Dunkin' Stix	1⅜-oz. piece	210	18.0
Gems:			
Chocolate coated	.5-oz. piece	65	7.0
Cinnamon sugar	.5-oz. piece	55	7.5
Coconut crunch	.5-oz. piece	60	8.0
Powdered sugar	.5-oz. piece	60	7.5
Jumbo:			
Plain	1.6-oz. piece	190	23.0
Cinnamon sugar	1.6-oz. piece	190	24.0
Sugar	1.7-oz. piece	210	27.0
Old fashioned:			
Cinnamon chip	2.2-oz. piece	280	32.0
Chocolate glazed	2.2-oz. piece	260	36.0
Chocolate iced	2.2-oz. piece	300	33.0
Glazed or orange crush	2.2-oz. piece	280	33.0
Powdered sugar	1.8-oz. piece	260	24.0
White iced	2.2-oz. piece	300	35.0
DRAMBUIE (Hiram Walker) (80 proof)	1 fl. oz.	110	11.0
DRUMSTICK, frozen:			
Ice Cream, in a cone:			
Topped with peanuts	1 piece	181	22.7
Topped with peanuts & cone bisque	1 piece	168	23.6

Food and Description	Measure or Quantity	Calories	Carbo-hydrates (grams)
Ice Milk, in a cone:			
Topped with peanuts	1 piece	163	24.3
Topped with peanuts & cone bisque	1 piece	150	25.2
DUCK, raw (USDA):			
Domesticated:			
Ready-to-cook	1 lb. (weighed with bone)	1213	0.
Meat only	4 oz.	187	0.
Wild:			
Dressed	1 lb. (weighed dressed)	613	0.
Meat only	4 oz.	156	0.
DULCITO, frozen (Hormel):			
Apple	4-oz. serving	290	44.0
Cherry	4-oz. serving	300	48.0

(USDA) = United States Department of Agriculture
(HHS/FAO) = Health and Human Services/Food and Agriculture Organization
* = prepared as package directs

Food and Description	Measure or Quantity	Calories	Carbo- hydrates (grams)

E

ECLAIR:
  Home recipe (USDA), with
    custard filling and chocolate

icing	4-oz. piece	271	26.3
Frozen (Rich's) chocolate	1 piece (2 oz.)	196	25.5

***ECTO* COOLER DRINK,**

canned (Hi-C)	6 fl. oz.	95	23.3

EEL (USDA):

Raw, meat only	4 oz.	264	0.
Smoked, meat only	4 oz.	374	0.

EGG (USDA) (See also **EGG SUBSTITUTE**):
  Chicken:
    Raw:

White only	1 large egg (1.2 oz.)	17	.3
White only	1 cup (9 oz.)	130	2.0
Yolk only	1 large egg (.6 oz.)	59	.1
Yolk only	1 cup (8.5 oz.)	835	1.4
Whole, small	1 egg (1.3 oz.)	60	.3
Whole, medium	1 egg (1.5 oz.)	71	.4
Whole, large	1 egg (1.8 oz.)	81	.4
Whole	1 cup (8.8 oz.)	409	2.3
Whole, extra large	1 egg (2. oz.)	94	.5
Whole, jumbo	1 egg (2.3 oz.)	105	.6
Cooked:			
Boiled	1 large egg (1.8 oz.)	81	.4
Fried in butter	1 large egg	99	.1
Omelet, mixed with milk and cooked in fat	1 large egg	107	1.5
Poached	1 large egg	78	.4

Food and Description	Measure or Quantity	Calories	Carbo-hydrates (grams)
Scrambled, mixed with milk & cooked in fat	1 large egg	111	1.5
Scrambled, mixed with milk & cooked in fat	1 cup (7.8 oz.)	381	5.3
Dried:			
Whole	1 cup (3.8 oz.)	639	4.4
White, powder	1 oz.	105	1.6
Yolk	1 cup (3.4 oz.)	637	2.4
Duck, raw	1 egg (2.8 oz.)	153	.6
Goose, raw	1 egg (5.8 oz.)	303	2.1
Turkey, raw	1 egg (3.1 oz.)	150	1.5

EGG BREAKFAST, frozen (Swanson) *Great Starts*:

Regular:

Omelet, with cheese sauce & ham	7-oz. pkg.	390	15.0
Reduced cholesterol with mini muffins	4¾-oz. pkg.	250	27.0
Scrambled:			
with bacon & home fries	5.6-oz. pkg.	340	16.0
with cheese & cinnamon pancakes	3.4-oz. pkg.	290	14.0
with home fries	4.6-oz. pkg.	260	14.0
& sausage,with home fries	6½-oz. pkg.	430	19.0
On a biscuit:			
With Canadian bacon & cheese	5.2-oz. pkg.	420	37.0
With sausage & cheese	5½-oz. pkg.	460	35.0
On a muffin:			
With beefsteak & cheese	4.9-oz. pkg.	360	27.0
With Canadian bacon & cheese	4.1-oz. pkg.	290	25.0

*EGG FOO YOUNG, dinner, canned:

(Chun King) stir fry	5-oz. serving	138	9.1
(La Choy)	1 patty + ¼ cup sauce	164	19.2

(USDA) = United States Department of Agriculture
(HHS/FAO) = Health and Human Services/Food and Agriculture Organization
* = prepared as package directs

Food and Description	Measure or Quantity	Calories	Carbo-hydrates (grams)
EGG NOG, dairy:			
(Borden)	½ cup	160	16.0
(Johanna)	½ cup	195	22.4
EGG NOG COCKTAIL			
(Mr. Boston) 15% alcohol	3 fl. oz.	177	18.9
EGGPLANT:			
Raw (USDA) whole	1 lb. (weighed whole)	92	20.6
Boiled (USDA) drained, diced	1 cup (7.1 oz.)	38	8.2
Frozen:			
(Buitoni) parmigiana	5-oz. serving	168	17.6
(Celentano):			
Parmigiana	½ of 16-oz. pkg.	280	23.0
Rollatines	11-oz. pkg.	320	36.0
(Mrs. Paul's) parmesan	5-oz. serving	240	18.0
EGG ROLL, frozen:			
(Chun King):			
Regular:			
Chicken	3½ oz. piece	210	31.0
Meat & shrimp	3½-oz. piece	214	30.0
Shrimp	3½-oz. piece	189	30.0
Restaurant style, pork	3-oz. piece	172	23.0
(La Choy):			
Chicken	.5-oz. piece	30	4.0
Lobster	.5-oz. piece	27	4.3
Lobster	3-oz. piece	180	25.0
Meat & shrimp	.5-oz. piece	27	4.0
Shrimp	3-oz. piece	160	24.0
EGG ROLL DINNER OR ENTREE, frozen:			
(La Choy) entree:			
Almond chicken	2 pieces	450	43.0
Beef & broccoli	2 pieces	380	45.0
Spicy oriental chicken	2 pieces	300	32.0
Sweet & sour pork	2 pieces	430	56.0
(Van de Kamp's) Cantonese	10½-oz. serving	560	80.0
EGG SUBSTITUTE:			
Egg Magic (Featherweight)	½ of envelope	60	1.0
Scramblers (Morningstar Farms)	1 egg substitute	35	1.5

Food and Description	Measure or Quantity	Calories	Carbo-hydrates (grams)
ELDERBERRY, fresh (USDA):			
Whole	1 lb. (weighed with stems)	307	69.9
Stems removed	4 oz.	82	18.6
EL POLLO LOCO **RESTAURANT:**			
Beans	3½-oz. serving	110	17.0
Chicken	2 pieces (4.8 oz. edible portion)	310	2.0
Cole slaw	2.8-oz. serving	80	5.0
Combo	16-oz. meal	720	70.0
Corn	3.3-oz. piece	110	20.0
Dole Whip	4½-oz. serving	90	19.0
Potato salad	4.3-oz. serving	140	15.0
Rice	2½-oz. serving	100	22.0
Salsa	1.8-oz. serving	10	1.0
Tortilla:			
Corn	3.3-oz. serving	210	42.0
Flour	3.3-oz. serving	280	45.0
ENCHANADA, frozen (Stouffer's) *Lean Cuisine:*			
Bean & beef	9¼-oz. meal	280	32.0
Chicken	9⅞-oz. meal	270	31.0
ENCHILADA OR ENCHILADA DINNER:			
Canned (Old El Paso) beef	1 enchilada	145	11.0
Frozen:			
Beef:			
(Banquet):			
Dinner	12-oz. dinner	500	72.0
Family Entree	2-lb. pkg.	1080	112.0
(Fred's Frozen Foods)			
Marquez	7½-oz. serving	304	23.5

(USDA) = United States Department of Agriculture
(HHS/FAO) = Health and Human Services/Food and Agriculture
Organization
* = prepared as package directs

Food and Description	Measure or Quantity	Calories	Carbo- hydrates (grams)
(Old El Paso):			
Dinner	11-oz. dinner	390	56.0
Entree	1 piece	210	16.0
(Patio)	13¼-oz. dinner	520	59.0
(Swanson)	13¾-oz. dinner	480	55.0
(Van de Kamp's):			
Dinner:			
Regular	12-oz. meal	390	45.0
Shredded	14¾-oz. meal	490	60.0
Entree:			
Regular	7½-oz. meal	250	20.0
Shredded	5½-oz. serving	180	15.0
(Weight Watchers)	9.1-oz. meal	300	25.0
Cheese:			
(Banquet)	12-oz. dinner	550	71.0
(Old El Paso):			
Dinner, festive	11-oz. dinner	590	51.0
Entree	1 piece	250	24.0
(Patio)	12¼-oz. dinner	380	59.0
(Van de Kamp's):			
Dinner	12-oz. dinner	390	45.0
Entree	7½-oz. pkg.	250	20.0
(Weight Watchers)	8.9-oz. meal	360	30.0
Chicken:			
(Old El Paso):			
Dinner, festive	11-oz. dinner	460	54.0
Entree:			
Regular	1 piece	226	20.0
With sour cream sauce	1 piece	280	18.0
(Weight Watchers)	9.37-oz. meal	330	26.0
ENCHILADA SAUCE:			
Canned:			
(El Molino) hot	1 T.	8	1.0
(La Victoria)	1 T.	5	1.0
(Old El Paso):			
Green chili	½ cup	36	7.2
Hot	½ cup	54	7.6
Mild	½ cup	50	7.2
(Rosarita)	3 oz.	19	4.0
Mix:			
*(Durkee)	½ cup	29	6.2
(French's)	1⅜-oz. pkg.	120	20.0

Food and Description	Measure or Quantity	Calories	Carbo-hydrates (grams)
ENCHILADA SEASONING MIX (Lawry's)	1.6-oz. pkg.	152	29.9
ENDIVE, CURLY, raw (USDA):			
Untrimmed	1 lb. (weighed untrimmed)	80	16.4
Trimmed	½ lb.	45	9.3
Cut up or shredded	1 cup (2.5 oz.)	14	2.9
ESCAROLE, raw (USDA):			
Untrimmed	1 lb. (weighed untrimmed)	80	16.4
Trimmed	½ lb.	46	9.2
Cut up or shredded	1 cup (2.5 oz.)	14	2.9
EULACHON OR SMELT, raw (USDA) meat only	4 oz.	134	0.
EXPRESSO COFFEE LIQUEUR (Mr. Boston) 26½% alcohol	1 fl. oz.	104	15.0

(USDA) = United States Department of Agriculture
(HHS/FAO) = Health and Human Services/Food and Agriculture Organization
* = prepared as package directs

Food and Description	Measure or Quantity	Calories	Carbo-hydrates (grams)

F

Food and Description	Measure or Quantity	Calories	Carbo-hydrates (grams)
FAJITA, frozen:			
(Healthy Choice):			
Beef	7-oz. meal	210	26.0
Chicken	7-oz. meal	200	25.0
(Weight Watchers):			
Beef	6¾-oz. meal	250	31.0
Chicken	6¾-oz. meal	230	30.0
FAJITA SEASONING			
MIX (Lawry's)	1.3-oz. pkg.	63	14.0
FARINA:			
(H-O) dry, regular	1 T. (.4 oz.)	40	8.5
Malt-O-Meal, dry:			
Regular	1 oz.	96	21.0
Quick cooking	1 oz.	100	22.2
*(Pillsbury) made with water and salt	⅔ cup	80	17.0
FAT, COOKING:			
(USDA):			
Lard	1 T. (.5 oz.)	115	0.
Vegetable oil	1 T. (1.4 oz.)	106	0.
Crisco:			
Regular	1 T. (.4 oz.)	110	0.
Butter flavor	1 T. (.5 oz.)	126	0.
(Mrs. Tucker's)	1 T.	120	0.
(Rokeach) neutral nyafat	1 T.	99	0.
Spry	1 T. (.4 oz.)	94	0.
FENNEL SEED (French's)	1 tsp. (2.1 grams)	8	1.3
FETTUCINI, frozen:			
(Armour) *Dining Lite,*			
& broccoli	9-oz. meal	290	33.0
(Green Giant) primavera	9½-oz. meal	230	26.0

Food and Description	Measure or Quantity	Calories	Carbo-hydrates (grams)
(Healthy Choice):			
Afredo	8-oz. meal	270	42.0
Chicken	8½-oz. meal	240	22.0
(Stouffer's) Alfredo	10-oz. pkg.	540	34.0
FIBER ONE, cereal			
(General Mills)	½ cup (1 oz.)	60	23.0
FIG:			
Fresh (USDA):			
Regular size	1 lb.	363	92.1
Small	1.3-oz. fig (1½″ dia.)	30	7.7
Candied (Bama)	1 T. (.7 oz.)	37	9.6
Canned, regular pack, solids & liq.: (USDA):			
Light syrup	4 oz.	74	19.1
Heavy syrup	3 figs & 2 T. syrup (4 oz.)	96	24.9
Heavy syrup	½ cup (4.4 oz.)	106	27.5
Extra heavy syrup	4 oz.	117	30.3
(Del Monte) whole	½ cup (4.3 oz.)	100	28.0
Canned, unsweetened or dietetic, solids & liq.:			
(USDA) water pack	4 oz.	54	14.1
(Diet Delight) Kadota	½ cup (4.4 oz.)	76	18.2
Dried (Sun-Maid):			
Calimyrna	½ cup (3.5 oz.)	250	58.0
Mission, regular or figlets	½ cup (3 oz.)	210	50.0
FIG JUICE (Sunsweet)	6 fl. oz.	120	30.0
FIGURINES (Pillsbury) all flavors	1 bar	100	10.0
FILBERT:			
(USDA):			
Whole	1 lb. (weighed in shell)	1323	34.9

(USDA) = United States Department of Agriculture
(HHS/FAO) = Health and Human Services/Food and Agriculture Organization
* = prepared as package directs

Food and Description	Measure or Quantity	Calories	Carbo- hydrates (grams)
Shelled	1 oz.	180	4.7
(Fisher) oil dipped, salted	½ cup (2 oz.)	360	5.4
FISH (See individual listings)			
***FISH BOUILLON** (Knorr)	8 fl. oz.	10	.4
FISH CAKE:			
Home recipe (USDA)	2 oz.	98	5.3
Frozen:			
(Captain's Choice)	2-oz. piece	130	14.0
(Mrs. Paul's) thins	1 piece	95	12.0
FISH & CHIPS, frozen:			
(Gorton's)	1 pkg.	1350	132.0
(Swanson):			
4-compartment dinner	10-oz. dinner	500	60.0
Homestyle Recipe	6½-oz. entree	340	37.0
(Van de Kamp's) batter dipped, french fried	7-oz. pkg.	440	35.0
FISH DINNER OR ENTREE, frozen (See also individual listings such as **COD DINNER**):			
(Banquet) platters	8¾-oz. dinner	450	33.0
(Gorton's):			
Fillet almondine	1 pkg.	340	2.0
Fillet, in herb butter	1 pkg.	190	3.0
(Kid Cuisine) nuggets	7-oz. meal	320	33.0
(Morton)	9¾-oz. dinner	370	46.0
(Mrs. Paul's):			
Dijon	8¾-oz. meal	200	17.0
Florentine	8-oz. meal	220	10.0
Mornay	9-oz. meal	230	12.0
(Stouffer's) *Lean Cuisine*, fillet:			
Divan	12⅜-oz. pkg.	260	17.0
Florentine	9-oz. pkg.	230	13.0
(Weight Watchers):			
Au gratin	9¼-oz. meal	200	11.0
Oven fried	7.1-oz. meal	300	27.0

FISH FILLET, frozen:

Food and Description	Measure or Quantity	Calories	Carbo-hydrates (grams)
(Captain's Choice):			
Crisp & crunchy	1 fillet	155	14.0
Fried, battered	3-oz. piece	240	10.0
(Frionor) *Bunch O' Crunch*, breaded	1½-oz. piece	140	3.8
(Gorton's):			
Regular:			
Batter dipped, crispy	1 piece	250	18.0
Crunchy	1 piece	175	9.5
Potato crisp	1 piece	170	10.0
Light Recipe:			
Lightly breaded	1 piece	180	16.0
Tempura batter	1 piece	200	8.0
(Mrs. Paul's):			
Batter dipped	1 fillet	165	14.0
Crispy crunchy	1 fillet	110	11.5
Crunchy batter	1 fillet	140	13.0
Light, in butter sauce	1 fillet	70	.5
FISH LOAF, Home recipe (USDA)	4 oz.	141	8.3
FISH NUGGET, frozen (Frionor) *Bunch O' Crunch*, breaded	.5-oz. piece	40	2.2
FISH SANDWICH, frozen (Frionor) *Bunch O' Crunch*, microwave	5-oz. sandwich	320	31.0
FISH STICKS, frozen:			
(Captain's Choice)	1 piece	76	7.0
(Frionor) *Bunch O' Crunch*, breaded	.7-oz. piece	58	3.5
(Gorton's):			
Batter dipped, crispy	1 piece	65	4.0
Crunchy, regular	1 piece	55	3.7
Potato crisp	1 piece	65	5.2
Value pack	1 piece	52	4.5

(USDA) = United States Department of Agriculture
(HHS/FAO) = Health and Human Services/Food and Agriculture Organization
* = prepared as package directs

Food and Description	Measure or Quantity	Calories	Carbohydrates (grams)
(Mrs. Paul's):			
Battered	1 piece	52	3.7
Crispy, crunchy:			
Battered	1 piece	47	4.5
Breaded	1 piece	35	3.5
FLOUNDER:			
Raw (USDA):			
Whole	1 lb. (weighed whole)	118	0.
Meat only	4 oz.	90	0.
Baked (USDA)	4 oz.	229	0.
Frozen:			
(Captain's Choice) fillet	3 oz.	99	0.
(Frionor) *Norway Gourmet*	4-oz. piece	60	0.
(Gorton's):			
Fishmarket Fresh	5 oz.	110	1.0
Microwave entree, stuffed	1 pkg.	350	21.0
(Mrs. Paul's) fillet:			
Crunchy batter	1 fillet	110	11.5
Light	1 fillet	240	20.0
FLOUR:			
(USDA):			
Buckwheat, dark, sifted	1 cup (3.5 oz.)	326	70.6
Buckwheat, light sifted	1 cup (3.5 oz.)	340	77.9
Cake:			
Unsifted, dipped	1 cup (4.2 oz.)	433	94.5
Unsifted, spooned	1 cup (3.9 oz.)	404	88.1
Carob or St. John's bread	1 oz.	51	22.9
Chestnut	1 oz.	103	21.6
Corn	1 cup (3.9 oz.)	405	84.5
Cottonseed	1 oz.	101	9.4
Fish, from whole fish	1 oz.	95	0.
Lima bean	1 oz.	95	17.9
Potato	1 oz.	100	22.7
Rice, stirred spooned	1 cup (5.6 oz.)	574	125.6
Rye:			
Light:			
Unsifted, spooned	1 cup (3.6 oz.)	361	78.7
Sifted, spooned	1 cup (3.1 oz.)	314	68.6
Medium	1 oz.	99	21.1

Food and Description	Measure or Quantity	Calories	Carbo-hydrates (grams)
Dark:			
Unstirred	1 cup (4.5 oz.)	419	87.2
Stirred	1 cup (4.5 oz.)	415	86.5
Soybean, defatted, stirred	1 cup (3.6 oz.)	329	38.5
Soybean, high fat	1 oz.	108	9.4
Sunflower seed, partially defatted	1 oz.	96	10.7
Wheat:			
All-purpose:			
Unsifted, dipped	1 cup (5 oz.)	521	108.8
Unsifted, spooned	1 cup (4.4 oz.)	459	95.9
Sifted, spooned	1 cup (4.1 oz.)	422	88.3
Bread:			
Unsifted, dipped	1 cup (4.8 oz.)	496	101.6
Unsifted, spooned	1 cup (4.3 oz.)	449	91.9
Sifted, spooned	1 cup (4.1 oz.)	427	87.4
Gluten:			
Unsifted, dipped	1 cup (5 oz.)	537	67.0
Sifted, spooned	1 cup (4.8 oz.)	514	64.2
Self-rising:			
Unsifted, dipped	1 cup (4.6 oz.)	458	96.5
Sifted, spooned	1 cup (3.7 oz.)	373	78.7
Whole wheat	1 oz.	94	20.1
(Aunt Jemima) self-rising	¼ cup (1 oz.)	109	23.6
Ballard:			
Self-rising	¼ cup	91	23.6
All-purpose	¼ cup (1 oz.)	100	21.8
Bisquick (Betty Crocker)	¼ cup (1 oz.)	120	18.5
(Drifted Snow)	¼ cup	100	21.8
(Elam's):			
Brown rice, whole grain, sodium & gluten free	¼ cup (1.2 oz.)	125	.2
Buckwheat, pure	¼ cup (¼ oz.)	131	27.2
Pastry, whole wheat	¼ cup (1.2 oz.)	122	24.9
Rye, whole grain	¼ cup	118	24.2
Soy, roasted, defatted	¼ cup (1.1 oz.)	108	9.8
3-in-1 mix	1 oz.	99	20.0
White, with wheat germ	¼ cup (1 oz.)	101	20.7
Whole wheat	¼ cup (1.1 oz.)	111	21.7

(USDA) = United States Department of Agriculture
(HHS/FAO) = Health and Human Services/Food and Agriculture Organization
* = prepared as package directs

Food and Description	Measure or Quantity	Calories	Carbo-hydrates (grams)
Gold Medal:			
All purpose or unbleached	¼ cup (1 oz.)	100	21.8
Better For Bread	¼ cup	100	20.7
Self-rising	¼ cup	95	20.8
Whole wheat	¼ cup	98	19.5
Pillsbury's Best:			
All-purpose or rye and wheat			
Bohemian style	¼ cup	100	21.5
Bread or rye, medium	1.4 cup	100	20.8
Self-rising	¼ cup	95	21.0
Shake & blend	1 T.	25	5.5
Whole wheat	¼ cup	100	21.0
Red Band:			
All purpose or unbleached	¼ cup	97	21.2
Self-rising	¼ cup	95	20.8
Wondra	¼ cup	100	21.8
FOLLE BLANC WINE (Louis M. Martini) 12.5% alcohol	3 fl. oz.	63	.2
FRANKEN*BERRY, cereal (General Mills)	1 cup (1 oz.)	110	24.0
FRANKFURTER, raw or cooked:			
(USDA), raw:			
Common type	1 frankfurter (10 per lb.)	140	.8
Meat	1 frankfurter (10 per lb.)	134	1.1
With cereal	1 frankfurter (10 per lb.)	112	.1
Cooked, common type	1 frankfurter (10 per lb.)	136	.7
(Eckrich):			
Beef	1.2-oz. frankfurter	110	2.0
Beef	1.6-oz. frankfurter	150	3.0
Beef	2-oz. frankfurter	190	3.0
Cheese	2-oz. frankfurter	190	3.0
Meat	1.2-oz. frankfurter	120	2.0

Food and Description	Measure or Quantity	Calories	Carbo-hydrates (grams)
Meat	1.6-oz. frankfurter	150	3.0
Meat	2.-oz. frankfurter	190	3.0
(Empire Kosher):			
Chicken	2-oz. frankfurter	106	1.0
Turkey	2-oz. frankfurter	107	1.0
Hebrew National:			
Beef	1.7-oz. frankfurter	149	<1.0
Collagen	2.3-oz. frankfurter	202	<1.0
Lite, beef	1.7-oz. frankfurter	120	<1.0
Natural casing	2-oz. frankfurter	175	<1.0
(Hormel):			
Beef	1 frankfurter (12-oz. pkg.)	100	1.0
Beef	1 frankfurter (1 lb. pkg.)	140	1.0
Chili, *Frank 'n Stuff*	1 frankfurter	165	2.0
Meat	1 frankfurter (12-oz. pkg.)	110	1.0
Meat	1 frankfurter (1-lb. pkg.)	140	1.0
Range Brand	1 frankfurter	170	1.0
Wrangler, smoked:			
Beef	1 frankfurter	170	2.0
Cheese	1 frankfurter	180	1.0
(Louis Rich):			
Turkey	1.5-oz. frankfurter	95	1.0
Turkey	1.6-oz. frankfurter	100	1.0
Turkey	2.-oz. frankfurter	125	1.0
(Ohse):			
Beef	1-oz. frankfurter	85	1.0

(USDA) = United States Department of Agriculture
(HHS/FAO) = Health and Human Services/Food and Agriculture Organization
* = prepared as package directs

Food and Description	Measure or Quantity	Calories	Carbohydrates (grams)
Wiener:			
Regular	1-oz. frankfurter	90	1.0
Chicken, beef & pork	1-oz. frankfurter	85	1.0
(Oscar Mayer):			
Bacon & cheddar	1.6-oz. frankfurter	139	1.0
Beef:			
Regular	1.6-oz. frankfurter	143	1.1
Jumbo	2-oz. frankfurter	179	1.4
Big One	4-oz. frankfurter	357	2.7
Cheese	1.6-oz. frankfurter	144	1.0
Little Wiener	2" frankfurter	28	.2
Wiener	1.6-oz. frankfurter	144	1.1
Wiener	2-oz. frankfurter	180	1.4
(Safeway) beef or meat	2-oz. frankfurter	170	1.0
(Smok-A-Roma):			
Beef	2-oz. frankfurter	170	1.0
Meat	2-oz. frankfurter	140	1.0
FRENCH TOAST, frozen			
(Aunt Jemima):			
Regular	1 slice (1½ oz.)	85	13.2
Cinnamon swirl	1 slice (1½ oz.)	97	13.6
FRENCH TOAST BREAKFAST, frozen (Swanson)			
Great Starts:			
Cinnamon swirl, with sausage	5½-oz. meal	390	37.0
Mini, with sausage	2½-oz. meal	190	22.0
Oatmeal, with lite links	4.6-oz. meal	310	35.0
With sausage	5½-oz. meal	380	35.0
FRITTERS:			
Home recipe (USDA):			
Clam	2" × 1¾" (1.4 oz.)	124	12.4
Corn	2" × 1½" (1.2 oz.)	132	13.9
Frozen (Mrs. Paul's) apple or corn	1 piece	120	17.5

Food and Description	Measure or Quantity	Calories	Carbo-hydrates (grams)
FROG LEGS, raw (USDA):			
Bone-in	1 lb. (weighed with bone)	215	0.
Meat only	4 oz.	83	0.
FROOT LOOPS, cereal (Kellogg's)	1 cup (1 oz.)	110	25.0
FROSTED RICE, cereal (Ralston Purina)	1 cup (1 oz.)	110	26.0
FROSTEE (Borden):			
Chocolate flavored	1 cup	200	30.0
Strawberry flavored	1 cup	180	27.0
FROSTING (See **CAKE ICING**)			
FROZEN DESSERT, dietetic (See also *TOFUTTI*):			
(Baskin-Robbins) chunky banana	½ cup	100	20.0
(Eskimo) bar, chocolate covered	2½-fl.-oz. bar	110	10.0
Mocha Mix (Presto):			
Bar, vanilla, chocolate covered	4 oz.	230	20.0
Bulk:			
Dutch chocolate	½ cup	140	16.0
Heavenly hash	½ cup	160	18.0
Mocha almond fudge	½ cup	150	19.0
Neapolitan or vanilla	½ cup	140	17.0
Peach	½ cup	130	19.0
Strawberry swirl or very berry	½ cup	140	20.0
Toasted almond	½ cup	150	17.0
FROZEN DINNER OR ENTREE (See individual listings such as **BEAN & FRANKFURTER DINNER;**			

(USDA) = United States Department of Agriculture
(HHS/FAO) = Health and Human Services/Food and Agriculture Organization
* = prepared as package directs

Food and Description	Measure or Quantity	Calories	Carbo-hydrates (grams)
BEEF DINNER OR ENTREE; LASAGNA, frozen; etc.)			
FRUIT (See individual listings such as **BANANA; FIG; KUMQUAT;** etc.)			
FRUIT, MIXED:			
Canned, solids & liq.:			
(Del Monte) Lite, chunky	½ cup	58	14.0
(Hunt's) *Snack Pack*	5-oz. container	120	31.0
Dried:			
(Sun-Maid/Sunsweet)	2 oz.	150	39.0
(Town House)	2 oz.	150	40.0
FRUIT BARS (General Mills)			
Fruit Corners:			
Regular:			
Cherry, grape or strawberry	1 bar	90	18.0
Orange pineapple or tropical	1 bar	90	17.0
Swirled	1 bar	90	18.0
FRUIT BITS, dried (Sun-Maid)	1 oz.	90	21.0
FRUIT 'N CHERRY JUICE			
(Tree Top):			
Canned	6 fl. oz.	80	21.0
*Frozen	6 fl. oz.	90	22.0
FRUIT 'N CITRUS JUICE			
(Tree Top):			
Canned	6 fl. oz.	100	24.0
*Frozen	6 fl. oz.	90	22.0
FRUIT COCKTAIL:			
Canned, regular pack, solids & liq.:			

Food and Description	Measure or Quantity	Calories	Carbo-hydrates (grams)
(USDA):			
Light syrup	4 oz.	68	17.8
Heavy syrup	½ cup (4.5 oz.)	97	25.2
Extra syrup	4 oz.	104	26.9
(Hunt's)	½ cup (4 oz.)	90	23.0
(Town House)	½ cup	90	24.0
Canned, dietetic or low calorie, solids & liq.:			
(Country Pure)	½ cup	50	14.0
(Diet Delight):			
Juice pack	½ cup (4.4 oz.)	50	14.0
Water pack	½ cup (4.3 oz.)	40	10.0
(Libby's) Lite, water pack	½ cup (4.4 oz.)	50	13.0
(S&W) *Nutradiet,* white or blue label	½ cup	40	10.0
FRUIT COMPOTE, canned (Rokeach)	½ cup (4 oz.)	120	31.0
FRUIT & CREAM BAR (Dole):			
Blueberry, peach or strawberry	1 bar	90	18.0
Chocolate-banana	1 bar	175	22.0
Chocolate-strawberry	1 bar	160	23.0
Raspberry	1 bar	90	19.0
FRUIT & FIBER, cereal (Post):			
Dates, raisins, walnuts with oat clusters	⅔ cup (1¼ oz.)	120	27.0
Tropical fruit with oat clusters	⅔ cup (1¼-oz.)	125	27.0
Whole wheat & bran flakes with peaches, raisins, almonds & oat clusters	⅔ cup (1¼ oz.)	121	266.0

(USDA) = United States Department of Agriculture
(HHS/FAO) = Health and Human Services/Food and Agriculture Organization
* = prepared as package directs

Food and Description	Measure or Quantity	Calories	Carbohydrates (grams)
FRUIT 'N GRAPE JUICE (Tree Top):			
Canned	6 fl. oz.	100	25.0
*Frozen	6 fl. oz.	110	27.0
FRUIT JUICE, canned (See individual listings such as *CRANAPPLE* JUICE DRINK; *ORANGE-GRAPEFRUIT JUICE; PINEAPPLE JUICE;* etc.)			
FRUIT 'N JUICE BAR:			
(Dole):			
Fresh Lites:			
Cherry, pineapple-orange & raspberry	1 bar	25	6.0
Lemon	1 bar	25	5.0
Fruit 'N Juice:			
Cherry or pineapple	1 bar	70	18.0
Peach passion fruit	1 bar	70	16.0
Pina colada	1 bar	80	15.0
Pineapple-orange-banana, raspberry or strawberry	1 bar	60	15.0
Sun Tops	1 bar	40	9.0
(Weight Watchers)	1.7-fl.-oz. bar	35	9.0
FRUIT & JUICE DRINK (Tree Top):			
Canned:			
Apple	6 fl. oz.	90	22.0
Berry	6 fl. oz.	80	21.0
Cherry	6 fl. oz.	100	24.0
Citrus	6 fl. oz.	90	22.0
Grape	6 fl. oz.	100	25.0
*Frozen:			
Apple	6 fl. oz.	90	23.0
Berry, cherry or citrus	6 fl. oz.	90	22.0
Grape	6 fl. oz.	110	27.0
FRUIT & NUT MIX (Estee)	1 piece	35	3.0

Food and Description	Measure or Quantity	Calories	Carbo-hydrates (grams)
FRUIT PUNCH:			
Canned:			
Bama (Borden)	8.45 fl.-oz. container	130	32.0
(Hi-C)	6 fl. oz.	96	23.7
(Lincoln) party	6 fl. oz.	90	23.0
(Minute Maid):			
Regular	8.45-fl.-oz. container	128	32.0
On the Go	10-fl.-oz. bottle	152	37.9
Chilled:			
(Minute Maid)	6 fl. oz.	91	22.7
(Sunkist)	8.45 fl. oz.	140	34.0
*Frozen (Minute Maid)	6 fl. oz.	91	22.7
*Mix:			
Regular (Funny Face)	8 fl. oz.	88	22.0
Dietetic, *Crystal Light* (General Foods)	8 fl. oz.	3	.1
FRUIT RINGS, cereal (Safeway)	1 oz.	110	26.0
FRUIT ROLLS:			
(Flavor Tree)	¾-oz. piece	80	18.0
Fruit Corners (General Mills):			
Apple, apricot, banana, cherry or grape	.5-oz. piece	50	12.0
Fruit punch	.5-oz. piece	60	12.0
(Sunkist)	.5-oz. piece	50	12.0
FRUIT SALAD:			
Canned, regular pack, solids & liq.:			
(USDA):			
Light syrup	4 oz.	67	17.6
Heavy syrup	½ cup (4.3 oz.)	85	22.0
Extra heavy syrup	4 oz.	102	26.5

(USDA) = United States Department of Agriculture
(HHS/FAO) = Health and Human Services/Food and Agriculture Organization
* = prepared as package directs

Food and Description	Measure or Quantity	Calories	Carbo-hydrates (grams)
(Dole) tropical, in light syrup	½ cup	70	17.0
(Libby's) heavy syrup	½ cup (4.4 oz.)	99	24.0
Canned, dietetic or low calorie, solids & liq.:			
(Diet Delight) juice pack	½ cup (4.4 oz.)	60	16.0
(S&W) *Nutradiet:*			
Juice pack, white label	½ cup	50	11.0
Water pack, blue label	½ cup	35	10.0
FRUIT SLUSH (Wyler's)	4 fl. oz.	157	39.3
FRUIT WRINKLES (General Mills) *Fruit Corners*	1 pouch	100	21.0
FRUITY YUMMY MUMMY, cereal (General Mills)	1 cup (1 oz.)	110	24.0

Food and Description	Measure or Quantity	Calories	Carbo-hydrates (grams)

G

GARFIELD AND FRIENDS
(General Mills):
Pouch:

1-2 Punch	.9-oz. pouch	100	21.0
Very strawberry	.9-oz. pouch	90	21.0
Roll	.5-oz. roll	50	12.0

GARLIC:
Raw (USDA):

Whole	2 oz. (weighed with skin)	68	15.4
Peeled	1 oz.	39	8.7
Flakes (Gilroy)	1 tsp.	13	2.6
Powder (French's)	1 tsp.	10	2.0
Salt (French's)	1 tsp.	4	1.0
Spread (Lawry's):			
Concentrate	1 T.	15	.2
Ready-to-use, bread spread	1 T.	94	2.0

GEFILTE FISH, canned:
(Manischewitz):

Fishlets	1 piece	8	4.4
Gefilte:			
Regular:			
12- or 24-oz. jar	3-oz. piece	53	4.4
4-lb. pkg.	2.7-oz. piece	48	4.4
Homestyle:			
12- or 24-oz. jar	3-oz. piece	55	6.2
4-lb. jar	2.7-oz. piece	50	6.2
Sweet:			
12- or 24-oz. jar	3-oz. piece	65	8.7
4-lb. jar	2.7-oz. piece	59	8.7

(USDA) = United States Department of Agriculture
(HHS/FAO) = Health and Human Services/Food and Agriculture Organization
* = prepared as package directs

Food and Description	Measure or Quantity	Calories	Carbo-hydrates (grams)
Whitefish & pike:			
Regular:			
12- or 24-oz. jar	3-oz. piece	49	4.8
4-lb. jar	2.7-oz. piece	44	4.8
Sweet:			
12- or 24-oz. jar	3-oz. piece	64	8.8
4-lb. jar	2.7-oz. piece	58	8.8
(Rokeach):			
Natural broth:			
12-oz. jar	2-oz. piece	46	3.0
24-oz. jar	2.6-oz. piece	60	4.0
Old Vienna:			
Regular:			
12-oz. jar	2-oz. piece	52	4.0
24-oz. jar	2.6-oz. piece	68	5.0
Jellied, whitefish & pike:			
12-oz. jar	2-oz. piece	54	4.0
24-oz. jar	2.6-oz. piece	70	5.0
Redi-Jell:			
12-oz. jar	2-oz. piece	46	3.0
24-oz. jar	2.6-oz. piece	60	4.0
Whitefish & pike, jellied broth:			
12-oz. jar	2-oz. piece	46	3.0
24-oz. jar	2.6-oz. piece	60	4.0
GELATIN, unflavored, dry:			
(USDA)	7-gram envelope	23	0.
Carmel Kosher	7-gram envelope	30	0.
(Knox)	1 envelope	25	0.
GELATIN DESSERT:			
Canned, dietetic (Dia-Mel; Louis Sherry)	4-oz. container	2	Tr.
*Powder:			
Regular:			
Carmel Kosher, all flavors	½ cup (4 oz.)	80	20.0
(Jell-O) all flavors	½ cup (4.9 oz.)	83	18.6
(Royal) all flavors	½ cup (4.9 oz.)	80	19.0
Dietetic:			
Carmel Kosher, all flavors	½ cup	8	0.
(D-Zerta) all flavors	½ cup (4.3 oz.)	7	.1
(Estee) all flavors	½ cup (4.2 oz.)	8	Tr.

Food and Description	Measure or Quantity	Calories	Carbo- hydrates (grams)
(Featherweight):			
Regular	½ cup	10	1.0
Artificially sweetened	½ cup	10	0.
(Jell-O) sugar free:			
Cherry	½ cup (4.3 oz.)	12	.1
Lime	½ cup	9	.1
Orange, raspberry or strawberry	½ cup	8	.1
(Louis Sherry)	½ cup	8	Tr.
(Royal)	½ cup	12	0.
GELATIN, DRINKING			
(Knox) orange	1 envelope	39	4.0
GIN, unflavored (See **DISTILLED LIQUOR**)			
GIN, SLOE:			
(DeKuyper)	1 fl. oz.	70	5.2
(Mr. Boston)	1 fl. oz.	68	4.7
GINGER, powdered (French's)	1 tsp.	6	1.2
GINGERBREAD:			
Home recipe (USDA)	1.9-oz piece (2″×2″×2″)	174	28.6
Mix:			
*(Betty Crocker):			
Regular	⅑ of pkg.	220	35.0
No cholesterol recipe	⅑ of pkg.	210	35.0
(Dromedary)	2″×2″ square (¹⁄₁₆ of pkg.)	100	19.0
(Pillsbury)	3″ square (⅑ of cake)	190	36.0
GOLDEN GRAHAMS, cereal (General Mills)	¾ cup (1 oz.)	110	24.0
GOOBER GRAPE (Smucker's)	1 T.	90	9.0

(USDA) = United States Department of Agriculture
(HHS/FAO) = Health and Human Services/Food and Agriculture Organization
* = prepared as package directs

Food and Description	Measure or Quantity	Calories	Carbo-hydrates (grams)
GOOD HUMOR (See ICE CREAM)			
GOOSE, domesticated (USDA):			
Raw	1 lb. (weighed ready-to-cook)	1172	0.
Roasted:			
Meat & skin	4 oz.	500	0.
Meat only	4 oz.	264	0.
GOOSEBERRY (USDA):			
Fresh	1 lb.	177	44.0
Fresh	1 cup (5.3 oz.)	58	14.6
Canned, water pack, solids & liq.	4 oz.	29	7.5
GOOSE GIZZARD, raw (USDA)	4 oz.	158	0.
GRAHAM CRACKER (See CRACKERS, PUFFS & CHIPS,** Graham)			
GRANOLA BAR:			
Nature Valley:			
Cinnamon or oats & honey	.8-oz. bar	120	17.0
Oat bran honey graham	.8-oz. bar	110	16.0
Peanut butter	.8-oz. bar	120	15.0
(Hershey's) chocolate covered:			
Chocolate chip	1.2-oz. piece	170	22.0
Cocoa creme	1.2-oz. piece	180	22.0
Cookies & creme	1.2-oz. piece	170	23.0
Peanut butter	1.2-oz. piece	180	19.0
GRANOLA CEREAL:			
Nature Valley:			
Cinnamon & raisin, fruit & nut or toasted oat	⅓ cup (1 oz.)	130	19.0
Coconut & honey	⅓ cup (1 oz.)	150	18.0

Food and Description	Measure or Quantity	Calories	Carbo-hydrates (grams)
Sun Country (Kretschmer):			
With almonds	¼ cup (1 oz.)	138	19.3
Honey almond	1 oz.	130	19.0
With raisins	¼ cup (1 oz.)	133	19.9
With raisins & dates	¼ cup (1 oz.)	130	20.0
GRANOLA SNACK:			
Kudos (M&M/Mars):			
Chocolate chip	1.25-oz. pkg.	180	21.0
Nutty fudge	1.3-oz. pkg.	190	19.0
Peanut butter	1.3-oz. pkg.	190	17.0
Nature Valley:			
Cinnamon or honey nut	1 pouch	140	19.0
Oats & honey	1 pouch	140	18.0
Peanut butter	1 pouch	140	17.0
GRAPE:			
Fresh:			
American type (slip skin), Concord, Delaware, Niagara, Catawba and Scuppernong:			
(USDA)	½ lb. (weighed with stem, skin & seeds)	98	22.4
(USDA)	½ cup (2.7 oz.)	33	7.5
(USDA)	3½" × 3" bunch (3.5 oz.)	43	9.9
European type (adherent skin), Malaga, Muscat, Tompson seedless, Emperor & Flame Tokay:			
(USDA)	½ lb. (weighed with stem & seeds)	139	34.9
(USDA) whole	20 grapes (¾" dia.)	52	13.5
(USDA) whole	½ cup (.3 oz.)	56	14.5
(USDA) halves	½ cup (.3 oz.)	56	14.4

(USDA) = United States Department of Agriculture
(HHS/FAO) = Health and Human Services/Food and Agriculture Organization
* = prepared as package directs

Food and Description	Measure or Quantity	Calories	Carbo-hydrates (grams)
Canned, solids & liq., (USDA) Thompson seedless, heavy syrup	4 oz.	87	22.7
Canned, dietetic pack, solids & liq.: (USDA) Thompson seedless, water pack	4 oz.	58	15.4
(Featherweight) water pack, seedless	½ cup	60	13.0
GRAPEADE, chilled or *frozen (Minute Maid)	6 fl. oz.	94	23.4
GRAPE-APPLE DRINK, canned (Mott's)	9.5-fl. oz. container	158	40.0
GRAPE DRINK: Canned: (Borden) *Bama*	8.45-fl.-oz. container	120	29.0
(Hi-C)	6 fl. oz.	96	23.7
(Johanna Farms) *Ssips*	8.45-fl-oz. container	130	32.0
(Lincoln)	6 fl. oz.	90	23.0
(Welchade)	6 fl. oz.	90	23.0
Chilled (Sunkist)	8.45 fl. oz.	140	33.0
*Mix: Regular (Funny Face)	8 fl. oz.	88	22.0
Dietetic (Sunkist)	8 fl. oz.	6	2.0
GRAPE JAM (Smucker's)	1 T. (.7 oz.)	53	13.7
GRAPE JELLY: Sweetened: (Borden) *Bama*	1 T.	45	12.0
(Empress)	1 T.	52	13.5
(Smucker's): Regular	1 T. (.5 oz.)	54	12.0
Goober Grape	1 T.	90	9.0
Dietetic: (Diet Delight)	1 T. (.6 oz.)	12	3.0
(Estee)	1 T.	6	0.
(Slenderella)	1 T.	21	6.0
(Weight Watchers)	1 T.	24	6.0

Food and Description	Measure or Quantity	Calories	Carbo-hydrates (grams)
GRAPE JUICE:			
Canned, unsweetened:			
(USDA)	½ cup (4.4 oz.)	83	20.9
(Ardmore Farms)	6 fl. oz.	99	24.9
(Borden) *Sippin' Pak*	8.45-fl.-oz. container	130	32.0
(Johanna Farms) *Tree Ripe*	8.45-fl.-oz. container	164	40.0
(Minute Maid)	8.45-fl. oz. container	150	37.4
(Town House)	6 fl. oz.	120	30.0
(Tree Top) sparkling	6 fl. oz.	120	29.0
*Frozen:			
(Minute Maid)	6 fl. oz.	99	13.3
(Welch's)	6 fl. oz.	100	25.0
GRAPE JUICE DRINK, chilled:			
(Sunkist)	8.45 fl. oz.	140	33.0
(Welch's)	6 fl. oz.	110	27.0
***GRAPE NUTS,** cereal (Post):*			
Regular	¼ cup (1 oz.)	105	23.0
Flakes	⅞ cup (1 oz.)	111	23.1
Raisin	¼ cup (1 oz.)	102	23.0
GRAPE PRESERVE OR JAM, sweetened (Welch's)	1 T.	52	13.5
GRAPEFRUIT:			
Fresh (USDA):			
White:			
Seeded type	1 lb. (weighed with seeds & skin)	86	22.4
Seedless type	1 lb. (weighed with skin)	87	22.6
Seeded type	½ med. grapefruit (3¾" dia., 8.5 oz.)	54	14.1
Pink and red:			

(USDA) = United States Department of Agriculture
(HHS/FAO) = Health and Human Services/Food and Agriculture Organization
* = prepared as package directs

Food and Description	Measure or Quantity	Calories	Carbo-hydrates (grams)
Seeded type	1 lb. (weighed with seeds & skin)	87	22.6
Seedless type	1 lb. (weighed with skin)	93	24.1
Seeded type	½ med. grapefruit (3¾" dia., 8.5 oz.)	46	12.0
Canned, syrup pack (Del Monte) solids & liq.:	½ cup	74	17.5
Canned, unsweetened or dietetic pack, solids & liq.:			
(USDA) water pack	½ cup (4.2 oz.)	36	9.1
(Del Monte) sections	½ cup	46	10.5
(Diet Delight) sections, juice pack	½ cup (4.3 oz.)	45	11.0
(Featherweight) sections, juice pack	½ of 8-oz. can	40	9.0
(S&W) *Nutradiet,* sections	½ cup	40	9.0
GRAPEFRUIT DRINK, canned (Lincoln)	6 fl. oz.	100	25.0
GRAPEFRUIT JUICE:			
Fresh (USDA) pink, red or white	½ cup (4.3 oz.)	46	11.3
Canned, sweetened:			
(Ardmore Farms)	6 fl. oz.	78	18.1
(Johanna Farms)	6 fl. oz.	76	18.0
(Libby's)	6 fl.oz.	70	17.0
(Minute Maid) On the Go	10-fl oz. bottle	130	30.7
(Mott's)	9.5-fl. oz. can	118	29.0
Canned, unsweetened:			
(Libby's)	6 fl. oz.	75	18.0
(Ocean Spray)	6 fl. oz.	70	16.2
(Town House)	6 fl. oz.	70	15.0
(Tree Top)	6 fl. oz.	80	19.0
Chilled (Sunkist)	6 fl. oz.	72	17.0
*Frozen (Minute Maid)	6 fl. oz.	83	19.7
GRAPEFRUIT JUICE COCKTAIL, canned (Ocean Spray) pink	6 fl. oz.	80	20.0

Food and Description	Measure or Quantity	Calories	Carbo-hydrates (grams)
GRAPEFRUIT-ORANGE JUICE COCKTAIL, canned, (Ardmore Farms)	6 fl. oz.	78	19.1
GRAPEFRUIT PEEL, CANDIED (USDA)	1 oz.	90	22.9
GRAVY, canned:			
Regular:			
Au jus (Franco-American)	2-oz. serving	10	2.0
Beef (Franco-American)	2-oz. serving	25	4.0
Brown (La Choy)	2-oz. serving	140	40.4
Chicken (Franco-American):			
Regular	2-oz. serving	45	3.0
Giblet	2-oz. serving	30	3.0
Cream (Franco-American)	2-oz. serving	35	4.0
Mushroom (Franco-American)	2-oz. serving	25	3.0
Pork (Franco-American)	2-oz. serving	40	3.0
Turkey:			
(Franco-American)	2-oz. serving	30	3.0
(Howard Johnson's) giblet	½ cup	55	5.5
Dietetic (Estee):			
Brown	¼ cup	14	3.0
Chicken & herb	¼ cup	20	4.0
GRAVYMASTER	1 tsp. (.2 oz.)	12	2.4
GRAVY MIX:			
Regular:			
Au jus:			
*(French's) *Gravy Makins*	½ cup	20	4.0
*(Lawry's)	½ cup	42	5.5
Brown:			
*(French's) *Gravy Makins*	½ cup	40	8.0
*(Knorr) classic	2 fl. oz.	25	3.1
*(Lawry's)	½ cup	47	18.2
*(Pillsbury)	½ cup	30	6.0

(USDA) = United States Department of Agriculture
(HHS/FAO) = Health and Human Services/Food and Agriculture Organization
* = prepared as package directs

Food and Description	Measure or Quantity	Calories	Carbohydrates (grams)
Chicken:			
*(French's) *Gravy Makins*	½ cup	50	8.0
(McCormick)	.85-oz. pkg.	82	13.4
*(Pillsbury)	½ cup	50	8.0
Homestyle:			
*(French's) *Gravy Makins*	½ cup	40	8.0
*(Pillsbury)	½ cup	30	6.0
Mushroom *(French's) *Gravy Makins*	½ cup	40	6.0
Onion:			
*(French's) *Gravy Makins*	½ cup	50	8.0
*(McCormick)	.85-oz. pkg.	72	9.8
Pork:			
(Durkee):			
*Regular	½ cup	35	7.0
Roastin' Bag	1.5-oz. pkg.	130	26.0
*(French's) *Gravy Makins*	½ cup	40	8.0
Pot roast (Durkee) *Roastin' Bag*, regular or onion	1.5-oz. pkg.	125	25.0
*Swiss steak (Durkee)	½ cup	22	5.4
Turkey:			
*(Durkee)	½ cup	47	7.0
*(French's) *Gravy Makins*	½ cup	50	8.0
*Dietetic (Estee):			
Brown	½ cup	28	6.0
Chicken, & herbs	½ cup	40	8.0

GRAVY WITH MEAT OR TURKEY, frozen

(Banquet):			
Cookin' Bag:			
Mushroom gravy & charbroiled beef patty	5-oz. pkg.	210	8.0
& salisbury steak	5-oz. pkg.	190	8.0
& sliced beef	4-oz. pkg.	100	5.0
& sliced turkey	5-oz. pkg.	100	5.0
Family Entree:			
Onion gravy & beef patties	¼ of 32-oz. pkg.	300	14.0
& salisbury steak	¼ of 32-oz. pkg.	300	12.0
& sliced beef	¼ of 32-oz. pkg.	160	8.0
& sliced turkey	¼ of 32-oz. pkg.	150	8.0

Food and Description	Measure or Quantity	Calories	Carbo-hydrates (grams)
GREENS, MIXED, canned, solids & liq.:			
(Allen's)	½ cup (4 oz.)	25	3.0
(Sunshine)	½ cup (4.1 oz.)	20	2.7
GRENADINE (Rose's) non-alcoholic	1 fl. oz.	65	6.0
GROUPER, raw (USDA):			
Whole	1 lb. (weighed whole)	170	0.
Meat only	4 oz.	99	0.
GUACAMOLE SEASONING MIX (Lawry's)	.7-oz. pkg.	60	12.6
GUAVA, COMMON, fresh (USDA):			
Whole	1 lb. (weighed untrimmed)	273	66.0
Whole	1 guava (2.8 oz.)	48	11.7
Flesh only	4 oz.	70	17.0
GUAVA, STRAWBERRY, fresh (USDA):			
Whole	1 lb. (weighed untrimmed)	289	70.2
Flesh only	4 oz.	74	17.9
GUAVA FRUIT DRINK, canned, *Mauna La'I*	6 fl. oz.	100	25.0
GUAVA JAM (Smucker's)	1 T.	53	13.5
GUAVA JELLY (Smucker's)	1 T.	53	13.5

(USDA) = United States Department of Agriculture
(HHS/FAO) = Health and Human Services/Food and Agriculture Organization
* = prepared as package directs

Food and Description	Measure or Quantity	Calories	Carbo-hydrates (grams)
GUAVA NECTAR (Libby's)	6 fl. oz.	70	17.0
GUAVA-PASSION FRUIT DRINK, canned, *Mauna La'l*	6 fl. oz.	100	25.0
GUINEA HEN, raw (USDA):			
Ready-to-cook	1 lb. (weighed ready-to-cook)	594	0.
Meat & skin	4 oz.	179	0.

Food and Description	Measure or Quantity	Calories	Carbo-hydrates (grams)

H

HADDOCK:
Raw (USDA) meat only	4 oz.	90	0.
Fried, breaded (USDA)	4″ × 3″ × ½″ fillet (3.5 oz.)	165	5.8
Smoked (USDA)	4-oz. serving	117	0.
Frozen:			
(Captain's Choice) fillet	3-oz. piece	95	0.
(Frionor) *Norway Gourmet*	4-oz. fillet	70	0.
(Gorton's):			
Fishmarket Fresh	4 oz.	90	0.
Microwave entree, in lemon butter	1 pkg.	360	19.0
(Mrs. Paul's):			
Crunchy batter	1 fillet	95	11.0
Light	1 fillet	110	7.5

HALIBUT:
Raw (USDA):			
Whole	1 lb. (weighed whole)	144	0.
Meat only	4 oz.	84	0.
Broiled (USDA)	4″ × 3″ × ½″ steak (4.4 oz.)	214	0.
Smoked (USDA)	4 oz.	254	0.
Frozen (Van de Kamp's) batter dipped, french fried	½ of 8-oz. pkg.	260	15.0

HAM (See also **PORK**):
Canned:			
(Hormel):			
Black Label (3- or 5-lb. size)	4 oz.	140	0.

(USDA) = United States Department of Agriculture
(HHS/FAO) = Health and Human Services/Food and Agriculture Organization
* = prepared as package directs

Food and Description	Measure or Quantity	Calories	Carbo-hydrates (grams)
Chopped	3 oz. (8-lb. ham)	240	1.0
Chunk	6¾-oz. serving	310	0.
Curemaster, smoked	4 oz.	140	1.0
EXL	4 oz.	120	0.
Holiday Glaze	4 oz. (3-lb. ham)	140	2.9
Patties	1 patty	180	0.
(Oscar Mayer) *Jubilee*, extra lean, cooked	1-oz. serving	31	.1
(Swift) *Premium*	1¾-oz. slice	111	.3
Deviled:			
(Hormel)	1 T.	35	0.
(Libby's)	1 T. (.5 oz.)	43	0.
(Underwood)	1 T. (.5 oz.)	49	Tr.
Packaged:			
(Carl Buddig) smoked	1-oz. slice	50	Tr.
(Eckrich):			
Chopped	1 oz.	45	1.0
Cooked or imported, Danish	1.2-oz. slice	30	1.2
Loaf	1 oz.	70	1.0
(Hormel):			
Black peppered, *Light & Lean*	1 slice	25	0.
Chopped	1 slice	44	0.
Cooked, *Light & Lean*	1 slice	25	0.
Glazed, *Light & Lean*	1 slice	25	0.
Red peppered, *Light & Lean*	1 slice	25	0.
Smoked, cooked, *Light & Lean*	1 slice	25	0.
(Ohse):			
Chopped	1 oz.	65	1.0
Cooked	1 oz.	30	1.0
Smoked, regular	1 oz.	45	1.0
Turkey ham	1 oz.	30	2.0
(Oscar Mayer):			
Chopped	1-oz. slice	64	.9
Cooked, smoked	1-oz. slice	34	0.
Jubilee boneless:			
Sliced	8-oz. slice	232	0.
Steak	2-oz. steak	59	0.1
(Smok-A-Roma):			
Chopped	1-oz. slice	55	1.0
Cooked or honey	1-oz. slice	30	1.0

Food and Description	Measure or Quantity	Calories	Carbo- hydrates (grams)
HAM & ASPARAGUS BAKE, frozen (Stouffer's)	9½-oz. meal	510	31.0
HAMBURGER (See BEEF, Ground; see also *MCDONALD'S; BURGER KING; DAIRY QUEEN; WHITE CASTLE;* etc.)			
*HAMBURGER MIX:			
*Hamburger Helper (General Mills):			
Beef noodle	⅕ of pkg.	320	26.0
Beef romanoff	⅕ of pkg.	350	30.0
Cheeseburger macaroni	⅕ of pkg.	370	28.0
Chili with beans	¼ of pkg.	350	25.0
Chili tomato	⅕ of pkg.	330	31.0
Hash	⅕ of pkg.	320	27.0
Lasagna	⅕ of pkg.	340	33.0
Pizza dish	⅕ of pkg.	360	37.0
Potatoes au gratin	⅕ of pkg.	320	28.0
Potato stroganoff	⅕ of pkg.	320	28.0
Rice oriental	⅕ of pkg.	340	38.0
Spaghetti	⅕ of pkg.	340	32.0
Stew	⅕ of pkg.	300	25.0
Tamale bake	⅕ of pkg.	380	39.0
Make a Better Burger (Lipton) mildly seasoned or onion	⅕ of pkg.	30	5.0
HAMBURGER SEASONING MIX:			
*(Durkee)	1 cup	663	7.5
(French's)	1-oz. pkg.	100	20.0
HAM & CHEESE:			
Canned (Hormel):			
Loaf	3 oz.	260	1.0
Patty	1 patty	190	0.

(USDA) = United States Department of Agriculture
(HHS/FAO) = Health and Human Services/Food and Agriculture
　　　　　　　Organization
* = prepared as package directs

Food and Description	Measure or Quantity	Calories	Carbohydrates (grams)
Packaged:			
(Eckrich) loaf	1-oz. serving	60	1.0
(Hormel) loaf	1-oz. slice	65	0.
(Ohse) loaf	1 oz.	65	2.0
(Oscar Mayer) spread	1 oz.	66	.6
HAM & CHEESE ON A BAGEL, frozen (Swanson)			
Great Starts	3-oz pkg.	240	28.0
HAM DINNER, frozen:			
(Armour) *Dinner Classics*	10¾-oz. dinner	270	36.0
(Banquet)	10-oz. dinner	400	43.0
(Le Menu) steak	10-oz. dinner	300	31.0
(Morton)	10-oz. dinner	290	49.0
HAM SALAD, canned (Carnation)	¼ of 7½-oz. can (1.9 oz.)	110	4.0
HAM SALAD SPREAD (Oscar Mayer)	1 oz.	59	3.6
HARDEE'S:			
Apple turnover	3.2-oz. piece	270	38.0
Big Cookie	1.7-oz. piece	260	31.0
Big Country Breakfast:			
Bacon	7.65-oz. meal	660	51.0
Country ham	8.96-oz. meal	670	52.0
Ham	8.85-oz. meal	620	51.0
Sausage	9.7-oz. meal	850	51.0
Biscuit:			
Bacon	3.3-oz. serving	360	34.0
Bacon & egg	4.4-oz. serving	410	35.0
Bacon, egg & cheese	4.8-oz. serving	460	35.0
Chicken	5.1-oz. serving	430	42.0
Country ham:			
Plain	3.8-oz. serving	350	35.0
& egg	4.9-oz. serving	400	35.0
'n gravy	7.8-oz. serving	440	45.0
Ham:			
Plain	3.7-oz. serving	320	34.0
With egg	4.9-oz. serving	370	35.0
With egg & cheese	5.3-oz. serving	420	35.0
Rise 'N Shine:			
Plain	2.9-oz. serving	320	34.0
Canadian bacon	5.7-oz. serving	470	35.0

Food and Description	Measure or Quantity	Calories	Carbo-hydrates (grams)
Sausage:			
Plain	4.2-oz. serving	440	34.0
With egg	5.3-oz. serving	490	35.0
Steak:			
Plain	5.2-oz. serving	500	46.0
With egg	6.3-oz. serving	550	47.0
Cheeseburger:			
Plain	4.3-oz. serving	320	33.0
Bacon	7.7-oz. serving	610	31.0
Quarter-pound	6.4-oz. serving	500	34.0
Chicken fillet sandwich	6.1-oz. sandwich	370	44.0
Chicken, grilled, sandwich	6.8-oz. sandwich	310	34.0
Chicken Stix:			
6-piece	3 ½-oz. serving	210	13.0
9-piece	5.3-oz. serving	310	20.0
Cool Twist:			
Cone:			
Chocolate:	4.2-oz. serving	200	31.0
Vanilla	4.2-oz. serving	190	28.0
Vanilla/chocolate	4.2-oz. serving	190	29.0
Sundae:			
Caramel	6-oz. serving	330	54.0
Hot fudge	5.9-oz. serving	320	45.0
Strawberry	5.9-oz. serving	260	43.0
Fisherman's Fillet, sandwich	7.3-oz. sandwich	500	49.0
Hamburger:			
Plain	3.9-oz. serving	270	33.0
Big Deluxe	7.6-oz. serving	500	32.0
Mushroom 'N Swiss	6.6-oz. serving	490	33.0
Hot dog, all beef	4.2-oz. serving	300	25.0
Hot ham 'n cheese	4.2-oz. sandwich	330	32.0
Margarine/butter blend	.2-oz. serving	35	0.
Pancakes, three:			
Plain	4.8-oz. serving	280	56.0
With sausage pattie	6.2-oz. serving	430	56.0
With bacon strips	5.3-oz. serving	350	56.0

(USDA) = United States Department of Agriculture
(HHS/FAO) = Health and Human Services/Food and Agriculture Organization
* = prepared as package directs

Food and Description	Measure or Quantity	Calories	Carbo- hydrates (grams)
Potato:			
French fries:			
Regular	2 ½-oz. order	230	30.0
Large	4-oz. order	360	48.0
Hash Rounds	2.8-oz. serving	230	24.0
Roast beef sandwich:			
Regular	4-oz. serving	260	31.0
Big Roast Beef	4.7-oz. serving	300	32.0
Salads:			
Chef	10.4-oz. serving	240	5.0
Chicken & pasta	14.6-oz. serving	230	23.0
Garden	8.5-oz. serving	210	3.0
Side	3.9-oz. serving	20	1.0
Shake:			
Chocolate	12 fl. oz.	460	85.0
Strawberry	12 fl. oz.	440	82.0
Vanilla	12 fl. oz.	400	66.0
Syrup, pancake	1 ½-oz. serving	120	31.0
Turkey club sandwich	7.3-oz. serving	390	32.0
HAWS, SCARLET, raw (USDA):			
Whole	1 lb. (weighed with core)	316	75.5
Flesh & skin	4 oz.	99	23.6
HEADCHEESE:			
(USDA)	1 oz.	76	.3
(Oscar Mayer)	1 oz.	55	0.
HEARTWISE, cereal (Kellogg's)	⅔ cup (1 oz.)	90	23.0
HEART OF PALM (See **SWAMP CABBAGE**)			
HERRING:			
Raw (USDA):			
Lake (See **LAKE HERRING**)			
Atlantic:			
Whole	1 lb. (weighed whole)	407	0.
Meat only	4 oz.	200	0.
Pacific, meat only	4 oz.	111	0.

Food and Description	Measure or Quantity	Calories	Carbohydrates (grams)
Canned:			
(USDA) in tomato sauce, solids & liq.	4-oz. serving	200	4.2
(Vita):			
Bismarck, drained	5-oz. jar	273	6.9
In cream sauce, drained	8-oz. jar	397	18.1
Matjis, drained	8-oz. jar	304	26.2
In wine sauce, drained	8-oz. jar	401	16.6
Pickled (USDA) Bismarck type	4-oz. serving	253	0.
Salted or brined (USDA)	4-oz. serving	247	0.
Smoked (USDA):			
Bloaters	4-oz. serving	222	0.
Hard	4-oz. serving	340	0.
Kippered	4-oz. serving	239	0.
HICKORY NUT (USDA):			
Whole	1 lb. (weighed in shell)	1068	20.3
Shelled	4 oz.	763	14.5
HOMINY, canned, solids & liq. (Allen's) golden or white	½ cup	80	16.0
HOMINY GRITS:			
Dry:			
(USDA):			
Degermed	1 oz.	103	22.1
Degermed	½ cup (2.8 oz.)	282	60.9
(Albers) quick, degermed	1½ oz.	150	33.0
(Aunt Jemima)	3 T. (1 oz.)	101	22.4
(Pocono) creamy	1 oz.	101	23.6
(Quaker):			
Regular or quick	1 T. (.33 oz.)	34	7.5
Instant:			
Regular	.8-oz. packet	79	17.7
With imitation bacon bits	1-oz. packet	101	21.6
With artificial cheese flavor	1-oz. packet	104	21.6

(USDA) = United States Department of Agriculture
(HHS/FAO) = Health and Human Services/Food and Agriculture Organization
* = prepared as package directs

Food and Description	Measure or Quantity	Calories	Carbo-hydrates (grams)
With imitation ham bits (3-Minute Brand) quick, enriched	1-oz. packet	99	21.3
	⅙ cup (1 oz.)	98	22.2
Cooked (USDA) degermed	⅔ cup (5.6 oz.)	84	18.0
HONEY, strained:			
(USDA)	½ cup (5.7 oz.)	494	134.1
(USDA)	1 T. (.7 oz.)	61	16.5
HONEY BUNCHES OF OATS, cereal (Post):			
With almonds	⅔ cup (1 oz.)	115	22.0
Honey roasted	⅔ cup (1 oz.)	111	23.0
HONEYCOMB, cereal (Post) crunch	1⅓ cups (1 oz.)	110	26.0
HONEYDEW, fresh (USDA):			
Whole	1 lb. (weighed whole)	94	22.0
Wedge	2″ × 7″ wedge (5.3 oz.)	31	7.2
Flesh only	4 oz.	37	8.7
Flesh only, diced	1 cup (5.9 oz.)	55	12.9
HONEY SMACKS, cereal (Kellogg's)	⅜ cup (1 oz.)	110	25.0
HORSERADISH:			
Raw, pared (USDA)	1 oz.	25	5.6
Prepared (Gold's)	1 tsp.	4	Tr.
HOT BITES, frozen (Banquet):			
Cheese, mozzarella nuggets	¼ of 10½-oz. pkg.	240	16.0
Chicken:			
Regular:			
Breast patties	¼ of 10½-oz. pkg.	210	13.0
Breast tenders:			
Regular	¼ of 10½-oz. pkg.	150	12.0
Southern fried	¼ of 10½-oz. pkg.	160	13.0

Food and Description	Measure or Quantity	Calories	Carbo-hydrates (grams)
Drum snackers	¼ of 10½-oz. pkg.	220	13.0
Nuggets:			
Plain	¼ of 10½-oz. pkg.	210	11.0
Cheddar	¼ of 10½-oz. pkg.	250	11.0
Hot & spicy	¼ of 10½-oz. pkg.	250	10.0
Sticks	¼ of 10½-oz. pkg.	220	11.0
Microwave:			
Breast pattie:			
Regular, & bun	4-oz. pkg.	310	32.0
Southern fried, & biscuit	4-oz. pkg.	320	37.0
Breast tenders	4-oz. pkg.	260	24.0
Nuggets, with sweet & sour sauce	4½-oz. pkg.	360	22.0
HOT DOG (See **FRANKFURTER**)			
HOT WHEELS, cereal (Ralston Purina)	1 cup (1 oz.)	110	24.0
HULA COOLER DRINK, canned (Hi-C)	6 fl. oz.	97	23.9
HULA PUNCH DRINK, canned (Hi-C)	6 fl. oz.	87	21.4
HYACINTH BEAN (USDA):			
Young bean, raw:			
Whole	1 lb. (weighed untrimmed)	140	29.1
Trimmed	4 oz.	40	8.3
Dry seeds	4 oz.	383	69.2

(USDA) = United States Department of Agriculture
(HHS/FAO) = Health and Human Services/Food and Agriculture Organization
* = prepared as package directs

Food and Description	Measure or Quantity	Calories	Carbo-hydrates (grams)

I

ICE CREAM (Listed below by flavor or by type, such as Cookie sandwich or *Whammy*. See also **FROZEN DESSERT**):

Food and Description	Measure or Quantity	Calories	Carbo-hydrates (grams)
Almond (Good Humor)	4 fl. oz.	350	29.4
Almond amaretto (Baskin-Robbins)	4 fl. oz.	280	26.0
Apple strudel (Lucerne)	½ cup	140	16.0
Banana Crumble (Lucerne)	½ cup	140	16.0
Blackberry pecan (Lucerne)	½ cup	150	20.0
Black walnut (Lucerne):			
Regular	½ cup	150	16.0
Gourmet, Ozark	½ cup	180	16.0
Brownie Sundae (Lucerne)	½ cup	140	16.0
Blueberry & cream (Häagen-Dazs)	4 fl. oz.	190	25.0
Bon Bon, nuggets (Carnation):			
Chocolate	1 piece	34	3.1
Vanilla	1 piece	33	2.8
Brittle bar (Häagen-Dazs)	1 bar	370	32.0
Bubble O Bill bar (Good Humor)	3 ½-fl.-oz. bar	149	17.0
Butter almond (Breyers)	½ cup	170	15.0
Butter Brickle (Snow Star)	½ cup	130	18.0
Butter pecan:			
(Breyers)	½ cup	180	15.0
(Good Humor)	4 fl. oz.	150	14.0
(Häagen-Dazs)	4 fl. oz.	290	29.0
(Lady Borden)	½ cup	180	16.0
(Lucerne) gourmet	½ cup	190	16.0
Calippo (Good Humor):			
Cherry	4 ½ fl. oz.	140	34.9
Lemon	4 ½ fl. oz.	112	27.6
Orange	4 ½ fl. oz.	110	27.2

Food and Description	Measure or Quantity	Calories	Carbo-hydrates (grams)
Cappuccino chip (Baskin-Robbins)	4 fl. oz.	310	31.0
Cherry Blossom (Lucerne)	½ cup	140	16.0
Cherry vanilla (Breyers)	4 fl. oz.	140	17.0
Chip crunch bar (Good Humor)	3-fl.-oz. bar	255	21.2
Chocolate:			
(Baskin-Robbins):			
Regular	4 fl. oz.	264	32.6
Chip	4 fl. oz.	260	27.0
Deluxe	4 fl. oz.	270	32.0
Mousse Royale	4 fl. oz.	293	36.3
World Class	4 fl. oz.	280	35.0
(Borden) Old Fashioned Recipe, Dutch	½ cup	130	16.0
(Häagen-Dazs):			
Regular	4 fl. oz.	270	24.0
Mint	4 fl. oz.	300	26.0
(Lucerne):			
Regular, German or *Our Natural*	½ cup	140	16.0
Dietary	½ cup	120	15.0
(Snow Star)	½ cup	120	16.0
Chocolate bar (Häagen-Dazs) dark chocolate coating	1 bar	360	35.0
Chocolate chip:			
(Häagen-Dazs)	4 fl. oz.	290	28.0
(Lucerne) regular or mint	½ cup	150	17.0
(Snow Star)	½ cup	130	16.0
Chocolate eclair (Good Humor)	3-fl.-oz. bar	187	22.6
Chocolate malt bar (Good Humor)	3-fl.-oz. bar	190	16.0
Chocolate marble (Lucerne)	½ cup	140	19.0
Chocolate marshmallow (Lucerne)	½ cup	140	20.0
Chocolate peanut butter:			
(Häagen-Dazs)	4 fl. oz.	330	25.0
(Lucerne)	½ cup	140	16.0

(USDA) = United States Department of Agriculture
(HHS/FAO) = Health and Human Services/Food and Agriculture Organization
* = prepared as package directs

Food and Description	Measure or Quantity	Calories	Carbo-hydrates (grams)
Chocolate raspberry truffle (Baskin-Robbins)	4 fl. oz.	310	35.0
Chocolate swirl (Borden)	½ cup	130	18.0
Chocoalte truffle (Lucurne) gourmet	½ cup	170	24.0
Coconut almond fudge (Lucerne)	½ cup	150	16.0
Coffee:			
(Breyers)	½ cup	140	15.0
(Häagen-Dazs)	4 fl. oz.	270	23.0
(Lucerne) regular	½ cup	140	16.0
Cookies & cream (Breyers)	4 fl. oz.	170	19.0
Cookie sandwich (Good Humor)	2.7-fl.-oz. piece	290	42.0
Crunch bar (Nestlé)	1 bar	180	15.0
Danish nut roll (Lucerne)	½ cup	145	16.0
Egg nog (Lucerne):			
Regular	½ cup	140	16.0
Gourmet	½ cup	160	19.0
Eskimo Pie:			
Chocolate fudge bar	1¾-fl.-oz. bar	60	14.0
Chocolate fudge bar	2½-fl.-oz. bar	90	20.0
Chocolate fudge bar	3-fl.-oz. bar	110	24.0
Dietary dairy bar, chocolate covered	2½-fl.-oz. bar	110	10.0
Old fashioned:			
Crispy	1 bar	290	24.0
Double chocolate	1 bar	280	25.0
Vanilla	1 bar	280	23.0
Original:			
Double chocolate	1 bar	140	12.0
Vanilla	1 bar	140	11.0
Pie:			
Regular:			
Chocolate	3-fl.-oz. bar	170	16.0
Crunch	3-fl.-oz. bar	170	15.0
Vanilla	3-fl.-oz. bar	170	14.0
Junior:			
Chocolate	1¾-fl.-oz. bar	100	10.0
Crunch	1¾-fl.-oz. bar	100	9.0
Vanilla	1¾-fl.-oz. bar	100	9.0
Thin mints	2-fl-oz. bar	130	10.0
Twin pops	1¾-fl.-oz. bar	40	10.0

Food and Description	Measure or Quantity	Calories	Carbohydrates (grams)
Twin pops	3-fl.-oz. bar	70	17.0
Fat Frog (Good Humor)	3-fl.-oz. bar	154	16.0
Fudge bar (Good Humor)	2½-fl.-oz. bar	127	26.5
Fudge cake (Good Humor)	6.3 fl. oz.	214	18.1
Fudge Royal (Sealtest)	½ cup	140	19.0
Grand Marnier (Baskin-Robbins)	4 fl. oz.	240	31.0
Halo bar (Good Humor)	2½-fl.-oz. bar	230	22.8
Heavenly Hash (Lucerne)	½ cup	150	18.0
Honey (Häagen-Dazs)	4 fl. oz.	250	22.0
Honey vanilla (Häagen-Dazs)	4 fl. oz.	240	8.0
Jumbo Jet Star (Good Humor)	4½ fl. oz.	84	19.5
King cone (Good Humor):			
Regular	5½ fl. oz.	290	40.9
Boysenberry	5 fl. oz.	340	51.6
Laser Blazer (Good Humor)	3 fl. oz.	131	23.1
Macadamia brittle (Häagen-Dazs)	4 fl. oz.	280	25.2
Macadamia nut (Häagen-Dazs)	4 fl. oz.	330	24.0
Maple nut (Lucerne)	½ cup	150	16.0
Maple walnut (Häagen-Dazs)	4 fl. oz.	310	18.0
Milky Pop (Good Humor)	1½-fl.-oz. pop	46	8.4
Mint chocolate chip (Breyers)	½ cup	170	18.0
Mocha double nut (Häagen-Dazs)	4 fl. oz.	290	22.0
Mocha fudge (Lucerne) nut	½ cup	150	17.0
Neapolitan (Lucerne)	½ cup	140	16.0
Oreo, cookies & cream:			
Chocolate, mint or vanilla	3 fl. oz.	140	16.0
Sandwich	1 sandwich	240	31.0
Stick	1 bar	220	19.0
Peach:			
(Breyers)	½ cup	140	19.0
(Häagen-Dazs)	4 fl. oz.	210	15.0
(Lucerne)	½ cup	140	16.0
Peach pie (Lucerne) southern	½ cup	130	17.0
Peanut butter (Lucerne)	½ cup	145	17.0

(USDA) = United States Department of Agriculture
(HHS/FAO) = Health and Human Services/Food and Agriculture Organization
* = prepared as package directs

Food and Description	Measure or Quantity	Calories	Carbo-hydrates (grams)
Peanut butter sundae (Lucerne):			
Regular	½ cup	140	16.0
Nut	½ cup	140	16.0
Peanut vanilla (Häagen-Dazs)	4 fl. oz.	280	19.0
Pecan pie (Lucerne) southern	½ cup	145	18.0
Peppermint stick (Lucerne)	½ cup	150	17.0
Pralines & Cream (Baskin-Robbins)	4-fl. oz.	280	35.0
Quik bar (Nestlé)	3-fl.-oz. bar	210	19.0
Ranch pecan (Lucerne)	½ cup	160	15.0
Raspberry & cream (Häagen-Dazs)	4 fl. oz.	180	26.0
Rocky road (Baskin-Robbins)	4 fl. oz.	300	39.0
Rum raisin (Häagen-Dazs)	4 fl. oz.	250	21.0
Sandwich (Lucerne)	1 sandwich	125	18.0
Shark (Good Humor)	3-fl. oz. pop	68	17.0
Strawberry:			
(Baskin-Robbins) very berry	4 fl. oz.	220	30.0
(Borden)	½ cup	130	18.0
(Breyers) natural	½ cup	130	17.0
(Häagen-Dazs)	4 fl.oz.	250	23.0
(Lucerne):			
Regular	½ cup	130	16.0
Gourmet	½ cup	140	17.0
(Snow Star)	½ cup	115	16.0
Strawberry cheesecake (Lucerne):			
Regular	½ cup	140	20.0
Gourmet	½ cup	155	18.0
Strawberry fudge bar (Good Humor)	2 ½-fl.-oz. bar	49	12.2
Strawberry shortcake (Good Humor)	3-fl.-oz. bar	176	23.8
Strawberry, vanilla, blueberry (Lucerne)	½ cup	140	17.0
Supreme (Good Humor):			
Regular	4 fl. oz.	375	32.9
Milk	4 fl. oz.	278	27.3
Tin Lizzy (Lucerne)	½ cup	140	19.0
Toasted almond bar (Good Humor)	3-fl.-oz. pop	212	24.3

Food and Description	Measure or Quantity	Calories	Carbo-hydrates (grams)
Vanilla:			
(Baskin-Robbins):			
Regular	4 fl.-oz. scoop	235	25.0
French	4 fl.-oz. scoop	280	25.0
(Borden) Old Fashioned			
Recipe	½ cup	130	15.0
(Eagle Brand)	½ cup	150	16.0
(Häagen-Dazs)	4 fl. oz.	260	23.0
(Land O' Lakes)	4 fl. oz.	140	16.0
(Lucerne):			
Regular, deluxe homestyle, *Our Natural* or real	½ cup	140	16.0
French	½ cup	150	16.0
Diabetic	½ cup	130	14.0
(Snow Star)	½ cup	130	16.0
Vanilla bar (Häagen-Dazs) with milk chocolate coating	1 bar	320	24.0
Vanilla sandwich (Good Humor)	3-fl.-oz. piece	191	31.1
Vanilla Swiss almond (Häagen-Dazs)	4 fl. oz.	290	24.0
Whammy (Good Humor) assorted	1.6-fl.-oz. piece	95	6.6
ICE CREAM CONE, cone only:			
(Baskin-Robbins):			
Sugar	1 piece	60	11.0
Waffle	1 piece	140	28.0
(Comet) sugar	1 piece (.35 oz.)	40	9.0
ICE CREAM CONES, cereal (General Mills)	¾ cup (1-oz.)	110	23.0
ICE CREAM CUP, cup only (Comet):			
Regular	1 cup	20	4.0
Chocolate	1 cup	25	5.0
*ICE CREAM MIX (Salada) any flavor	1 cup	310	31.0

(USDA) = United States Department of Agriculture
(HHS/FAO) = Health and Human Services/Food and Agriculture
                Organization
* = prepared as package directs

Food and Description	Measure or Quantity	Calories	Carbo-hydrates (grams)
ICE CREAM & SHERBET (See **SHERBET OR SORBET & ICE CREAM**)			
ICE MILK:			
(USDA):			
Hardened	1 cup (4.6 oz.)	199	29.3
Soft-serve	1 cup (6.3 oz.)	266	39.2
(Borden):			
Chocolate	½ cup	100	18.0
Strawberry or vanilla	½ cup	90	17.0
(Dean):			
Count Calorie, 2.1% fat	1 cup (4.8 oz.)	155	17.1
5% fat	1 cup (4.9 oz.)	227	35.0
(Land O' Lakes) vanilla	4 fl. oz.	110	17.0
(Lucerne):			
Regular:			
Caramel nut	½ cup	105	19.0
Chocolate:			
Regular or marble	½ cup	110	19.0
Chip	½ cup	100	18.0
Pecan crunch or vanilla	½ cup	100	18.0
Rocky road	½ cup	110	19.0
Strawberry	½ cup	95	18.0
Triple treat	½ cup	100	19.0
Light:			
Chocoalte	½ cup	120	20.0
Vanilla	½ cup	110	19.0
(Weight Watchers) *Grand Collection*:			
Chocolate:			
Regular or fudge	½ cup	110	18.0
Chip or swirl	½ cup	120	19.0
Fudge marble	½ cup	120	19.0
Neapolitan	½ cup	110	18.0
Pecan pralines 'n creme	½ cup	120	20.0
Strawberries 'n creme	½ cup	120	21.0
Vanilla	½ cup	100	16.0
ICE TEASERS (Nestlé)	8 fl. oz.	6	1.0
ICING (See **CAKE ICING**)			

Food and Description	Measure or Quantity	Calories	Carbo-hydrates (grams)

INSTANT BREAKFAST (See individual brand name or company listings)

IRISH WHISKEY (See **DISTILLED LIQUOR**)

(USDA) = United States Department of Agriculture
(HHS/FAO) = Health and Human Services/Food and Agriculture Organization
* = prepared as package directs

Food and Description	Measure or Quantity	Calories	Carbo-hydrates (grams)

J

JACKFRUIT, fresh (USDA):

Food and Description	Measure or Quantity	Calories	Carbo-hydrates (grams)
Whole	1 lb. (weighed with seeds & skin)	124	32.5
Flesh only	4 oz.	111	28.8

JACK-IN-THE-BOX **RESTAURANT:**

Food and Description	Measure or Quantity	Calories	Carbo-hydrates (grams)
Breakfast Jack	4.4-oz. serving	307	30.0
Breadstick, sesame	.6-oz. serving	70	12.0
Burger:			
Regular	3.6-oz. serving	267	28.0
Cheeseburger:			
Regular	4-oz. serving	315	33.0
Bacon	8.1-oz. serving	705	48.0
Double	5¼-oz. serving	467	33.0
Ultimate	9.9-oz. serving	942	33.0
Jumbo Jack:			
Regular	7.8-oz. serving	584	42.0
With cheese	8.5-oz. serving	677	46.0
Monterey Burger	9.9-oz. serving	865	72.0
Swiss & bacon	6.6-oz. serving	678	34.0
Cheesecake	3.5-oz. serving	309	29.0
Chicken fajita pita sandwich	6.7-oz. serving	292	29.0
Chicken fillet sandwich, grilled	7.2-oz. serving	408	33.0
Chicken strips	1 piece	87	7.0
Chicken supreme sandwich	8.1-oz. serving	575	34.0
Coffee, black	8 fl. oz.	2	.5
Egg, scrambled, platter	8.8-oz. serving	662	52.0
Egg roll	1 piece	135	14.0
Fish supreme sandwich	8-oz. sandwich	554	47.0
French fries:			
Regular	2.4-oz. order	221	27.0
Large	3.8-oz. order	353	43.0
Jumbo	4.8-oz. order	442	54.0
Jelly, grape	.5-oz. serving	38	9.0
Ketchup	1 serving	10	2.0
Mayonnaise	1 serving	152	.5
Milk, low fat	8 fl. oz.	122	12.0

Food and Description	Measure or Quantity	Calories	Carbo-hydrates (grams)
Milk shake:			
Chocolate	10-oz. serving	320	55.0
Strawberry	10-oz. serving	320	55.0
Vanilla	10-oz. serving	320	57.0
Mustard	1 serving	8	.7
Onion rings	3.8-oz. serving	382	39.0
Orange juice	6.5-oz. serving	80	20.0
Pancake platter	8.1-oz. serving	612	87.0
Salad:			
Chef	11.7-oz. salad	325	10.0
Mexican chicken	15.2-oz. salad	443	31.0
Side	3.9-oz. salad	51	Tr.
Taco	14.8-oz. salad	641	34.0
Salad dressing:			
Regular:			
Blue cheese	1.2-oz. serving	131	7.0
Buttermilk	1.2-oz. serving	181	4.0
1000 Island	1.2-oz. serving	156	6.0
Dietetic or low calorie,			
French	1.2-oz. serving	80	13.0
Sauce:			
A-1	1.8-oz. serving	35	9.0
BBQ	.9-oz. serving	39	9.4
Guacamole	.9-oz. serving	55	1.8
Mayo-mustard	.8-oz. serving	124	2.0
Mayo-onion	.8-oz. serving	143	1.0
Salsa	.9-oz. serving	8	2.0
Seafood cocktail	1-oz. serving	32	6.8
Sweet & sour	1-oz. serving	40	11.0
Sausage crescent	5.5-oz. serving	585	28.0
Shrimp	1 piece (.3 oz.)	27	2.2
Soft drink:			
Sweetened:			
Coca-Cola Classic	12 fl. oz.	144	36.0
Dr Pepper	12 fl. oz.	144	37.0
Root beer, *Ramblin'*	12 fl. oz.	176	46.0
Sprite	12 fl. oz.	144	36.0
Dietetic, *Coca-Cola*	12 fl. oz.	Tr.	.3
Supreme crescent	5.1-oz. serving	547	27.0
Syrup, pancake	1.5-oz. serving	121	30.0

(USDA) = United States Department of Agriculture
(HHS/FAO) = Health and Human Services/Food and Agriculture
                 Organization
* = prepared as package directs

Food and Description	Measure or Quantity	Calories	Carbohydrates (grams)
Taco:			
Regular	2.9-oz. serving	191	16.0
Super	4.8-oz. serving	288	21.0
Taquito	1-oz. piece	73	8.0
Tea, iced, plain	12 fl. oz.	3	.8
Tortilla chips	1 oz.	139	18.0
Turnover, hot apple	4.2-oz. piece	410	45.0
JACK MACKEREL, raw (USDA) meat only	4 oz.	162	0.
JAM, sweetened (See also individual listings by flavor) (USDA)	1 T. (.7 oz.)	54	14.0
JELL-O FRUIT BARS	1 bar	45	11.0
JELL-O GELATIN POPS:			
Cherry, grape, orange, or strawberry	1.7-oz. pop	37	8.5
Raspberry	1.7-oz. pop	34	7.7
JELL-O PUDDING POPS:			
Chocolate, chocolate-caramel swirl, chocolate with chocolate chips & vanilla with chocolate chips	1 bar	80	13.0
Chocolate covered chocolate & vanilla	1 bar	130	14.0
Chocolate-vanilla swirl & vanilla	1 bar	70	12.0
JELLY, sweetened (See also individual flavors) (Crosse & Blackwell) all flavors	1 T.	51	12.8
JERUSALEM ARTICHOKE (USDA):			
Unpared	1 lb. (weighed with skin)	207	52.3
Pared	4 oz.	75	18.9
JOHANNISBERG RIESLING WINE (Louis M. Martini)	3 fl. oz.	59	1.3

Food and Description	Measure or Quantity	Calories	Carbo-hydrates (grams)
JUICE (See individual listings)			
JUJUBE OR CHINESE DATE (USDA):			
Fresh, whole	1 lb. (weighed with seeds)	443	116.4
Fresh, flesh only	4 oz.	119	31.3
Dried, whole	1 lb. (weighed with seeds)	1159	297.1
Dried, flesh only	4 oz.	325	83.5
JUST RIGHT, cereal (Kellogg's):			
with fiber nuggets	⅔ cup (1 oz.)	100	24.0
with fruit & nuts	¾ cup (1.3 oz.)	140	30.0

(USDA) = United States Department of Agriculture
(HHS/FAO) = Health and Human Services/Food and Agriculture Organization
* = prepared as package directs

Food and Description	Measure or Quantity	Calories	Carbo-hydrates (grams)

K

KABOOM, cereal (General Mills) | 1 cup (1 oz.) | 110 | 23.0 |

KALE:

Food and Description	Measure or Quantity	Calories	Carbo-hydrates (grams)
Raw (USDA) leaves only	1 lb. (weighed untrimmed)	154	26.1
Boiled, leaves only (USDA)	4 oz.	44	6.9
Canned (Allen's) chopped, solids & liq.	½ cup (4.1 oz.)	25	2.0
Frozen, chopped:			
(Bel-Air)	3.3 oz.	25	5.0
(Birds Eye)	⅓ of 10-oz. pkg.	31	4.6
(Frosty Acres)	3.3-oz. serving	25	5.0
(McKenzie)	⅓ of 10-oz. pkg.	30	5.0

KARO SYRUP (See **SYRUP**)

KENMEI, cereal (Kellogg's):

Plain	¾ cup (1 oz.)	110	24.0
Almond & raisin	¾ cup (1.4 oz.)	150	31.0

KFC (KENTUCKY FRIED CHICKEN)

Biscuit, buttermilk	2.3-oz. serving	235	28.0
Chicken:			
Original Recipe:			
Breast:			
Center	1 piece	260	8.8
Side	1 piece	245	9.0
Drumstick	1 piece	152	3.0
Thigh	1 piece	287	8.0
Wing	1 piece	172	5.0

Food and Description	Measure or Quantity	Calories	Carbohydrates (grams)
Extra Tasty Crispy:			
Breast:			
Center	1 piece	344	15.0
Side	1 piece	379	15.0
Drumstick	1 piece	205	7.0
Thigh	1 piece	414	15.0
Wing	1 piece	231	8.0
Hot & Spicy:			
Breast:			
Center	1 piece	382	16.0
Side	1 piece	398	18.0
Drumstick	1 piece	207	10.0
Thigh	1 piece	412	16.0
Wing	1 piece	244	9.0
Skinfree Crispy:			
Breast:			
Center	1 piece	244	11.0
Side	1 piece	278	11.0
Drumstick	1 piece	154	8.0
Thigh	1 piece	235	9.0
Chicken Littles	1.7-oz. sandwich	169	13.8
Chicken nugget, *Kentucky Nuggets*	1 piece	46	2.2
Chicken sandwich, *Colonel's*	1 sandwich	482	39.0
Cole slaw	3.2-oz. serving	114	13.2
Corn on the cob	2.6-oz. serving	90	16.0
Hot wings	1 piece	78	3.0
Potatoes:			
French fries	2.7-oz. regular order	244	31.0
Mashed & gravy	3½-oz. serving	71	11.9
Sauce:			
Barbecue	1-oz. serving	35	7.1
Honey	.5-oz. serving	49	12.1
Mustard	1-oz. serving	36	6.0
Sweet & sour	1-oz. serving	58	13.0

KETCHUP (See CATSUP)

(USDA) = United States Department of Agriculture
(HHS/FAO) = Health and Human Services/Food and Agriculture Organization
* = prepared as package directs

Food and Description	Measure or Quantity	Calories	Carbo-hydrates (grams)
KIDNEY (USDA):			
Beef, braised	4 oz.	286	.9
Calf, raw	4 oz.	128	.1
Lamb, raw	4 oz.	119	1.0
KIELBASA (See **SAUSAGE,** Polish-style)			
KINGFISH, raw (USDA):			
Whole	1 lb. (weighed whole)	210	0.
Meat only	4 oz.	119	0.
KIPPER SNACKS (King David Brand) Norwegian	3¼-oz. can	195	0.
KIWIFRUIT (Calavo)	1 fruit (5-oz. edible portion)	45	9.0
KIX, cereal (General Mills)	1½ cups (1 oz.)	110	24.0
KNOCKWURST (See **SAUSAGE**)			
KOHLRABI (USDA):			
Raw:			
Whole	1 lb. (weighed with skin, without leaves)	96	21.9
Diced	1 cup (4.8 oz.)	40	9.1
Boiled:			
Drained	4 oz.	27	6.0
Drained	1 cup (5.5 oz.)	37	8.2
KOO KOOS (Dolly Madison)	1½-oz. piece	190	25.0
KOOL-AID (General Foods):			
Canned, *Kool Aid Koolers*:			
Cherry or mountainberry punch	8.45 fl. oz.	142	37.6
Grape	8.45 fl. oz.	136	35.5
Orange	8.45 fl. oz.	115	30.1
Rainbow punch or strawberry	8.45 fl. oz	135	35.6
Sharkleberry Fin	8.45 fl. oz.	140	36.8
Tropical punch	8.45 fl. oz.	132	34.9

Food and Description	Measure or Quantity	Calories	Carbo-hydrates (grams)
*Mix:			
Unsweetened, sugar to be added	8 fl. oz.	98	25.0
Pre-sweetened:			
Regular:			
Grape	8 fl. oz.	80	21.0
Orange, surfin berry punch	8 fl. oz.	79	20.0
Sunshine punch	8 fl. oz.	83	21.0
Dietetic:			
Rainbow punch	8 fl. oz.	4	Tr.
Raspberry	8 fl. oz.	2	Tr.
All others	8 fl. oz.	3	Tr.
KRISPIES, cereal (Kellogg's):			
Plain	1 cup (1 oz.)	110	25.0
Frosted	¾ cup (1 oz.)	110	26.0
Fruity marshmallow	1¼ cups (1.3 oz.)	140	32.0
KUMQUAT, fresh (USDA):			
Whole	1 lb. (weighed with seeds)	274	72.1
Flesh & skin	4 oz.	74	19.4

(USDA) = United States Department of Agriculture
(HHS/FAO) = Health and Human Services/Food and Agriculture Organization
* = prepared as package directs

Food and Description	Measure or Quantity	Calories	Carbohydrates (grams)

L

LAKE HERRING (See also **HERRING**), raw (USDA):

Whole	1 lb.	226	0.
Meat only	4 oz.	109	0.

LAKE TROUT, raw (USDA):

Whole	1 lb. (weighed whole)	404	0.
Meat only	4 oz.	191	0.

LAKE TROUT OR SISCOWET (See also **TROUT**), raw (USDA):

Less than 6.5 lb.:			
Whole	1 lb. (weighed whole)	404	0.
Meat only	4 oz.	273	0.
More than 6.5 lb.:			
Whole	1 lb. (weighed whole)	856	0.
Meat only	4 oz.	594	0.

LAMB, choice grade (USDA):

Chop, broiled:			
Loin. One 5-oz. chop (weighed before cooking with bone) will give you:			
Lean & fat	2.8 oz.	280	0.
Lean only	2.3 oz.	122	0.
Rib. One 5-oz. chop (weighed before cooking with bone) with give you:			
Lean & fat	2.9 oz.	334	0.
Lean only	2 oz.	118	0.
Fat, separable, cooked	1 oz.	201	0.

Food and Description	Measure or Quantity	Calories	Carbo-hydrates (grams)
Leg:			
Raw, lean & fat	1 lb. (weighed with bone)	845	0.
Roasted, lean & fat	4 oz.	316	0.
Roasted, lean only	4 oz.	211	0.
Shoulder:			
Raw, lean & fat	1 lb. (weighed with bone)	1092	0.
Roasted, lean & fat	4 oz.	383	0.
Roasted, lean only	4 oz.	232	0.
LAMB'S QUARTERS (USDA):			
Raw, trimmed	1 lb.	195	33.1
Boiled, drained	4 oz.	36	5.7
LARD:			
(USDA)	1 cup (6.2 oz.)	1849	0.
(USDA)	1 T. (.5 oz.)	117	0.
LASAGNA:			
Dry:			
(Buitoni) pre-cooked	1 sheet	48	8.9
(Mueller's)	2 oz.	210	42.0
Frozen:			
(Armour) *Dining Lite*:			
Cheese	9-oz. meal	260	36.0
Meat sauce	9-oz. meal	260	33.0
(Banquet) *Family Entree* with meat sauce	28-oz. pkg.	1080	120.0
(Buitoni):			
Alforno	8-oz. meal	327	31.8
Cheese, sorrentino	8-oz. serving	286	37.4
Individual portion	9-oz. serving	342	30.9
With meat sauce	5-oz. serving	212	23.4
(Celentano):			
Regular	½ of 16-oz. pkg.	370	32.0
Regular	¼ of 25-oz. pkg.	300	25.0
Primavera	11-oz. pkg.	330	34.0
(Healthy Choice) with meat sauce	9-oz. meal	260	37.0

(USDA) = United States Department of Agriculture
(HHS/FAO) = Health and Human Services/Food and Agriculture Organization
* = prepared as package directs

Food and Description	Measure or Quantity	Calories	Carbo-hydrates (grams)
(Le Menu) healthy style, entree:			
Garden vegetable	10½-oz. meal	260	35.0
With meat sauce	10-oz. meal	290	36.0
(Mrs. Paul's) seafood, light	9½-oz. meal	290	39.0
(Stouffer's)			
Regular:			
Plain	10 ½-oz. meal	360	33.0
Vegetable	10 ½-oz. meal	420	23.0
Lean Cuisine:			
With meat sauce	10 ¼-oz. meal	270	24.0
Tuna, with spinach noodles & vegetables	9¾-oz. meal	270	29.0
Zucchini	11-oz. meal	260	28.0
(Swanson) *Homestyle Recipe*, with meat sauce	10½-oz. meal	400	39.0
(Weight Watchers):			
Gardena	11-oz. meal	330	35.0
Italian cheese	11-oz. meal	380	38.0
Meat sauce	11-oz. meal	330	33.0
Mix (Golden Grain) Stir-N-Serv	⅕ of pkg.	150	28.0
LATKES, frozen (Empire Kosher):			
Mini	3 oz.	190	20.0
Rounds	2 ½ oz.	120	20.0
Triangles	3 oz.	140	12.0
LEEKS, raw (USDA):			
Whole	1 lb. (weighed untrimmed)	123	26.4
Trimmed	4 oz.	59	12.7
LEMON, fresh (USDA):			
Whole	2⅛″ lemon (109 grams)	**22**	**11.7**
Peeled	2⅛″ lemon (74 grams)	**20**	**6.1**
LEMONADE:			
Canned:			
(Ardmore Farms)	6 fl. oz.	89	22.5
Country Time	6 fl. oz.	69	17.2
(Hi-C)	6 fl. oz.	77	19.3

Food and Description	Measure or Quantity	Calories	Carbo-hydrates (grams)
(Johanna Farms) *Ssips*	8.45-fl.-oz. container	85	21.0
Kool-Aid Koolers	8.45-fl.-oz. container	120	31.5
Chilled (Minute Maid) regular or pink	6 fl. oz.	81	21.3
*Frozen:			
Country Time, regular or pink	6 fl. oz.	68	18.0
Minute Maid,	6 fl. oz.	77	20.1
(Sunkist)	6 fl. oz.	92	24.2
*Mix:			
Regular:			
Country Time, regular or pink	6 fl. oz.	68	20.6
(4C)	8 fl. oz.	80	20.0
(Funny Face)	8 fl. oz.	88	22.0
Kool-Aid, regular or pink:			
Sugar to be added	6 fl. oz.	73	18.8
Pre-sweetened with sugar	6 fl. oz.	65	16.3
Lemon Tree (Lipton)	6 fl. oz.	68	16.5
(Minute Maid)	6 fl. oz.	80	20.0
(Wyler's):			
Regular	8 fl. oz.	91	19.6
Wild strawberry	8 fl. oz.	80	20.7
Dietetic:			
Crystal Light	6 fl. oz.	4	.2
Kool-Aid	6 fl. oz.	3	.2
LEMONADE BAR (Sunkist)	3 fl. oz. bar	68	17.6
*LEMONADE PUNCH, mix			
Country Time, regular	8 fl. oz.	82	20.0
LEMON JUICE:			
Fresh (USDA)	1 T. (.5 oz.)	4	1.2
Plastic container, *ReaLemon*	1 T. (.5 oz.)	3	.5

(USDA) = United States Department of Agriculture
(HHS/FAO) = Health and Human Services/Food and Agriculture Organization
* = prepared as package directs

Food and Description	Measure or Quantity	Calories	Carbo-hydrates (grams)
*Frozen (Sunkist) unsweetened	1 fl. oz.	7	2.0
*LEMON-LIMEADE DRINK, MIX:			
Regular:			
(Minute Maid)	6 fl. oz.	80	20.0
Country Time	6 fl. oz.	65	16.2
Dietetic, *Crystal Light*	6 fl. oz.	4	.2
LEMON PEEL, CANDIED (USDA)	1 oz.	90	22.9
LEMON & PEPPER SEASONING:			
(Lawry's)	1 tsp.	6	1.2
(McCormick)	1 tsp.	7	.8
LENTIL:			
Whole:			
Dry:			
(USDA)	½ lb.	771	136.3
(USDA)	1 cup (6.7 oz.)	649	114.8
(Sinsheimer)	1 oz.	95	17.0
Cooked (USDA) drained	½ cup (3.6 oz.)	107	19.5
Split (USDA) dry	½ lb.	782	140.2
LETTUCE (USDA):			
Bibb, untrimmed	1 lb.	47	8.4
Bibb, untrimmed	7.8-oz. head (4″ dia.)	23	4.1
Boston, untrimmed	1 lb.	47	8.4
Boston, untrimmed	7.8-oz. head (4″ dia.)	23	4.1
Butterhead varieties (See Bibb; Boston)			
Cos (See Romaine)			
Dark green (See Romaine)			
Grand Rapids	1 lb. (weighed untrimmed)	52	10.2
Great Lakes	1 lb. (weighed untrimmed)	56	12.5

Food and Description	Measure or Quantity	Calories	Carbo-hydrates (grams)
Great Lakes, trimmed	1 lb. head (4¾" dia.)	59	13.2
Iceberg:			
Untrimmed	1 lb.	56	12.5
Trimmed	1 lb. head (4¾" dia.)	59	13.2
Leaves	1 cup (2.3 oz.)	9	1.9
Chopped	1 cup (2 oz.)	8	1.7
Chunks	1 cup (2.6 oz.)	10	2.1
Looseleaf varieties (See Salad Bowl)			
New York	1 lb. (weighed untrimmed)	56	12.5
New York	1 lb. head (4¾" dia.)	59	13.2
Romaine:			
Untrimmed	1 lb.	52	10.2
Trimmed, shredded & broken into pieces	½ cup	4	.8
Salad Bowl	1 lb. (weighed untrimmed)	52	10.2
Salad Bowl	2 large leaves (1.8 oz.)	9	1.8
Simpson	1 lb. (weighed untrimmed)	52	10.2
Simpson	2 large leaves (1.8 oz.)	9	1.8
White Paris (See Romaine)			
LIFE, cereal (Quaker) regular or cinnamon	⅔ cup (1 oz.)	105	19.7
LIME, fresh (USDA) peeled fruit	2" dia. lime (1.8 oz.)	15	4.9
***LIMEADE,** frozen (Minute Maid)	6 fl. oz.	71	19.2

(USDA) = United States Department of Agriculture
(HHS/FAO) = Health and Human Services/Food and Agriculture Organization
* = prepared as package directs

Food and Description	Measure or Quantity	Calories	Carbohydrates (grams)
LIME JUICE, *ReaLime*	1 T.	2	.5
LINGCOD, raw (USDA):			
Whole	1 lb. (weighed whole)	130	0.
Meat only	34 oz.	95	0.
LINGUINI, frozen:			
(Healthy Choice) with shrimp	9½-oz. meal	230	40.0
(Mrs. Paul's) with shrimp & clams, light	10-oz. meal	240	36.0
(Stouffer's) *Lean Cuisine*	9⅝-oz. meal	270	35.0
(Weight Watchers) seafood	9-oz. meal	210	27.0
LIQUEUR (See individual kinds such as **CREME DE BANANA; PEACH LIQUEUR;** etc.)			
LIQUOR (See **DISTILLED LIQUOR**)			
LITCHI NUT (USDA):			
Fresh:			
Whole	4 oz. (weighed in shell with seeds)	44	11.2
Flesh only	4 oz.	73	18.6
Dried:			
Whole	4 oz. (weighed in shell with seeds)	145	36.9
Flesh	2 oz.	157	40.1
LIVER:			
Beef:			
(USDA):			
Raw	1 lb.	635	24.0
Fried	4 oz.	260	6.0
(Swift) packaged, True-Tender, sliced, cooked	⅕ of 1-lb. pkg.	141	3.1
Calf (USDA):			
Raw	1 lb.	635	18.6
Fried	4 oz.	296	4.5

Food and Description	Measure or Quantity	Calories	Carbohydrates (grams)
Chicken:			
Raw	1 lb.	585	13.2
Simmered	4 oz.	187	3.5
Goose, raw (USDA)	1 lb.	826	24.5
Hog (USDA):			
Raw	1 lb.	594	11.8
Fried	4 oz.	273	2.8
Lamb (USDA):			
Raw	1 lb.	617	13
LIVERWURST SPREAD, canned:			
(Hormel)	1 oz.	70	0.
(Underwood)	2.4 oz.	220	3.0
LOBSTER:			
Raw (USDA):			
Whole	1 lb. (weighed whole)	107	.6
Meat only	4-oz.	103	.6
Cooked, meat only (USDA)	4-oz.	108	.3
Canned (USDA) meat only	4-oz.	108	.3
Frozen, South African rock lobster	2-oz. tail	65	.1
LOBSTER NEWBURG:			
Home recipe (USDA)	4 oz.	220	5.8
Frozen (Stouffer's)	6½ oz.	380	9.0
LOBSTER PASTE, canned (USDA)	1 oz.	51	.4
LOBSTER SALAD, home recipe (USDA)	4 oz.	125	2.6
LOGANBERRY (USDA):			
Fresh:			
Untrimmed	1 lb. (weighed with caps)	267	64.2

(USDA) = United States Department of Agriculture
(HHS/FAO) = Health and Human Services/Food and Agriculture Organization
* = prepared as package directs

Food and Description	Measure or Quantity	Calories	Carbo- hydrates (grams)
Trimmed	1 cup (5.1 oz.)	89	21.5
Canned, solids & liq.:			
Extra heavy syrup	4 oz.	101	25.2
Heavy syrup	4 oz.	101	25.2
Juice pack	4 oz.	61	14.4
Light syrup	4 oz.	79	19.5
Water pack	4 oz.	45	10.7
LONGAN (USDA):			
Fresh:			
Whole	1 lb. (weighed with shell & seeds)	147	38.0
Flesh only	4 oz.	69	17.9
Dried:			
Whole	1 lb. (weighed with shell & seeds)	467	120.8
Flesh only	4 oz.	324	83.9
LONG ISLAND TEA COCKTAIL (Mr. Boston)			
12½% alcohol	3 fl. oz.	93	9.0
LONG JOHN SILVER'S:			
Catfish:			
Dinner	13.2-oz. serving	860	90.0
Fillet	2½-oz. piece	180	10.0
Catsup	.4-oz. packet	15	3.0
Chicken plank:			
Dinner:			
3-piece	13-oz. serving	830	88.0
4-piece	14.6-oz. serving	940	94.0
Single piece	1.6-oz. piece	110	6.0
Children's meals:			
Chicken planks	7.1-oz. serving	510	52.0
Fish	6½-oz. serving	440	49.0
Fish & chicken planks	8.1-oz. serving	550	55.0
Chowder, clam, with cod	7-oz. serving	140	10.0
Clam:			
Breaded	2.3-oz. serving	240	26.0
Dinner	12.8-oz. serving	980	122.0
Cod, entree:			

Food and Description	Measure or Quantity	Calories	Carbo-hydrates (grams)
Baked:			
Regular	5.8-oz. serving	150	21.0
Delight	6-oz. serving	180	4.0
Supreme	6.2-oz. serving	190	3.0
Broiled	5.4-oz. serving	160	2.0
Cole slaw, drained on fork	3.4-oz. serving	140	20.0
Corn on the cob, with whirl	6.6-oz. ear	270	38.0
Cracker, *Club*	.2-oz. package	35	5.0
Fish, battered	2.6-oz. piece	150	9.0
Fish dinner, 3-piece	16.1-oz. serving	960	97.0
Fish dinner, home-style:			
3-piece	13.1-oz. serving	880	97.0
4-piece	14.8-oz. serving	1,010	106.0
6-piece	18.1-oz. serving	1,260	124.0
Fish & fryes, entree:			
2-piece	10-oz. serving	660	68.0
3-piece	12.6-oz. serving	810	77.0
Fish, homestyle	1.6-oz. piece	125	9.0
Fish & more	13.4-oz. entree	800	88.0
Fish sandwich, homestyle	6.9-oz. serving	510	58.0
Fish sandwich platter, homestyle	13.4-oz. serving	870	108.0
Flounder, broiled	5.1-oz. piece	180	0.
Gumbo, with cod & shrimp bobs	7-oz. serving	120	4.0
Halibut steak, broiled	4.1-oz. serving	140	0.
Hushpuppie	.8-oz. piece	70	10.0
Pie:			
Lemon meringue	4.2-oz. slice	260	47.0
Pecan	4.4-oz. slice	530	70.0
Potato:			
Baked, without topping	7.1-oz. serving	150	33.0
Fryes	3-oz. serving	220	30.0
Rice pilaf	3-oz. serving	150	32.0
Roll, dinner, plain	.9-oz. piece	70	12.0
Salad:			
Garden	8.7-oz. serving	170	13.0
Ocean chef	11.3-oz. serving	250	19.0
Seafood, entree	11.9-oz. serving	270	36.0
Side	4.3-oz. serving	20	5.0

(USDA) = United States Department of Agriculture
(HHS/FAO) = Health and Human Services/Food and Agriculture
                Organization
* = prepared as package directs

Food and Description	Measure or Quantity	Calories	Carbo-hydrates (grams)
Salad dressing:			
Regular:			
Bleu cheese	1.5-oz. packet	120	22.0
Ranch	1.5-oz. packet	140	27.0
Sea salad	1.6-oz. packet	140	20.0
Dietetic, Italian	1.6-oz. packet	18	2.0
Salmon, broiled	4.4-oz. piece	180	0.
Sauce:			
Honey mustard	1.2-oz. packet	60	13.0
Seafood	1.2-oz. packet	45	8.0
Sweet & sour	1.2-oz. packet	60	13.0
Tartar	1-oz. packet	80	13.0
Seafood platter	14.1-oz. entree	970	109.0
Shrimp, battered	.5-oz. piece	40	2.0
Shrimp, breaded	2.2-oz. serving	190	20.0
Shrimp dinner, battered:			
6-piece	11.1-oz. serving	740	82.0
9-piece	12.6-oz. serving	860	88.0
Shrimp feast, breaded:			
13-piece	12.6-oz. serving	880	110.0
21-piece	14.8-oz. serving	1070	130.0
Shrimp, fish & chicken dinner	13.4-oz. dinner	840	89.0
Shrimp & fish dinner	12.3-oz. dinner	770	85.0
Shrimp scampi, baked	5.7-oz. serving	160	7.0
Vegetables, mixed	4-oz. serving	60	9.0
Vinegar, malt	.4-oz. packet	2	0.
LOQUAT, fresh, flesh only (USDA)	2 oz.	27	7.0
LUCKY CHARMS, cereal (General Mills)	1 cup (1 oz.)	110	24.0
LUNCHEON MEAT (See also individual listings such as **BOLOGNA; HAM;** etc.):			
All meat (Oscar Mayer)	1-oz. slice	95	.7
Banquet loaf (Eckrich)	¾-oz. slice	50	1.0
Bar-B-Que Loaf:			
(Eckrich)	1-oz. slice	35	1.0
(Oscar Mayer)	1-oz. slice	46	1.7
Beef, jellied (Hormel) loaf	1 slice	45	0.
Gourmet loaf (Eckrich):			

Food and Description	Measure or Quantity	Calories	Carbo-hydrates (grams)
Regular	1-oz. slice	35	2.0
Smorgas Pac	¾-oz. slice	25	2.0
Ham & cheese (See **HAM & CHEESE**)			
Honey loaf:			
(Eckrich):			
Regular	1-oz. slice	40	3.0
Smorgas Pac	¾-oz. slice	30	2.0
Smorgas Pac	1-oz. slice	35	3.0
(Hormel)	1 slice	45	.5
(Oscar Mayer)	1-oz. slice	34	1.1
Iowa Brand (Hormel)	1 slice	45	0.
Jalapeño loaf (Oscar Mayer)	1-oz. slice	72	2.4
Liver cheese (Oscar Mayer)	1.3-oz. slice	114	.5
Liver loaf (Hormel)	1 slice	80	6.5
Macaroni-cheese loaf (Eckrich)	1-oz. slice	70	3.0
Meat loaf (USDA)	1-oz. serving	57	.9
New England Brand sliced sausage:			
(Eckrich)	1-oz. slice	35	1.0
(Oscar Mayer)	.8-oz. slice	29	.4
Old fashioned loaf:			
(Eckrich):			
Regular	1-oz. slice	70	3.0
Smorgas Pac	¾-oz. slice	50	2.0
(Oscar Mayer)	1-oz. slice	62	2.3
Olive loaf:			
(Eckrich)	1-oz. slice	80	2.0
(Hormel)	1 slice	55	2.5
(Oscar Mayer)	1-oz. slice	60	3.1
Peppered loaf:			
(Eckrich)	1-oz. slice	40	1.0
(Oscar Mayer)	1-oz. slice	39	1.3
Pickle loaf:			
(Eckrich):			
Regular	1-oz. slice	80	2.0
Smorgas Pac	¾-oz. slice	50	1.0
(Hormel) *Light & Lean*	1 slice	50	1.5
(Ohse)	1 oz.	60	2.0

(USDA) = United States Department of Agriculture
(HHS/FAO) = Health and Human Services/Food and Agriculture Organization
* = prepared as package directs

Food and Description	Measure or Quantity	Calories	Carbo-hydrates (grams)
Pickle & pimiento loaf (Oscar Mayer)	1-oz. slice	62	3.7
Picnic loaf (Oscar Mayer)	1-oz. slice	60	1.2
Spiced (Hormel)	1 slice	75	.5
LUNG, raw (USDA):			
Beef	1 lb.	435	0.
Calf	1 lb.	481	0.
Lamb	1 lb.	467	0.

Food and Description	Measure or Quantity	Calories	Carbo-hydrates (grams)

M

MACADAMIA NUT (Royal Hawaiian) | 1 oz. | 197 | 4.5

MACARONI:
Dry:

(USDA)	1 oz.	105	21.3
Spinach (Creamette) ribbons	1 oz.	105	21.0
Whole wheat (Pritikin)	1 oz.	110	18.0

Cooked (USDA):

8-10 minutes, firm	4 oz.	168	34.1
14-20 minutes, tender	4 oz.	126	26.

MACARONI & BEEF:
Canned (Franco-American)

BeefyO's, in tomato sauce	7½-oz. can	220	30.0

Frozen:

(Morton)	10-oz. meal	245	30.4
(Stouffer's) & tomatoes	11½-oz. meal	340	30.0
(Swanson) 3-compartment	12-oz. dinner	370	48.0

MACARONI & CHEESE:

Canned (Franco-American)	7⅜-oz. can	170	24.0

Frozen:
(Banquet):

Casserole	8-oz. pkg.	350	36.0
Dinner	10-oz. dinner	420	36.0
Family Entree	2-lb. pkg.	1160	128.0

(Birds Eye):

Classics	½ of 10-oz. pkg.	236	24.0
For One	5¾-oz. pkg.	304	27.0
(Celentano) baked	½ of 12-oz. pkg.	290	29.0
(Green Giant) one serving	5½-oz. pkg.	230	28.0

(USDA) = United States Department of Agriculture
(HHS/FAO) = Health and Human Services/Food and Agriculture Organization
* = prepared as package directs

Food and Description	Measure or Quantity	Calories	Carbo-hydrates (grams)
(Morton):			
Casserole	20-oz. casserole	648	91.2
Dinner	11-oz. dinner	278	45.8
Family Meal	2-lb. pkg.	1043	143.7
(Stouffer's)	6-oz. serving	250	22.0
(Swanson)			
3-compartment	12¼-oz. dinner	370	48.0
Mix:			
(Golden Grain) deluxe	¼ of 7¼-oz. pkg.	190	35.0
*(Kraft):			
Regular, plain or spiral	¼ of box	190	36.0
Velveeta	¼ of pkg.	270	32.0
*(Town House)	1 cup	370	51.0
MACARONI & CHEESE LOAF, packaged (Ohse)	1 oz.	60	4.0
MACARONI & CHEESE PIE, frozen (Swanson)	7-oz. pie	200	24.0
***MACARONI SALAD,** mix (Betty Crocker) creamy	⅙ of pkg.	200	20.0
MACE (French's)	1 tsp.	10	.8
MACKEREL (See also **SPANISH MACKEREL**) (USDA):			
Atlantic:			
Raw:			
Whole	1 lb. (weighed whole)	468	0.
Meat only	4 oz.	217	0.
Broiled with butter	8½″ × 2½″ × ½″ fillet (3.7 oz.)	268	0.
Canned, solids & liq.	4 oz.	208	0.
Pacific:			
Raw:			
Dressed	1 lb. (weighed with bones & skin)	519	0.
Meat only	4 oz.	180	0.
Canned, solids & liq.	4 oz.	204	0.
Salted	4 oz.	346	0.
Smoked	4 oz.	248	0.

Food and Description	Measure or Quantity	Calories	Carbohydrates (grams)
MADEIRA WINE (Leacock) 19% alcohol	3 fl. oz.	120	6.3
MAHI MAHI (Captain's Choice) frozen	3-oz. fillet	73	0.
MALT, dry (USDA)	1 oz.	104	21.9
MALTED MILK MIX (Carnation):			
Chocolate	3 heaping tsps. (.7 oz.)	85	18.0
Natural	3 heaping tsps. (.7 oz.)	88	15.8
MALT LIQUOR:			
Colt 45	12 fl. oz.	156	11.1
Elephant	12 fl. oz.	212	17.1
Kingsbury, no alcohol	12 fl. oz.	60	12.8
Mickey's	12 fl. oz.	156	11.1
Schlitz	12 fl. oz.	88	7.2
MALT-O-MEAL, cereal:			
Regular	1 T. (.3 oz.)	33	7.3
Chocolate-flavored	1 T. (.3 oz.)	33	7.0
MAMEY OR MAMMEE APPLE, fresh (USDA)	1 lb. (weighed with skin & seeds)	143	35.2
MANDARIN ORANGE (See **TANGERINE**)			
MANGO, fresh (USDA):			
Whole	1 lb. (weighed with seeds & skin)	201	51.1
Flesh only, diced or sliced	½ cup	54	13.8

(USDA) = United States Department of Agriculture
(HHS/FAO) = Health and Human Services/Food and Agriculture Organization
* = prepared as package directs

Food and Description	Measure or Quantity	Calories	Carbohydrates (grams)
MANHATTAN COCKTAIL			
(Mr. Boston) 20% alcohol	3 fl. oz.	123	12.3
MANICOTTI, frozen:			
(Buitoni):			
Plain	5½-oz. serving	310	26.0
Florentine	1 piece (2½ oz.)	142	14.3
(Celentano):			
Plain	2 pieces (7 oz.)	380	34.0
With sauce	2 pieces (8 oz.)	300	22.0
(Le Menu) 3-cheese	11¾-oz. dinner	390	44.0
(Weight Watchers) cheese	9¼-oz. dinner	300	28.0
MANWICH (Hunt's):			
Dry mix:			
Mix only	.25 oz	20	5.0
*Sandwich	1 serving	320	31.0
Extra thick & chunky:			
Sauce only	2½ oz.	60	15.0
*Sandwich	1 serving	330	36.0
Mexican:			
Sauce only	2½ oz.	35	9.0
*Sandwich	1 serving	310	30.0
MAPLE SYRUP (See **SYRUP,** Maple)			
MARGARINE, salted or unsalted:			
Regular:			
(USDA)	1 lb.	3266	1.8
(USDA)	1 cup (8 oz.)	1633	.9
(Autumn) soft or stick	1 T.	80	0.
(Blue Bonnet) soft or stick	1 T. (.5 oz.)	90	0.
(Chiffon):			
Soft	1 T.	90	0.
Stick	1 T.	100	0.
(Fleischmann's) soft or stick	1 T. (.5 oz.)	100	0.
(Golden Mist)	1 T.	100	0.
(Holiday)	1 T. (.5 oz.)	102	0.
I Can't Believe It's Not Butter, any type	1 T. (.5 oz.)	90	0.

Food and Description	Measure or Quantity	Calories	Carbo-hydrates (grams)
(Imperial) soft or stick	1 T. (.5 oz.)	102	Tr.
(Land O' Lakes)	1 T.	100	0.
(Mazola)	1 T.	100	0.
(Parkay)	1 T.	100	0.
(Promise) soft or stick	1 T.	90	Tr.
Imitation or dietetic:			
Country Morning:			
Regular:			
Stick	1 T.	100	0.
Tub	1 T.	90	0.
Light	1 T.	60	0.
Imperial:			
Regular	1 T.	50	Tr.
Light	1 T.	60	Tr.
(Land O' Lakes):			
Tub, 64% soy oil spread	1 T.	75	0.
Stick, sweet cream	1 T.	90	0.
Mazola	1 T.	50	Tr.
(Weight Watchers):			
Regular	1 T.	60	0.
Corn oil	1 T.	50	0.
Whipped:			
(Blue Bonnet)	1 T. (9 grams)	70	0.
(Chiffon)	1 T.	70	0.
(Fleischmann's)	1 T.	70	0.
(Imperial)	1 T. (9 grams)	45	0.
(Parkay) cup	1 T.	67	Tr.

MARGARITA COCKTAIL
(Mr. Boston) 12½% alcohol:

Regular	3 fl. oz.	105	10.8
Strawberry	3 fl. oz.	138	18.9

MARGARITA COCKTAIL MIX:
Dry (Holland House):

Regular	.5-oz. pkg.	57	14.0
Strawberry	.6-oz. pkg.	66	16.0

(USDA) = United States Department of Agriculture
(HHS/FAO) = Health and Human Services/Food and Agriculture Organization
* = prepared as package directs

Food and Description	Measure or Quantity	Calories	Carbo-hydrates (grams)
*Frozen (Bacardi):			
Water only	4 fl. oz.	49	12.4
Made with liquor	4 fl. oz.	82	12.4
Liquid (Holland House):			
Regular	1 fl. oz.	27	6.0
Strawberry	1 fl. oz.	31	7.0
MARINADE MIX:			
Chicken (Adolph's)	1-oz. packet	64	14.4
Meat:			
(Adolph's)	.8-oz. pkg.	38	8.5
(Durkee)	1-oz. pkg.	47	9.0
(French's)	1-oz. pkg.	80	16.0
(Kikkoman)	1-oz. pkg.	64	12.5
MARJORAM (French's)	1 tsp. (1.2 grams)	4	.8
MARMALADE:			
Sweetened:			
(USDA)	1 T. (.7 oz.)	51	14.0
(Empress)	1 T.	52	13.5
(Keiller)	1 T.	60	15.0
(Smucker's)	1 T. (.7 oz.)	54	12.0
Dietetic:			
(Estee; Louis Sherry)	1 T. (.6 oz.)	6	0.
(Featherweight)	1 T.	16	4.0
(S&W) *Nutradiet*, red label	1 T.	12	3.0
MARSHMALLOW (See CANDY, GENERIC and regular)			
MARSHMALLOW FLUFF	1 heaping tsp.	59	14.4
MARSHMALLOW KRISPIES, cereal (Kellogg's)	1¼ cups (1.3 oz.)	140	32.0
MARTINI COCKTAIL (Mr. Boston) 20% alcohol:			
Gin, extra dry	3 fl. oz.	99	Tr.
Vodka	3 fl. oz.	102	Tr.

Food and Description	Measure or Quantity	Calories	Carbo-hydrates (grams)
MATZO:			
(Goodman's):			
Diet-10s	1 sq.	109	23.0
Unsalted	1 matzo (1 oz.)	109	23.0
(Horowitz-Margareten)			
unsalted	1 matzo	135	28.2
(Manischewitz):			
Regular:			
Plain	1 piece	110	24.0
American	1-oz. piece	115	22.0
Egg	1 piece	108	26.6
Egg & onion	1 piece	112	23.0
Miniature	1 piece	9	20.0
Tam Tams	1 piece	15	DNA
Wheat	1 piece	9	1.8
Dietetic:			
Tam Tams	1 piece	14	DNA
Thins	1 piece	91	19.0
MATZO MEAL (Manischewitz)	½ cup	267	DNA
MAYONNAISE:			
Real:			
(Bama)	1 T.	100	0.
(Bennett's)	1 T.	110	1.0
(Luzianne) *Blue Plate*	1 T.	100	1.0
Hellmann's (Best Foods)	1 T. (.5 oz.)	100	.1
(Kraft)	1 T.	100	0.
(Nu Made)	1 T.	100	0.
(Rokeach)	1 T.	100	0.
Imitation or dietetic:			
Hellmann's Lite (Best Foods)	1 T.	50	1.0
(Luzianne) *Blue Plate*	1 T.	50	1.0
(Estee)	1 T. (.5 oz.)	50	1.0
Heart Beat (GFA)	1 T.	40	1.0
(Nu Made)	1 T.	40	1.0
(Weight Watchers)	1 T.	50	1.0

(USDA) = United States Department of Agriculture
(HHS/FAO) = Health and Human Services/Food and Agriculture Organization
* = prepared as package directs

Food and Description	Measure or Quantity	Calories	Carbo-hydrates (grams)
MAYPO, cereal:			
30-second	¼ cup (.8 oz.)	89	16.4
Vermont style	¼ cup (1.1 oz.)	121	22.0
McDONALD'S:			
Apple pie	2.9-oz. serving	260	30.0
Bacon bits	.1 oz.	16	.1
Big Mac	1 hamburger	560	42.5
Biscuit:			
Plain, with spread	2.6-oz. piece	260	31.9
With bacon, egg & cheese	5.5-oz. piece	440	33.3
With sausage	4.3-oz. piece	440	31.9
With sausage & egg	6.2-oz. piece	520	32.6
Cheeseburger	1 cheeseburger	310	31.2
Chicken McNuggets	1 serving (4 oz.)	290	16.5
Chicken McNuggets sauce:			
Barbecue	1.1-oz. serving	50	12.1
Honey	.5-oz. serving	45	11.5
Hot mustard	1-oz. serving	70	8.2
Sweet & sour	1.1-oz. serving	60	13.8
Cookies:			
Chocolate chip	1 package	330	41.9
McDonaldland	1 package	290	47.1
Danish:			
Apple	4-oz. piece	390	51.2
Cheese, iced	3.9-oz. piece	390	42.3
Cinnamon raisin	3.9-oz. piece	440	57.5
Raspberry	4.1-oz. piece	410	61.5
Egg McMuffin	1 serving	290	28.1
Egg, scrambled	1 serving	140	1.2
English muffin, with butter	1 muffin	170	26.7
Filet-O-Fish	1 sandwich	440	37.9
Grapefruit juice	6 fl. oz.	80	17.9
Hamburger	1 hamburger	260	30.6
Hot cakes with butter & syrup	1 serving	410	74.4
McD.L.T. sandwich	8¼-oz. serving	580	36.0
McLean Deluxe	1 sandwich	320	35.0
Milk shake:			
Chocolate	10.7 fl. oz.	390	62.6
Strawberry	10.7 fl. oz.	350	55.7
Vanilla	10.7 fl. oz.	380	63.2
Orange juice	6 fl. oz.	80	18.5
Potato:			
Fried	1 reg. order	220	26.6
Hash browns	1.9-oz. piece	130	14.9

Food and Description	Measure or Quantity	Calories	Carbo-hydrates (grams)
Quarter Pounder:			
Plain	5.8-oz. serving	410	34.1
With cheese	6.8-oz. serving	520	35.1
Salad:			
Chef	10-oz. serving	230	7.5
Chicken, chunky	8.6-oz. serving	140	5.0
Garden	7.5-oz. serving	110	6.2
Side	4.1-oz. serving	60	3.3
Salad dressing:			
Regular:			
Bleu cheese	.5-oz. serving	70	1.2
Caesar	.5-oz. serving	60	.6
French	.5-oz. serving	58	2.7
Peppercorn	.5-oz. serving	80	.5
Ranch	.5-oz. serving	83	1.3
1000 Island	.5-oz. serving	78	2.4
Dietetic:			
Ranch	.5-oz. serving	40	5.2
Vinaigrette	.5-oz. serving	15	2.0
Sausage	1.9-oz. piece	180	0.
Sausage McMuffin:			
Plain	4.1-oz. piece	370	27.3
With egg	5.8-oz. piece	440	27.9
Soft drink:			
Sweetened:			
*Coca-Cola,*classic	12 fl. oz.	144	38.0
*Coca-Cola,*classic	16 fl. oz.	190	50.0
*Coca-Cola,*classic	22 fl. oz.	264	70.0
Orange drink	12 fl. oz.	133	33.0
Orange drink	16 fl. oz.	177	44.0
Orange drink	22 fl. oz.	243	60.0
Sprite	12 fl. oz.	144	36.0
Sprite	16 fl. oz.	190	48.0
Sprite	22 fl. oz.	264	66.0
Dietetic, *Diet Coke*	12 fl. oz.	1	.3
Sundae:			
Caramel	6.1-oz. sundae	340	58.4
Hot fudge	6-oz. sundae	310	49.6
Strawberry	6-oz. sundae	280	48.3
Vanilla soft-serve, with cone	3 fl. oz.	140	21.9

(USDA) = United States Department of Agriculture
(HHS/FAO) = Health and Human Services/Food and Agriculture
            Organization
* = prepared as package directs

Food and Description	Measure or Quantity	Calories	Carbo-hydrates (grams)
MEATBALL SEASONING MIX:			
*(Durkee) Italian	1 cup	619	4.5
(French's)	¼ of 1.5-oz. pkg.	35	7.0
MEATBALL STEW:			
Canned (Hormel) *Dinty Moore*	⅓ of 24-oz. can	240	15.0
Frozen (Stouffer's) *Lean Cuisine*	10-oz. meal	250	20.0
MEATBALL, SWEDISH, frozen:			
(Armour) *Dinner Classics*	11¼-oz. meal	330	23.0
(Stouffer's) with parsley noodles	11-oz. meal	480	37.0
MEAT LOAF DINNER, frozen:			
(Armour) *Dinner Classics*	11¼-oz. dinner	360	32.0
(Banquet):			
Cookin' Bag	4-oz. meal	200	8.0
Dinner	11-oz. meal	440	27.0
(Morton)	10-oz. dinner	310	26.0
(Swanson) 4-compartment	10¾-oz. dinner	360	41.0
MEAT LOAF SEASONING MIX:			
(Bell's)	4½-oz. serving	300	14.0
(Contadina)	3¾-oz. pkg.	360	72.4
MEAT TENDERIZER:			
Regular (Adolph's; McCormick)	1 tsp.	2	.5
Seasoned (McCormick)	1 tsp.	5	.8
MELBA TOAST, salted (Old London):			
Garlic, onion or white rounds	1 piece	10	1.8
Pumpernickel, rye, wheat or white	1 piece	17	3.4
Sesame, flat	1 piece	18	3.0
MELON (See individual kinds)			
MELON BALLS, in syrup, frozen (USDA)	½ cup (4.1 oz.)	72	18.2

Food and Description	Measure or Quantity	Calories	Carbo-hydrates (grams)
MENHADEN, Atlantic, canned			
(USDA) solids & liq.	4 oz.	195	0.
MENUDO, canned (Old El Paso)	½ can	476	14.0
MERLOT WINE (Louis M.			
Martini) 12½% alcohol	3 fl. oz.	63	TR.
MEXICAN DINNER, frozen:			
(Banquet) dinner:			
Regular	12-oz. dinner	490	62.0
Combination	12-oz. dinner	520	72.0
(Morton)	10-oz. dinner	300	44.0
(Patio):			
Regular	13¼-oz. meal	540	64.0
Fiesta	12¼-oz. meal	470	55.0
(Swanson):			
4-course	14¼-oz. dinner	490	62.0
Hungry Man	20¼-oz. dinner	820	88.0
MILK, CONDENSED,			
sweetened, canned:			
(USDA)	1 T. (.7 oz.)	61	10.4
(Carnation)	1 fl. oz.	123	20.8
Eagle Brand (Borden)	1 T. (.7 oz.)	60	10.4
(Milnot) *Dairy Sweet*	1 fl. oz.		
	(1.3 oz.)	119	19.3
MILK, DRY:			
Whole (USDA) packed cup	1 cup (5.1 oz.)	728	55.4
*Nonfat, instant:			
(USDA)	8 fl. oz.	82	10.8
(Alba):			
Regular	8 fl. oz.	81	11.6
Chocolate flavor	8 fl. oz.	80	12.9
(Carnation)	8 fl. oz.	80	12.0
(Lucerne)	8 fl. oz.	80	12.0

(USDA) = United States Department of Agriculture
(HHS/FAO) = Health and Human Services/Food and Agriculture
Organization
* = prepared as package directs

Food and Description	Measure or Quantity	Calories	Carbo-hydrates (grams)
MILK, EVAPORATED:			
Regular:			
(Carnation)	½ cup (4 fl. oz.)	170	12.2
(Lucerne)	½ cup	170	12.0
(Pet)	½ cup (4 fl. oz.)	170	12.0
Filled, *Dairymate*	½ cup	150	12.0
Low fat (Carnation)	½ cup	110	12.0
Skimmed:			
(Carnation)	½ cup	100	14.0
Pet 99	½ cup	100	14.0
MILK, FRESH:			
Buttermilk:			
(Friendship) lowfat	1 cup	120	12.0
(Johanna Farms)	1 cup	120	11.0
(Land O' Lakes)	8 fl. oz.	110	12.0
(Lucerne):			
Regular	8 fl. oz.	120	12.0
Bulgarian or old time	8 fl. oz.	150	11.0
Chocolate:			
(Borden) *Dutch Blend*, lowfat	1 cup	180	25.0
(Hershey's) lowfat	1 cup	190	29.0
(Johanna Farms):			
Regular	1 cup	200	26.0
Lowfat	1 cup	150	26.0
(Land O' Lakes) lowfat:			
½%	8 fl. oz.	150	26.0
with *Nutrasweet*	8 fl. oz.	110	14.0
(Lucerne) lowfat	1 cup	180	26.0
(Nestlé) *Quik*	1 cup	220	30.0
White:			
Whole (3.25% butterfat) (USDA)	1 cup	159	12.0
Lowfat:			
(Borden):			
1% milkfat	1 cup	100	11.0
2% milkfat, *Hi-Protein Brand*	1 cup	140	13.0
(Johanna Farms):			
1% lowfat, protein fortified	1 cup	110	13.0
2% lowfat, *Mighty Milk*	1 cup	140	13.0

Food and Description	Measure or Quantity	Calories	Carbo-hydrates (grams)
(Land O' Lakes):			
1% milkfat	8 fl. oz.	100	12.0
2% milkfat	8 fl. oz.	120	11.0
(Lucerne):			
Acidophilus or 2-10	8 fl. oz.	140	13.0
½%, 1% or 1½% milkfat	8 fl. oz.	90	11.0
2% milkfat	8 fl. oz.	120	11.0
Skim:			
(Land O' Lakes)	8 fl. oz.	90	12.0
(Weight Watchers)	1 cup	90	13.0
MILK, GOAT (USDA) whole	1 cup	163	11.2
MILK, HUMAN (USDA)	1 oz. (by wt.)	22	2.7
MILNOT	½ cup	151	12.2
MINERAL WATER (See also **VICHY WATER**)	any quantity	0	0.
MINI-WHEATS, cereal (Kellogg's):			
Regular	¼-oz. biscuit	25	6.0
Bite size	½ cup (1 oz.)	100	24.0
MINT, LEAVES, raw, trimmed (HEW/FAO)	½ oz.	4	.8
MIRACLE WHIP (See **SALAD DRESSING,** Mayonnaise-type)			
MOLASSES:			
Barbados (USDA)	1 T. (.7 oz.)	51	13.3
Blackstrap (USDA)	1 T. (.7 oz.)	40	10.4
Dark (Brer Rabbit)	1 T. (.7 oz.)	33	10.6
Light (USDA)	1 T. (.7 oz.)	48	12.4
Medium (USDA)	1 T.	44	11.4
Unsulphured (Grandma's)	1 T.	60	15.0

(USDA) = United States Department of Agriculture
(HHS/FAO) = Health and Human Services/Food and Agriculture Organization
* = prepared as package directs

Food and Description	Measure or Quantity	Calories	Carbo-hydrates (grams)
MORNING FUNNIES, cereal			
(Ralston Purina)	1 cup (1 oz.)	110	25.0
MORTADELLA, sausage			
(USDA)	1 oz.	89	.2
MOUSSE:			
Frozen (Weight Watchers):			
Chocolate	2½-oz. serving	170	24.0
Praline pecan	½ of 5.4-oz. pkg.	190	27.0
Raspberry	2½-oz. serving	150	21.0
*Mix:			
Regular (Knorr):			
Unflavored	½ cup	80	8.0
Chocolate:			
Dark	½ cup	90	10.0
Milk	½ cup	90	11.0
White	½ cup	80	10.0
Dietetic:			
(Estee):			
Amaretto	½ cup	70	10.0
Chocolate or orange	½ cup	70	9.0
Lite Whip (TKI Foods):			
Chocolate:			
Skim milk	½ cup	70	10.0
Whole milk	½ cup	80	10.0
Lemon:			
Skim milk	½ cup	60	9.0
Whole milk	½ cup	70	9.0
Vanilla:			
Skim milk	½ cup	50	7.0
Whole milk	½ cup	70	9.0
*(Weight Watchers):			
Cheesecake or raspberry	½ cup	60	12.0
Chocolate:			
Regular	½ cup	60	9.0
White	½ cup	60	6.0
MUESLI, cereal (Ralston Purina):			
Raisins, dates & almonds	½ cup (1.45 oz.)	140	32.0
Raisins, peaches & pecan or raisins, walnuts & cranberries	½ cup (1.45 oz.)	150	30.0

Food and Description	Measure or Quantity	Calories	Carbo-hydrates (grams)
MÜESLIX, cereal (Kellogg's):			
Crispy blend	⅔ cup (1½ oz.)	160	33.0
Golden Crunch	½ cup (1.2 oz.)	120	25.0
MUFFIN:			
Blueberry:			
Home recipe (USDA)	1.4-oz. muffin	112	16.8
(Pepperidge Farm)	1.9-oz. muffin	170	27.0
Bran:			
Home recipe (USDA)	1.4-oz. muffin	104	17.2
(Pepperidge Farm)	1 muffin	170	30.0
Corn:			
Home recipe (USDA) prepared with whole-ground cornmeal	1.4-oz. muffin	115	17.0
(Pepperidge Farm)	1.9-oz. muffin	180	27.0
English:			
Millbrook (Interstate Brands):			
Regular	2-oz. muffin	130	23.0
Cinnamon raisin	2-oz. muffin	130	24.0
Sourdough	2-oz. muffin	120	23.0
Whole wheat	2-oz. muffin	120	23.0
(Mrs. Wright's)	2-oz. muffin	130	27.0
(Pepperidge Farm):			
Plain or cinnamon apple	1 muffin	140	27.0
Cinnamon chip	1 muffin	160	28.0
Cinnamon raisin	1 muffin	150	29.0
Sourdough	1 muffin	135	27.0
(Pritikin)	2.3-oz. muffin	150	28.0
(Roman Meal)	2.3-oz. muffin	150	29.8
Sunmaid (Interstate Brands) raisin	2.3-oz. muffin	180	33.0
(Thomas'):			
Regular or frozen	2-oz. muffin	133	25.7
Honey wheat	2-oz. muffin	135	27.0
Raisin	2.2-oz. muffin	153	30.4
Sourdough	2-oz. muffin	133	25.8
Granola (Mrs. Wright's)	2.3-oz. muffin	150	29.0
Oatbran (Pepperidge Farm) with apple	1 muffin	190	29.0

(USDA) = United States Department of Agriculture
(HHS/FAO) = Health and Human Services/Food and Agriculture Organization
* = prepared as package directs

Food and Description	Measure or Quantity	Calories	Carbo-hydrates (grams)
Plain (USDA) home recipe	1.4-oz. muffin	118	16.9
Raisin cinnamon (Mrs. Wright's)	2.3-oz. muffin	150	31.0
MUFFIN MIX:			
*Apple cinnamon (Betty Crocker):			
Regular	¹⁄₁₂ of pkg.	120	18.0
No cholesterol recipe	¹⁄₁₂ of pkg.	110	18.0
*Banana nut (Betty Crocker)	¹⁄₁₂ of pkg.	150	21.0
Blueberry:			
*(Betty Crocker) wild:			
Regular	1 muffin	120	18.0
No cholesterol recipe	1 muffin	110	18.0
(Duncan Hines):			
Bakery style	¹⁄₁₂ of pkg.	184	32.7
Wild	¹⁄₁₂ of pkg.	98	17.0
*Gold Medal	¹⁄₆ of pkg.	170	26.0
*Carrot nut (Betty Crocker)	¹⁄₁₂ of pkg.	150	22.0
*Chocolate chip (Betty Crocker)	¹⁄₁₂ of pkg.	150	22.0
Regular	¹⁄₁₂ of pkg.	150	22.0
No cholesterol recipe	¹⁄₁₂ of pkg.	140	22.0
*Cinnamon streusel (Betty Crocker)	¹⁄₁₀ of pkg.	200	27.0
Cinnamon swirl (Duncan Hines) bakery style	1 muffin	195	34.1
Corn:			
*(Dromedary)	1 muffin	120	20.0
*(Flako)	1 muffin	140	23.0
*Gold Medal	¹⁄₆ of pkg.	130	24.0
Cranberry orange nut (Duncan Hines) bakery style	¹⁄₁₂ of pkg.	184	27.1
*Honey bran, Gold Medal	¹⁄₆ of pkg.	170	25.0
*Oat, Gold Medal	¹⁄₆ of pkg.	150	23.0
Oat bran:			
*(Betty Crocker):			
Regular	¹⁄₈ of pkg.	190	25.0
No cholesterol recipe	¹⁄₈ of pkg.	180	25.0
(Duncan Hines):			
Blueberry	¹⁄₁₂ of pkg.	97	16.2
& honey	¹⁄₁₂ of pkg.	129	20.7
*Oatmeal raisin (Betty Crocker):			
Regular	¹⁄₁₂ of pkg.	140	22.0
No cholesterol recipe	¹⁄₁₂ of pkg.	130	22.0

Food and Description	Measure or Quantity	Calories	Carbo-hydrates (grams)
Pecan nut (Duncan Hines) bakery style	¹/₁₂ of pkg.	211	27.3
MUSCATEL WINE (Gallo) 14% alcohol	3 fl. oz.	86	7.9
MUSHROOM:			
Raw (USDA):			
Whole	½ lb. (weighed untrimmed)	62	9.7
Trimmed, sliced	½ cup (1.2 oz.)	10	1.5
Canned (Green Giant) solids & liq., whole or sliced,	¼ cup	12	2.0
Frozen (Birds Eye)	⅓ of 8-oz. pkg.	19	4.0
MUSHROOM, CHINESE, dried (HEW/FAO):			
Dry	1 oz.	81	18.9
Soaked, drained	1 oz.	12	2.4
MUSKELLUNGE, raw (USDA):			
Whole	1 lb. (weighed whole)	242	0.
Meat only	4 oz.	234	0.
MUSKMELON (See CANTALOUPE; CASABA; HONEYDEW; etc.)			
MUSKRAT, roasted (USDA)	4 oz.	174	0.
MUSSEL (USDA):			
Atlantic & Pacific, raw:			
In shell	1 lb. (weighed in shell)	153	7.2
Meat only	4 oz.	108	3.7
Pacific, canned, drained	4 oz.	129	1.7

(USDA) = United States Department of Agriculture
(HHS/FAO) = Health and Human Services/Food and Agriculture
           Organization
* = prepared as package directs

Food and Description	Measure or Quantity	Calories	Carbo- hydrates (grams)
MUSTARD:			
Powdered (dry) (French's)	1 tsp. (1.5 grams)	9	.3
Prepared:			
Brown (French's; Gulden's)	1 tsp.	5	.3
Chinese (Chun King)	1 tsp.	5	.3
Cream salad (French's)	1 tsp.	3	.3
Dijon, *Grey Poupon*	1 tsp. (.2 oz.)	6	Tr.
Horseradish (French's)	1 tsp. (.2 oz.)	5	.3
Medford (French's)	1 tsp.	5	.3
Onion (French's)	1 tsp.	8	1.6
Yellow (Gulden's)	1 tsp.	5	.4
MUSTARD GREENS:			
Raw (USDA) whole	1 lb. (weighed untrimmed)	98	17.8
Boiled (USDA) drained	1 cup (7.8 oz.)	51	8.8
Canned (Allen's) chopped, solids & liq.	½ cup (4.1 oz.)	20	2.0
Frozen, chopped:			
(Bel-Air)	3.3 oz.	20	3.0
(Birds Eye)	⅓ of 10-oz. pkg.	25	3.2
(Frosty Acres)	3.3-oz. serving	20	3.0
MUSTARD SPINACH (USDA):			
Raw	1 lb.	100	17.7
Boiled, drained, no added salt	4-oz. serving	18	3.2

Food and Description	Measure or Quantity	Calories	Carbo-hydrates (grams)

N

NATHAN'S:
French fries	1 reg. order	550	60.0
Hamburger	4½-oz. sandwich	360	18.0
Hot dog	3.4-oz. serving	290	19.0

NATURAL CEREAL:
Familia:
Regular	½ cup (1.8 oz.)	187	34.8
With bran	½ cup (1.7 oz.)	166	29.0
With granola	½ cup (2.0 oz.)	257	37.2
No added salt	½ cup (1.8 oz.)	181	32.1

Heartland:
Plain, coconut or raisin	¼ cup (1 oz.)	130	18.0
Trail mix	¼ cup (1 oz.)	120	19.0

Nature Valley:
Cinnamon & raisin	⅓ cup (1 oz.)	120	20.0
Fruit & nut or toasted oat	⅓ cup (1 oz.)	130	19.0

NATURE SNACKS (Sun-Maid):
Carob Crunch	1 oz.	143	16.8
Carob Peanut	1¼ oz.	190	18.0
Carob Raisin or Yogurt Raisin	1¼ oz.	160	25.0
Nuts Galore	1 oz.	170	5.0
Raisin Crunch or Rocky Road	1 oz.	126	19.1
Sesame Nut Crunch	1 oz.	154	14.6
Tahitian Treat or Yogurt Crunch	1 oz.	123	19.4
Yogurt Peanut	1¼ oz.	200	18.0

NECTARINE, fresh (USDA):
Whole	1 lb. (weighed with pits)	267	71.4

(USDA) = United States Department of Agriculture
(HHS/FAO) = Health and Human Services/Food and Agriculture Organization
* = prepared as package directs

Food and Description	Measure or Quantity	Calories	Carbo-hydrates (grams)
Flesh only	4 oz.	73	19.4
NINTENDO CEREAL SYSTEM, cereal (Ralston Purina)	1 cup (1 oz.)	110	25.0
NOODLE (See also **SPAGHETTI**). Plain noodle products are essentially the same in caloric value and carbohydrate content on the same weight basis. The longer they are cooked, the more water is absorbed and this affects the nutritive values. Also, the longer they are cooked, the amount of calories decreases somewhat. (USDA):			
Dry	1 oz.	110	20.4
Dry, 1½″ strips	1 cup (2.6 oz.)	283	52.6
Cooked	1 oz.	35	6.6
NOODLES & BEEF:			
Canned (Hormel) *Short Orders*	7½-oz. can	230	16.0
Frozen (Banquet)	2-lb. pkg.	800	88.0
NOODLES & CHICKEN:			
Canned (Hormel) *Dinty Moore, Short Orders*	7½-oz. can	210	15.0
Frozen (Swanson)	10½-oz. dinner	280	45.0
NOODLES, CHOW MEIN:			
(Chun King)	1 oz.	139	16.5
(La Choy)	½ cup (1 oz.)	150	16.0
NOODLE MIX:			
(Lipton) & Sauce:			
Alfredo:			
Regular	¼ of pkg.	131	20.4
Carbonara	¼ of pkg.	126	20.2
Beef	¼ of pkg.	120	21.7
Butter	¼ of pkg.	142	21.7
Butter & herb	¼ of pkg.	136	21.8
Cheese	¼ of pkg.	136	23.9
Chicken	¼ of pkg.	125	21.8
Parmesan	¼ of pkg.	138	20.2
Sour cream & chive	¼ of pkg.	142	22.6

Food and Description	Measure or Quantity	Calories	Carbohydrates (grams)
Stroganoff	¼ of pkg.	110	19.1
Noodle Roni, parmesano	⅕ of 6-oz. pkg.	130	21.0
NOODLES, RICE (La Choy)	1 oz.	130	21.0
NOODLE ROMANOFF, frozen (Stouffer's)	⅓ of 12-oz. pkg.	170	15.0
NUT (See specific variety such as **CASHEW NUT; COCONUT; PEANUT;** etc.)			
NUT, MIXED:			
Dry roasted:			
(Flavor House) salted	1 oz.	172	5.4
(Planters)	1 oz.	160	7.0
Oil roasted (Planters) with or without peanuts	1 oz.	180	6.0
NUT & HONEY CRUNCH, cereal (Kellogg's)	⅔ cup (1 oz.)	110	24.0
NUT & HONEY CRUNCH Os, cereal (Kellogg's)	⅔ cup (1 oz.)	110	22.0
NUTMEG (French's)	1 tsp. (1.9 grams)	11	.9
NUTRIFIC, cereal (Kellogg's)	1 cup (1.3 oz.)	120	28.0
NUTRI-GRAIN, cereal (Kellogg's):			
Almond raisin	⅔ cup (1.4 oz.)	140	31.0
Raisin bran	1 cup (1.4 oz.)	130	31.0
Wheat	⅔ cup (1 oz.)	100	24.0

Food and Description	Measure or Quantity	Calories	Carbohydrates (grams)

0

Food and Description	Measure or Quantity	Calories	Carbohydrates (grams)
OATBAKE, cereal (Kellogg's)	⅓ (1 oz.)	110	21.0
OAT FLAKES, cereal (Post)	⅔ cup (1 oz.)	107	21.5
OATMEAL:			
Dry:			
Regular:			
(USDA)	½ cup (1.2 oz.)	140	44.5
(Elam's):			
Scotch style or stone ground	1 oz.	108	18.2
Steel cut, whole grain	¼ cup (1.6 oz.)	174	30.4
(H-O) old fashioned	1 T. (.14 oz.)	14	2.6
(Safeway)	1 oz.	100	18.0
(3-Minute Brand)	⅓ cup (1 oz.)	160	24.0
Instant:			
(H-O):			
Regular, boxed	1 T.	15	2.6
Regular, packets	1-oz. packet	105	17.9
With bran & spice	1½-oz. packet	157	29.0
Country apple & brown sugar	1.1-oz. packet	121	22.7
With maple & brown sugar flavor	1½-oz. packet	160	31.8
Sweet & mellow	1.4-oz. packet	149	28.7
Oatmeal Swirlers (General Mills):			
Apple cinnamon	1.7-oz. pkg.	160	24.0
Cherry or strawberry	1.7-oz. pkg.	150	32.0
Cinnamon spice or maple brown sugar	1.6-oz. pkg.	160	35.0
Milk chocolate	1.7-oz. pkg	170	37.0
(3-Minute Brand):			
Regular	1-oz.-pkg.	160	26.0
Apple cinnamon	1⅜-oz. pkg.	210	37.0
Cinnamon & spice	1½-oz. pkg.	240	41.0
Maple & brown sugar	1½-oz. pkg.	220	38.0

Food and Description	Measure or Quantity	Calories	Carbo-hydrates (grams)
Total (General Mills):			
Regular	1.2-oz. pkg.	110	22.0
Apple cinnamon	1¼-oz. pkg.	150	32.0
Cinnamon raisin	1.8-oz. pkg.	170	38.0
Maple brown sugar	1.6-oz. pkg.	160	34.0
Cooked:			
Regular (USDA)	1 cup (8.5 oz.)	132	23.3
Quick:			
(Harvest Brand)	⅓ cup (1 oz.)	110	18.1
(H-O)	½ cup (1.2 oz.)	129	22.2
(Quaker)	⅓ cup (1 oz.)	109	18.5
(Ralston Purina)	⅓ cup (1 oz.)	110	18.0
(Safeway)	1 oz.	100	18.0
Total (General Mills)	1 oz.	90	18.0
OCTOPUS, raw (USDA) meat only	4 oz.	83	0.
OIL, SALAD OR COOKING:			
(USDA) all kinds, including olive	1 T. (.5 oz.)	124	0.
(USDA) all kinds, including olive	½ cup (3.9 oz.)	972	0.
(Bertoli) olive	1 T.	120	0.
(Calavo) avocado	1 T.	120	0.
(Country Pure) canola	1 T.	120	0.
Crisco, Fleischmann's; Mazola	1 T. (.5 oz.)	120	0.
(Golden Thistle; *Goya*)	1 T. (.5 oz.)	130	0.
Mrs. Tucker's, corn or soybean	1 T.	130	0.
(Planters) peanut or popcorn	1 T.	130	0.
Sunlite; Wesson	1 T.	120	0.
OKRA:			
Raw (USDA) whole	1 lb. (weighed untrimmed)	140	29.6
Boiled (USDA) drained:			
Whole	½ cup (3.1 oz.)	26	5.3
Pods	8 pods (3 oz.)	25	5.1
Slices	½ cup (2.8 oz.)	23	4.8

(USDA) = United States Department of Agriculture
(HHS/FAO) = Health and Human Services/Food and Agriculture Organization
* = prepared as package directs

Food and Description	Measure or Quantity	Calories	Carbo-hydrates (grams)
Frozen:			
(Bel-Air):			
Cut	3.3 oz.	25	6.0
Whole	3.3 oz.	30	7.0
(Birds Eye)			
Whole, baby	⅓ of 10-oz. pkg.	36	6.7
Cut	⅓ of 10-oz. pkg.	30	5.7
(Frosty Acres):			
Cut	3.3-oz. serving	25	6.0
Whole	3.3-oz. serving	30	7.0
(McKenzie):			
Cut	3.3 oz.	30	6.0
Whole	3.3 oz.	35	7.0
(Ore-Ida) breaded	3 oz.	170	17.0
OLIVE:			
Greek style (USDA):			
With pits, drained	1 oz.	77	2.0
Pitted, drained	1 oz.	96	2.5
Green (USDA)	1 oz.	33	.4
Ripe, by variety (USDA):			
Ascalano, any size, pitted & drained	1 oz.	37	.7
Manzanilla, any size	1 oz.	37	.7
Mission	3 small or 2 large	18	.3
Mission, slices	½ cup (2.2 oz.)	26	6.1
Ripe, by size (Lindsay):			
Colossal	1 olive	9	.6
Extra large	1 olive	6	.3
Jumbo	1 olive	7	.5
Large	1 olive	6	.4
Medium	1 olive	3	.2
Super colossal	1 olive	11	.8
ONION (See also **ONION, GREEN; ONION, WELCH**):			
Raw (USDA):			
Whole	1 lb. (weighed untrimmed)	157	35.9
Whole	3.9-oz. onion (2½″ dia.)	38	8.7

Food and Description	Measure or Quantity	Calories	Carbo-hydrates (grams)
Chopped	½ cup (3 oz.)	33	7.5
Chopped	1 T. (.4 oz.)	4	1.0
Grated	1 T. (.5 oz.)	5	1.2
Slices	½ cup (2 oz.)	21	4.9
Boiled, drained (USDA):			
Whole	½ cup (3.7 oz.)	30	6.8
Whole, pearl onions	½ cup (3.2 oz.)	27	6.0
Halves or pieces	½ cup (3.2 oz.)	26	5.8
Canned, O & C (Durkee):			
Boiled	1-oz. serving	8	2.0
In cream sauce	1-oz. serving	143	17.0
Dehydrated:			
Flakes:			
(USDA)	1 tsp. (1.3 grams)	5	1.1
(Gilroy)	1 tsp.	5	1.2
Powder (Gilroy)	1 tsp.	9	2.0
French fried (Durkee), canned	¼ cup (13 grams)	80	5
Frozen:			
(Bel-Air) chopped	1 oz.	8	2.0
(Birds Eye):			
Chopped	1 oz.	8	2.0
Small, whole	¼ of 16-oz. pkg.	44	9.6
Small, with cream sauce	⅓ of 9-oz. pkg.	118	11.2
(Frosty Acres) chopped	1 oz.	8	2.0
(Mrs. Paul's) rings, breaded & fried	½ of 5-oz. pkg.	190	19.0
(Ore-Ida) chopped	2 oz.	20	4.0
ONION, COCKTAIL (Vlasic) lightly spiced	1 oz.	4	1.0
ONION, GREEN, raw (USDA):			
Whole	1 lb. (weighed untrimmed)	157	35.7
Bulb & entire top	1 oz.	10	2.3
Bulb without green top	3 small onions (.9 oz.)	11	2.6
Slices, bulb & white portion of top	½ cup (1.8 oz.)	22	5.2
Tops only	1 oz.	8	1.6

(USDA) = United States Department of Agriculture
(HHS/FAO) = Health and Human Services/Food and Agriculture Organization
* = prepared as package directs

Food and Description	Measure or Quantity	Calories	Carbo-hydrates (grams)
ONION, WELCH, raw (USDA):			
Whole	1 lb. (weighed untrimmed)	100	19.2
Trimmed	4 oz.	39	7.4
ONION BOUILLON:			
(Herb-Ox):			
Cube	1 cube	10	1.3
Packet	1 packet	14	2.1
MBT	1 packet	16	2.0
(Wyler's)	1 tsp.	10	1.0
ONION SALT (French's)	1 tsp.	6	1.0
ONION SOUP (See **SOUP,** Onion)			
OPOSSUM (USDA) roasted, meat only	4 oz.	251	0.
ORANGE, fresh (USDA):			
California Navel:			
Whole	1 lb. (weighed with rind & seeds)	157	39.3
Whole	6.3-oz. orange (2⅘″ dia.)	62	15.5
Sections	1 cup (8.5 oz.)	123	30.6
California Valencia:			
Whole	1 lb. (weighed with rind & seeds)	174	42.2
Fruit, including peel	6.3-oz. orange (2⅝″ dia.)	72	27.9
Sections	1 cup (8.6 oz.)	123	29.9
Florida, all varieties:			
Whole	1 lb. (weighed with rind & seeds)	158	40.3
Whole	7.4-oz. orange (3″ dia.)	73	18.6
Sections	1 cup (8.5 oz.)	113	28.9
ORANGE, MANDARIN (See **TANGERINE**)			

Food and Description	Measure or Quantity	Calories	Carbo-hydrates (grams)
ORANGE DRINK:			
Canned:			
(Ardmore Farms)	6 fl. oz.	86	20.9
(Borden) *Bama*	8.45-fl.-oz. container	120	29.0
(Hi-C)	6 fl. oz.	95	23.3
(Johanna Farms) *Ssips*	8.45-fl.-oz. container	130	32.0
(Lincoln)	6 fl. oz.	90	23.0
*Mix:			
Regular:			
(Funny Face)	8 fl. oz.	88	22.0
(Town House)	6 fl. oz.	90	22.0
Dietetic:			
Crystal Light	6 fl. oz.	4	.4
(Sunkist)	8 fl. oz.	8	2.0
ORANGE EXTRACT (Virginia Dare) 79% alcohol	1 tsp.	22	0.
ORANGE FRUIT JUICE BLEND, canned (Mott's)	9.5 fl. oz.	139	34.0
ORANGE-GRAPEFRUIT JUICE:			
Canned:			
(Del Monte):			
Sweetened	6 fl. oz.	91	21.1
Unsweetened	6 fl. oz.	79	18.3
(Libby's) unsweetened	6 fl. oz.	80	19.0
*Frozen (Minute Maid) unsweetened	6 fl. oz.	76	19.1
ORANGE JUICE:			
Fresh (USDA):			
California Navel	½ cup (4.4 oz.)	60	14.0
California Valencia	½ cup (4.4 oz.)	58	13.0
Florida, early or midseason	½ cup (4.4 oz.)	50	11.4
Florida Temple	½ cup (4.4 oz.)	67	16.0
Florida Valencia	½ cup (4.4 oz.)	56	13.0

(USDA) = United States Department of Agriculture
(HHS/FAO) = Health and Human Services/Food and Agriculture Organization
* = prepared as package directs

Food and Description	Measure or Quantity	Calories	Carbo-hydrates (grams)
Canned, unsweetened:			
(USDA)	½ cup (4.4 oz.)	60	13.9
(Ardmore Farms)	6 fl. oz.	84	20.1
(Borden) *Sippin' Pak*	8.45-fl.-oz. container	110	26.0
(Johanna Farms)	6 fl. oz.	84	19.5
(Land O' Lakes)	6 fl. oz.	90	22.0
(Ocean Spray)	6 fl. oz.	90	18.0
(Town House)	6 fl. oz.	82	21.0
(Tree Top)	6 fl. oz.	90	22.0
Canned, sweetened:			
(USDA)	6 fl. oz.	66	15.4
(Del Monte)	6 fl. oz.	76	17.4
Chilled:			
(Citrus Hill):			
Regular	6 fl. oz.	90	20.0
Lite	6 fl. oz.	60	14.0
(Minute Maid):			
Regular	6 fl. oz.	91	21.9
Calcium fortified	6 fl. oz.	93	21.9
Reduced acid	6 fl. oz.	89	21.9
(Sunkist)	6 fl. oz.	76	17.7
*Dehydrated crystals (USDA)	½ cup (4.4 oz.)	57	13.4
*Frozen:			
(USDA)	½ cup (4.4 oz.)	56	13.3
(Citrus Hill):			
Regular	6 fl. oz.	90	20.0
Lite	6 fl. oz.	60	14.0
(Minute Maid) regular	6 fl. oz.	91	21.9
(Sunkist)	6 fl. oz.	84	20.1
ORANGE JUICE BAR, frozen (Sunkist)	3-fl.-oz. bar	72	17.6
ORANGE PEEL, CANDIED (USDA)	1 oz.	90	22.9
ORANGE-PINEAPPLE-BANANA JUICE, canned (Land O' Lakes)	6 fl. oz.	100	24.0
ORANGE-PINEAPPLE DRINK, canned (Lincoln)	6 fl. oz.	90	23.0

Food and Description	Measure or Quantity	Calories	Carbo-hydrates (grams)
ORANGE-PINEAPPLE JUICE, canned (Land O' Lakes)	6 fl. oz.	90	23.0
OREGANO (French's)	1 tsp.	6	1.0
OVEN FRY (General Foods):			
Chicken:			
Extra crispy	4.2-oz. pkg.	461	82.4
Homestyle flour	3.2-oz. pkg.	339	60.5
Pork, *Shake & Bake,* extra crispy	4.2-oz. pkg.	482	83.1
OYSTER:			
Raw (USDA):			
Eastern, meat only	19–31 small or 13–19 med.	158	8.2
Pacific & Western, meat only	6–9 small or 4–6 med. (8.5 oz.)	218	15.4
Canned (Bumble Bee) shelled, whole, solids & liq.	1 cup (8.5 oz.)	218	15.4
Fried (USDA) dipped in milk, egg & breadcrumbs	4 oz.	271	21.1
OYSTER STEW (USDA):			
Home recipe:			
1 part oysters to 1 part milk by volume	1 cup (8.5 oz., 6–8 oysters)	245	14.2
1 part oysters to 2 parts milk by volume	1 cup (8.5 oz.)	233	10.8
1 part oysters to 3 parts milk by volume	1 cup (8.5 oz.)	206	11.3
Frozen:			
Prepared with equal volume milk	1 cup (8.5 oz.)	201	14.2
Prepared with equal volume water	1 cup (8.5 oz.)	122	8.2

(USDA) = United States Department of Agriculture
(HHS/FAO) = Health and Human Services/Food and Agriculture Organization
* = prepared as package directs

Food and Description	Measure or Quantity	Calories	Carbo- hydrates (grams)

P

Food and Description	Measure or Quantity	Calories	Carbo- hydrates (grams)
PAC-MAN, cereal (General Mills)	1 cup (1 oz.)	110	25.0
PANCAKE, frozen:			
(Pillsbury) microwave:			
Regular	1 pancake	80	15.7
Blueberry	1 pancake	83	16.3
Buttermilk	1 pancake	87	17.0
Harvest wheat	1 pancake	80	19.0
(Swanson) *Great Starts*:			
With bacon	4½-oz. meal	400	43.0
& sausage	6-oz. meal	460	52.0
Silver dollar & sausage	3¾-oz. meal	310	37.0
Whole wheat, & lite links	5½-oz. meal	350	39.0
*PANCAKE BATTER, frozen (Aunt Jemima):			
Plain	4″ pancake	70	14.1
Blueberry or buttermilk	4″ pancake	68	13.8
Buttermilk	4″ pancake	68	14.2
*PANCAKE & WAFFLE MIX:			
Plain:			
(Aunt Jemima):			
Original	4″ pancake	73	8.7
Complete	4″ pancake	80	15.7
Bisquick Shake 'N Pour:			
Regular	4″ pancake	87	16.0
Complete	1 waffle	140	25.5
Fastshake (Little Crow)	½ container	266	50.0
(Mrs. Butterworth's):			
Regular	4″ pancakes	73	13.4
Complete	4″ pancake	63	12.3
(Pillsbury) *Hungry Jack*:			
Extra Lights, regular	4″ pancake	70	10.0
Panshakes	4″ pancake	83	14.3

Food and Description	Measure or Quantity	Calories	Carbo-hydrates (grams)
*Apple cinnamon, *Bisquick Shake 'N Pour*	4" pancake	90	16.3
Blueberry (Pillsbury) *Hungry Jack*	4" pancake	107	9.7
Buttermilk:			
(Betty Crocker):			
Regular	4" pancake	93	13.0
Complete	4" pancake	70	13.7
(Mrs. Butterworth's)	4" pancake	63	12.3
(Pillsbury) *Hungry Jack:*			
Regular	4" pancake	80	9.7
Complete	4" pancake	63	13.0
Dietetic:			
(Estee)	3" pancake	33	7.0
(Featherweight) low sodium	4" pancake	43	8.0

PANCAKE & WAFFLE SYRUP (See **SYRUP,** Pancake & Waffle)

PANCREAS, raw (USDA):

Beef, lean only	4 oz.	160	0.
Calf	4 oz.	183	0.
Hog or hog sweetbread	4 oz.	274	0.

PAPAW, fresh (USDA):

Whole	1 lb. (weighed with rind & seeds)	289	57.2
Flesh only	4 oz.	96	19.1

PAPAYA, fresh (USDA):

Whole	1 lb. (weighed with skin & seeds)	119	30.4
Cubed	1 cup (6.4 oz.)	71	18.2

PAPAYA JUICE, canned (HEW/FAO) | 4 oz. | 77 | 19.6 |

(USDA) = United States Department of Agriculture
(HHS/FAO) = Health and Human Services/Food and Agriculture
        Organization
* = prepared as package directs

Food and Description	Measure or Quantity	Calories	Carbohydrates (grams)
PAPRIKA, domestic (French's)	1 tsp.	7	1.1
PARSLEY, fresh (USDA):			
Whole	½ lb.	100	19.3
Chopped	1 T. (4 grams)	2	.3
PARSLEY FLAKES, dehydrated (French's)	1 tsp. (1.1 grams)	4	.6
PARSNIP (USDA):			
Raw, whole	1 lb. (weighed unprepared)	293	67.5
Boiled, drained, cut in pieces	½ cup (3.7 oz.)	70	15.8
PASSION FRUIT, fresh (USDA):			
Whole	1 lb. (weighed with shell)	212	50.0
Pulp & seeds	4 oz.	102	24.0
PASSION FRUIT JUICE, fresh (HEW/FAO)	4 oz.	50	11.5
PASTA ACCENTS, frozen (Green Giant):			
Creamy cheddar	⅙ of 16-oz. pkg.	100	12.0
Garden herb	⅙ of 16-oz. pkg.	80	11.0
Garlic or primavera	⅙ of 16-oz. pkg.	110	13.0
PASTA DINNER OR ENTREE:			
Canned (Franco-American):			
Circus O's:			
With meatballs	7⅜-oz. can	210	25.0
In tomato & cheese sauce	7⅜-oz. can	170	33.0
Sporty O's:			
With meatballs	7⅜-oz. can	210	25.0
In tomato & cheese sauce	7⅜-oz. can	170	33.0
Frozen:			
(Birds Eye):			
Continental	5-oz. serving	164	16.0
Marinara	5-oz. serving	115	21.0
Primavera	5-oz. serving	204	21.7
(Celetano) & cheese, baked	6-oz. serving	280	41.0

Food and Description	Measure or Quantity	Calories	Carbo-hydrates (grams)
(Green Giant):			
Dijon	9½-oz. meal	260	21.0
Florentine	9½-oz. meal	230	27.0
Marinara	6-oz. meal	180	29.0
Parmesan	5½-oz. meal	170	24.0
(Stouffer's):			
Carbonara	9¾-oz. meal	620	34.0
Casino	9¼-oz. meal	300	44.0
Mexicali	10-oz. meal	490	36.0
Oriental	9⅞-oz. meal	300	25.0
Primavera	10⅝-oz. meal	270	13.0
(Weight Watchers):			
Primavera	8½-oz. meal	260	22.0
Rigati	11-oz. meal	290	30.0
PASTA SALAD, frozen			
(Birds Eye) Italian style	5-oz. serving	170	22.2
*PASTA & SAUCE, mix			
(Lipton):			
Cheddar broccoli with fusilli	¼ of pkg.	135	23.9
Cheese supreme	¼ of pkg.	139	23.8
Garlic, creamy	¼ of pkg.	144	25.3
Mushroom & chicken	¼ of pkg.	124	23.4
Mushroom, creamy	¼ of pkg.	143	24.8
Oriental with fusilli	¼ of pkg.	130	25.5
Tomato, herb	¼ of pkg.	130	26.0
PASTINA, DRY (USDA):			
Carrot	1 oz.	105	21.5
Egg	1 oz.	109	20.4
Spinach	1 oz.	104	21.2
PASTRAMI, packaged:			
(Carl Buddig) smoked, sliced	1 oz.	40	Tr.
Hebrew National, 1st cut	1 oz.	44	<1.0
(Oscar Mayer)	.6-oz. slice	16	.1
PASTRY SHEET, PUFF, frozen			
(Pepperidge Farm)	1 sheet	1040	88.0

(USDA) = United States Department of Agriculture
(HHS/FAO) = Health and Human Services/Food and Agriculture Organization
* = prepared as package directs

Food and Description	Measure or Quantity	Calories	Carbo-hydrates (grams)
PASTRY SHELL, frozen:			
(Pepperidge Farm) regular	1 shell (1.7 oz.)	210	16.0
(Pet-Ritz)	3" shell	150	12.0
PÂTÉ:			
De foie gras (USDA)	1 T. (.5 oz.)	69	.7
Liver:			
(Hormel)	1 T.	35	.3
(Sell's)	½ of 4.8-oz. can	223	2.7
PEA, GREEN:			
Raw (USDA):			
In pod	1 lb. (weighed in pod)	145	24.8
Shelled	1 lb.	381	65.3
Shelled	½ cup (2.4 oz.)	58	9.9
Boiled (USDA) drained	½ cup (2.9 oz.)	58	9.9
Canned, regular pack:			
(USDA):			
Alaska, early or June:			
Solids & liq.	½ cup (4.4 oz.)	82	15.5
Solids only	½ cup (3 oz.)	76	14.4
Sweet:			
Solids & liq.	½ cup (4.4 oz.)	71	12.9
Solids only	½ cup (3 oz.)	69	12.9
Drained liquid	4 oz.	25	4.9
(Green Giant)	½ cup	50	12.0
(Larsen) *Freshlike*	½ cup (4.4 oz.)	50	10.0
(Town House)	½ cup	70	14.0
Canned, dietetic pack:			
(USDA):			
Alaska, early or June:			
Solids & liq.	4 oz.	62	11.1
Solids only	4 oz.	88	16.2
Sweet:			
Solids & liq.	4 oz.	53	9.5
Solids only	4 oz.	82	14.7
(Del Monte) no salt added, sweet, solids & liq.	½ cup (4.3 oz.)	60	11.0
(Diet Delight) solids & liq.	½ cup (4.3 oz.)	50	8.0
(Larsen) *Fresh-Lite*, no salt added	½ cup (4.4 oz.)	50	10.0
Frozen:			
(Bel-Air)	3.3 oz.	80	13.0

Food and Description	Measure or Quantity	Calories	Carbo- hydrates (grams)
(Birds Eye):			
Regular	⅓ of 10-oz. pkg.	78	13.3
In butter sauce	⅓ of 10-oz. pkg.	85	12.6
In cream sauce	⅓ of 8-oz. pkg.	84	14.3
Tiny, tender, deluxe	⅓ of 10-oz. pkg.	64	10.7
(Frosty Acres):			
Regular	3.3-oz. serving	80	13.0
Tiny	3.3-oz. serving	60	11.0
(Green Giant):			
Early June:			
Butter sauce, One Serving	4½-oz. pkg.	90	16.0
Harvest Fresh	½ cup (3 oz.)	60	13.0
Polybag	½ cup (2.7 oz.)	50	11.0
Sweet:			
Regular, Harvest Fresh or polybag	½ cup	50	11.0
Butter sauce	½ cup (4 oz.)	80	14.0
(Le Sueur) early, in butter sauce	⅓ of 10-oz. pkg.	67	11.7
(McKenzie):			
Regular	3.3 oz.	80	13.0
Tiny	3.3 oz.	60	10.0
PEA, CHOWDER, frozen:			
(Birds Eye)	⅕ of 16-oz. pkg.	130	22.6
(McKenzie)	3-oz. serving	130	23.0
(Southland)	⅕ of 16-oz. pkg.	130	23.0
PEA, MATURE SEED, dry			
(USDA):			
Whole	1 lb.	1542	272.5
Whole	1 cup	680	120.6
Split	1 lb.	1579	284.4
Split	1 cup (7.2 oz.)	706	127.3
Cooked, split, drained solids	½ cup (3.4 oz.)	112	20.2

(USDA) = United States Department of Agriculture
(HHS/FAO) = Health and Human Services/Food and Agriculture Organization
* = prepared as package directs

Food and Description	Measure or Quantity	Calories	Carbo-hydrates (grams)
PEA & CARROT:			
Canned, regular pack, solids & liq.:			
(Larsen) *Freshlike*	½ cup (4.6 oz.)	50	12.0
(Veg-All)	½ cup	50	12.0
Canned, dietetic pack, solids & liq.:			
(Diet Delight)	½ cup (4.3 oz.)	40	6.0
(Larsen) *Freshlike*, no salt added	½ cup (4.6 oz.)	50	12.0
Frozen:			
(Bel-Air)	3.3 oz.	60	11.0
(Birds Eye)	⅓ of 10-oz. pkg.	61	11.2
(Frosty Acres)	3.3-oz. serving	60	11.0
(McKenzie)	3.3-oz. serving	60	11.0
PEA & ONION:			
Canned (Larsen)	½ cup	60	12.0
Frozen (Birds Eye)	⅓ of 10-oz. pkg.	67	11.7
PEA POD:			
Raw (USDA) edible podded or Chinese	1 lb. (weighed untrimmed)	228	51.7
Boiled (USDA) drained	4 oz.	49	10.8
Frozen (La Choy)	6-oz. pkg.	70	12.0
PEA PUREE, canned (Larsen) no salt added	½ cup	50	10.0
PEACH:			
Fresh (USDA):			
Whole, without skin	1 lb. (weighed unpeeled)	150	38.3
Whole	4-oz. peach (2" dia.)	38	9.6
Diced	½ cup (4.7 oz.)	51	12.9
Sliced	½ cup (3 oz.)	31	8.2
Canned, regular pack, solids & liq.:			
(USDA):			
Extra heavy syrup	4 oz.	110	28.5
Heavy syrup	2 med. halves & 2 T. syrup (4.1 oz.)	91	23.5

Food and Description	Measure or Quantity	Calories	Carbo-hydrates (grams)
Juice pack	4 oz.	51	13.2
Light syrup	4 oz.	66	17.1
(Del Monte):			
Cling:			
Halves or slices	½ cup (4 oz.)	80	22.0
Spices	3½ oz.	80	20.0
Freestone	½ cup (4 oz.)	90	23.0
(Hunt's) halves or slices	4 oz.	80	23.0
(Town House)	½ cup	100	25.0
Canned, dietetic pack, solids & liq.:			
(Country Pure) halves or pieces	½ cup	50	14.0
(Del Monte) Lite:			
Cling	½ cup (4 oz.)	50	13.0
Freestone	½ cup (4 oz.)	60	13.0
(Diet Delight) Cling:			
Juice pack	½ cup (4.4 oz.)	50	14.0
Water pack	½ cup (4.3 oz.)	30	2.0
Dehydrated (USDA):			
Uncooked	1 oz.	96	24.9
Cooked, with added sugar, solids & liq.	½ cup (5.4 oz.)	184	47.6
Dried (USDA):			
Uncooked	½ cup	231	60.1
Cooked:			
Unsweetened	½ cup	111	28.9
Sweetened	½ cup (5.4 oz.)	181	46.8
Frozen (Birds Eye) quick thaw	5-oz. serving	141	34.1
PEACH, STRAINED, canned (Larsen) no salt added	½ cup	65	17.0
PEACH BUTTER (Smucker's)	1 T. (.7 oz.)	45	12.0
PEACH DRINK, canned (Hi-C)	6 fl. oz.	101	24.8

(USDA) = United States Department of Agriculture
(HHS/FAO) = Health and Human Services/Food and Agriculture Organization
* = prepared as package directs

Food and Description	Measure or Quantity	Calories	Carbo-hydrates (grams)
PEACH JUICE, canned (Smucker's)	8 fl. oz.	120	30.0
PEACH LIQUEUR (DeKupyer)	1 fl. oz.	82	8.3
PEACH NECTAR, canned (Ardmore Farms)	6 fl. oz.	90	23.4
PEACH PARFAIT, frozen (Pepperidge Farm) dessert light	4½-oz. serving	150	24.0
PEACH PRESERVE OR JAM:			
Sweetened (Smucker's)	1 T. (.7 oz.)	54	12.0
Dietetic (Dia-Mel)	1 T.	6	0.
PEANUT:			
Raw (USDA):			
In shell	1 lb. (weighed in shell)	1868	61.6
With skins	1 oz.	160	5.3
Without skins	1 oz.	161	5.0
Roasted:			
(USDA):			
Whole	1 lb. (weighed in shell)	1769	62.6
Chopped	½ cup	404	13.0
Halves	½ cup	421	13.5
(Adams):			
Regular	1 oz.	170	5.0
Butter toffee	1 oz.	140	20.0
(Beer Nuts)	1 oz.	180	7.0
(Eagle):			
Fancy Virginia	1 oz.	180	6.0
Honey Roast	1 oz.	170	7.0
Lightly salted	1 oz.	170	5.0
(Fisher):			
In shell, salted	1 oz.	105	3.7
Shelled:			
Dry roasted, salted or unsalted	1 oz.	160	6.0
Oil roasted, salted	1 oz.	166	5.3
(Party Pride)	1 oz.	170	5.0

Food and Description	Measure or Quantity	Calories	Carbo-hydrates (grams)
(Planters):			
Dry roasted	1 oz. (jar)	160	6.0
Oil roasted	¾-oz. bag	170	5.0
(Tom's):			
In shell	1 oz.	120	3.4
Shelled:			
Dry roasted	1 oz.	160	5.0
Hot flavored	1 oz.	170	4.0
Redskin or toasted	1 oz.	170	5.0
Spanish, roasted:			
(Adams)	1 oz.	170	5.0
(Frito-Lay's)	1 oz.	168	6.6
(Planters):			
Dry roasted	1 oz. (jar)	175	3.4
Oil roasted	1 oz. (can)	182	3.4

PEANUT BUTTER:

Food and Description	Measure or Quantity	Calories	Carbo-hydrates (grams)
Regular:			
(Algood) *Cap'n Kid*	1 T.	85	3.0
(Bama)	1 T.	100	3.0
(Estee) low sodium	1 T.	100	3.0
(Home Brands)	1 T.	105	2.5
Jif, creamy or extra crunchy	1 T.	93	2.7
(Peter Pan):			
Crunchy	1 T. (.6 oz.)	95	2.9
Smooth	1 T. (.6 oz.)	95	2.5
(Skippy) creamy or super chunk	1 T.	95	2.1
(Smucker's) Goober Grape	1 T.	90	9.0
Dietetic:			
(Adams) low sodium	1 T. (.6 oz.)	95	2.5
(Algood)	1 T.	95	3.0
(Estee)	1 T.	100	3.0
(Home Brands):			
Lightly salted or unsalted	1 T.	105	2.5
No sugar added	1 T.	90	3.0
(Smucker's) no salt added	1 T.	100	3.0

(USDA) = United States Department of Agriculture
(HHS/FAO) = Health and Human Services/Food and Agriculture Organization
* = prepared as package directs

Food and Description	Measure or Quantity	Calories	Carbo-hydrates (grams)
PEANUT BUTTER BOPPERS (General Mills):			
Cookie crunch or fudge chip	1 bar	170	15.0
Fudge graham	1 bar	160	15.0
Honey crisp	1 bar	160	14.0
Peanut crunch	1 bar	170	13.0
PEANUT BUTTER MORSELS:			
(Nestlé)	1 oz.	160	12.0
(Reese's)	1 oz.	153	21.3
PEAR:			
Fresh (USDA):			
Whole	1 lb. (weighed with stems & core)	252	63.2
Whole	6.4-oz. pear (3″ × 2½″ dia.)	101	25.4
Quartered	1 cup (6.8 oz.)	117	29.4
Slices	½ cup (2.9 oz.)	50	12.5
Canned, regular pack, solids & liq.: (USDA):			
Extra heavy syrup	4 oz.	104	26.8
Heavy syrup	½ cup	87	22.3
Juice pack	4 oz.	52	13.4
Light syrup	4 oz.	69	17.7
(Hunt's) halves	4 oz.	90	22.0
(Town House) Bartlett, halves or sliced	½ cup	95	24.5
(Libby's) halves, heavy syrup	½ cup (4.5 oz.)	102	25.1
Canned, dietetic pack, solids & liq.:			
(Country Pure) halves or slices	½ cup	60	15.0
(Diet Delight):			
Juice pack	½ cup	60	16.0
Water pack	½ cup	35	9.0
(Libby's) water pack	½ cup	60	15.0
(S&W) *Nutradiet*, halves, quarters or slices, white or blue label	½ cup	35	10.0
Dried (Sun-Maid)	½ cup (3.5 oz.)	260	70.0

Food and Description	Measure or Quantity	Calories	Carbo-hydrates (grams)
PEAR, CANDIED (USDA)	1 oz.	86	21.5
PEAR, STRAINED, canned (Larsen) no salt added	½ cup	65	17.0
PEAR-APPLE JUICE (Tree Top) canned or frozen	6 fl. oz.	90	23.0
PEAR-GRAPE JUICE (Tree Top) canned or frozen	6 fl. oz.	100	26.0
PEAR NECTAR, canned:			
(Ardmore Farms)	6 fl. oz.	96	24.6
(Libby's)	6 fl. oz.	100	25.0
PEAR-PASSION FRUIT NECTAR, canned (Libby's)	6 fl. oz.	60	14.0
PEBBLES, cereal (Post):			
Cocoa	⅞ cup (1 oz.)	117	24.4
Fruity	⅞ cup (1 oz.)	116	24.5
PECAN:			
In shell (USDA)	1 lb. (weighed in shell)	1652	35.1
Shelled (USDA):			
Whole	1 lb.	3116	66.2
Chopped	½ cup (1.8 oz.)	357	7.6
Chopped	1 T. (7 grams)	48	1.0
Halves	12—14 halves (.5 oz.)	96	2.0
Halves	½ cup (1.9 oz.)	371	7.9
Oil dipped (Fisher) salted	¼ cup	410	8.9
Roasted, dry:			
(Fisher) salted	1 oz.	170	3.0
(Flavor House)	1 oz.	195	4.1
(Planters)	1 oz.	206	3.5
PEPPER, BANANA (Vlasic) hot rings	1 oz.	4	1.0

(USDA) = United States Department of Agriculture
(HHS/FAO) = Health and Human Services/Food and Agriculture Organization
* = prepared as package directs

Food and Description	Measure or Quantity	Calories	Carbo-hydrates (grams)
PEPPER, BLACK (French's):			
Regular	1 tsp. (2.3 grams)	9	1.5
Seasoned	1 tsp.	8	1.0
PEPPER, CHERRY (Vlasic)			
mild	1 oz.	8	2.0
PEPPER, CHILI:			
Raw, green (USDA) without seeds	4 oz.	42	10.3
Canned:			
(La Victoria):			
Marinated	1 T.	4	1.0
Nacho	1 T.	2	1.0
(Old El Paso) green, chopped or whole	1 oz.	7	1.4
(Ortega):			
Green, diced, strips or whole	1 oz.	10	2.6
Jalapeño, diced or whole	1 oz.	9	1.7
(Vlasic) Jalapeño	1 oz.	8	2.0
PEPPER, STUFFED:			
Home recipe (USDA) with beef & crumbs	2¾" × 2½" pepper with 1⅛ cups stuffing	314	31.1
Frozen:			
(Celentano) red, with beef, in sauce	12½-oz. pkg.	290	21.0
(Stouffer's) green with beef in tomato sauce	7¾-oz. serving	200	19.0
PEPPER, SWEET:			
Raw (USDA):			
Green:			
Whole	1 lb. (weighed untrimmed)	82	17.9
Without stem & seeds	1 med. pepper (2.6 oz.)	13	2.9
Chopped	½ cup (2.6 oz.)	16	3.6
Slices	½ cup (1.4 oz.)	9	2.0

Food and Description	Measure or Quantity	Calories	Carbo-hydrates (grams)
Red:			
Whole	1 lb. (weighed untrimmed)	112	25.8
Without stem & seeds	1 med. pepper (2.2 oz.)	19	2.4
Boiled, green, without salt, drained	1 med. pepper (2.6 oz.)	13	2.8
Frozen:			
(Bel-Air) green, diced	1 oz.	6	1.0
(Frosty Acres):			
Green	1-oz. serving	6	1.0
Red & green	2-oz. serving	15	2.0
(Larsen) green	1 oz.	6	1.0
(Southland):			
Green, diced	2-oz. serving	10	2.0
Red & green, cut	2-oz. serving	15	2.0
PEPPER & ONION, frozen			
(Southland)	2-oz. serving	15	2.0
PEPPER STEAK, frozen:			
(Armour):			
Classic Lite, beef	11¼-oz. meal	220	29.0
Dining Lite, oriental	9-oz. meal	260	33.0
(Healthy Choice) beef:			
Dinner	11-oz. dinner	290	35.0
Entree	9½-oz. entree	250	36.0
(La Choy) *Fresh & Lite*, with rice & vegetables	10-oz. meal	280	33.1
(Le Menu)	11½-oz. meal	370	36.0
(Stouffer's)	10½-oz. pkg.	330	36.0
*PEPPER STEAK MIX (Chun King) stir fry	6-oz. serving	249	8.6
PEPPERONI:			
(Eckrich)	1-oz. serving	135	1.0
(Hormel):			
Regular, chub, *Rosa* or *Rosa Grande*	1 oz.	140	0.

(USDA) = United States Department of Agriculture
(HHS/FAO) = Health and Human Services/Food and Agriculture Organization
* = prepared as package directs

Food and Description	Measure or Quantity	Calories	Carbohydrates (grams)
Canned bits	1 T.	35	0.
Leoni Brand	1 oz.	130	0.
Packaged, sliced	1 slice	40	0.
PERCH, OCEAN:			
Raw Atlantic, (USDA):			
Whole	1 lb. (weighed whole)	124	0.
Meat only	4 oz.	108	0.
Pacific, raw, whole	1 lb. (weighed whole)	116	0.
Frozen:			
(Captain's Choice)	3-oz. fillet	103	0.
(Frionor) *Norway Gourmet*	4-oz. piece	120	0.
(Gorton's) *Fishmarket Fresh*	4 oz.	140	2.0
(Van de Kamp's):			
Regular batter, dipped, french fried	2-oz. piece	135	10.0
Light & crispy	2-oz. piece	170	10.0
Today's Catch	4 oz.	110	0.
PERNOD (Julius Wile)	1 fl. oz.	79	1.1
PERSIMMON (USDA):			
Japanese or Kaki, fresh:			
With seeds	4.4-oz. piece	79	20.1
Seedless	4.4-oz. piece	81	20.7
Native, fresh, flesh only	4-oz. serving	144	38.0
PETIT SIRAH WINE (Louis M. Martini):			
Regular, 12½% alcohol	3 fl. oz.	61	.2
White, 12.3% alcohol	3 fl. oz.	54	Tr.
PHEASANT, raw (USDA) meat only	4-oz. serving	184	0.
PICKLE:			
Cucumber, fresh or bread & butter			
(USDA)	3 slices (.7 oz.)	15	3.8
(Fannings)	1.2-oz. serving	17	3.9
(Featherweight) low sodium	1-oz. pickle	12	3.0

Food and Description	Measure or Quantity	Calories	Carbo-hydrates (grams)
(Vlasic):			
Chips	1-oz. serving	30	7.0
Chunks	1-oz. serving	25	6.0
Stix	1-oz. serving	18	5.0
Dill:			
(USDA)	4.8-oz. pickle	15	3.0
(Claussen) halves	2 oz.	7	1.3
(Featherweight) low sodium, whole kosher	1-oz. serving	4	1.0
(Smucker's):			
Candied sticks	4" piece (.8 oz.)	45	11.0
Hamburger, sliced	1 slice (.13 oz.)	Tr.	0.
Polish, whole	3½" pickle (1.8 oz.)	8	1.0
Spears	3½" spear (1.4 oz.)	6	1.0
(Vlasic):			
No garlic	1-oz. serving	4	1.0
Original	1-oz. serving	2	1.0
Hamburger (Vlasic) chips	1-oz. serving	2	1.0
Hot & spicy (Vlasic) garden mix	1-oz. serving	4	1.0
Kosher dill:			
(Featherweight) low sodium	1-oz. serving	4	1.0
(Smucker's):			
Baby	2¾"-long pickle	4	.5
Slices	1 slice (.1 oz.)	Tr.	0.
Whole	3½"-long pickle (.5 oz.)	8	1.0
(Vlasic):			
Deli	1-oz. serving	4	1.0
Spear, regular or half-the-salt	1-oz. serving	4	1.0
Sour (USDA) cucumber	1 oz.	3	.6
Sweet:			
(Nalley's) *Nubbins*	1-oz. serving	28	7.9
(Smucker's):			
Candied mix	1 piece (.3 oz.)	14	3.3
Gherkins	2" long pickle (9 grams)	15	3.5

(USDA) = United States Department of Agriculture
(HHS/FAO) = Health and Human Services/Food and Agriculture Organization
* = prepared as package directs

Food and Description	Measure or Quantity	Calories	Carbo-hydrates (grams)
Slices	1 slice (.2 oz.)	11	2.3
Whole	2½" long pickle	18	4.0
(Vlasic) butter chips, half-the-salt	1-oz. serving	30	7.0
Sweet & sour (Claussen) slices	1 slice	3	.8

PIE:
Regular, non-frozen:
  Apple:

Food and Description	Measure or Quantity	Calories	Carbo-hydrates (grams)
Home recipe (USDA), 2-crust	⅙ of 9" pie	404	60.2
(Dolly Madison)	4½-oz. pie	490	59.0
Banana, home recipe (USDA), cream or custard, 1-crust	⅙ of 9" pie	336	46.7
Blackberry, home recipe (USDA) 2-crust	⅙ of 9" pie	384	54.4
Blueberry:			
Home recipe (USDA), 2-crust	⅙ of 9" pie	382	55.1
(Dolly Madison)	4½-oz. pie	430	56.0
Boston cream (USDA), home recipe, 1-crust	¹⁄₁₂ of 8" pie	208	34.4
Butterscotch (USDA), home recipe, 1-crust	⅙ of 9" pie	406	58.2
Cherry:			
Home recipe (USDA), 2-crust	⅙ of 9" pie	412	60.7
(Dolly Madison):			
Regular	4½-oz. pie	470	53.0
N' cream	4½-oz. pie	440	63.0
Chocolate (Dolly Madison):			
Regular	4½-oz. pie	560	74.0
Pudding	4½-oz. pie	500	53.0
Chocolate chiffon (USDA) home recipe, made with vegetable shortening, 1-crust	⅙ of 9" pie	459	61.2
Chocolate meringue (USDA), home recipe, made with vegetable shortening, 1-crust	⅙ of 9" pie	353	46.9
Coconut custard (USDA), home recipe, 1-crust	⅙ of 9" pie	357	37.8
Lemon (Dolly Madison)	4½-oz. pie	460	60.0

Food and Description	Measure or Quantity	Calories	Carbo-hydrates (grams)
Lemon meringue (USDA) 1-crust	⅙ of 9″ pie	357	52.8
Mince, home recipe, (USDA) 2-crust	⅙ of 9″ pie	428	65.1
Peach (Dolly Madison)	4½-oz. pie	460	54.0
Pecan, home recipe (USDA) 1-crust, made with lard or vegetable shortening	⅙ of 9″ pie	577	70.8
Pineapple, home recipe (USDA) 1- crust, made with lard or vegetable shortening	⅙ of 9″ pie	344	48.8
Pineapple custard, home recipe (USDA) made with lard or vegetable shortening	⅙ of 9″ pie (5.4 oz.)	400	60.2
Pumpkin, home recipe (USDA) 2-crust, made with lard or vegetable shortening	⅙ of 9″ pie (5.4 oz.)	321	37.2
Raisin, home recipe (USDA) 2-crust, made with lard or vegetable shortening	⅙ of 9″ pie (5.6 oz.)	427	67.9
Rhubarb, home recipe (USDA) 2-crust, made with lard or vegetable shortening	⅙ of 9″ pie (5.6 oz.)	400	60.4
Strawberry, home recipe (USDA) made with lard or vegetable shortening-1-crust	⅙ of 9″ pie (5.6 oz.)	313	48.8
Vanilla (Dolly Madison) pudding	4½-oz. pie	500	52.0
Frozen: Apple: (Banquet) family size	⅙ of 20-oz. pie	250	37.0
(Mrs. Smith's): Regular: Plain	⅛ of 8″ pie (3¼ oz.)	220	31.0
Plain	⅛ of 10″ pie (5¾ oz.)	390	55.0

(USDA) = United States Department of Agriculture
(HHS/FAO) = Health and Human Services/Food and Agriculture Organization
* = prepared as package directs

Food and Description	Measure or Quantity	Calories	Carbo-hydrates (grams)
Dutch	⅛ of 8″ pie (3¼ oz.)	250	37.0
Dutch	⅛ of 10″ pie (5¾ oz.)	430	64.0
Natural Juice:			
Plain	⅛ of 9″ pie (4.6 oz.)	370	45.0
Dutch	⅛ of 9″ pie (5.11 oz.	380	56.0
Pie In Minutes	⅛ of 25-oz. pie	210	29.0
(Pet-Ritz)	⅙ of 26-oz. pie	330	53.0
(Weight Watchers)	3½-oz. serving	200	39.0
Banana cream:			
(Banquet)	⅙ of 14-oz. pie	180	21.0
(Pet-Ritz)	⅙ of 14-oz. pie	170	22.0
Blackberry (Banquet)	⅙ of 20-oz. pie	270	40.0
Blueberry:			
(Banquet)	⅙ of 20-oz. pie	270	40.0
(Mrs. Smith's):			
Regular	⅛ of 8″ pie (3¼ oz.)	210	30.0
Natural Juice	⅛ of 9″ pie (4.6 oz.)	350	49.0
Pie In Minutes	⅛ of 26-oz. pie	220	32.0
(Pet-Ritz)	⅙ of 26-oz. pie	370	50.0
Cherry:			
(Banquet) family size	⅙ of 24-oz. pie	250	36.0
(Mrs. Smith's) Regular:			
Small	⅛ of 26-oz. pie	220	31.0
Large	⅛ of 46-oz. pie	390	55.0
Natural Juice	⅛ of 36.8-oz. pie	350	49.0
Pie In Minutes	⅛ of 25-oz. pie	220	32.0
(Pet-Ritz)	⅙ of 26-oz. pie	300	48.0
Chocolate cream:			
(Banquet)	⅙ of 14-oz. pie	185	24.0
(Pet-Ritz)	⅙ of 14-oz. pie	190	27.0
Chocolate mocha (Weight Watchers)	2¾-oz. serving	160	23.0
Coconut cream:			
(Banquet)	⅙ of 14-oz. pie	187	22.0
(Pet-Ritz)	⅙ of 14-oz. pie	190	27.0
Coconut custard (Mrs.			

Food and Description	Measure or Quantity	Calories	Carbo-hydrates (grams)
Smith's):			
8″ pie	⅛ of 25-oz. pie	180	22.0
10″ pie	⅛ of 44-oz. pie	280	36.0
Custard, egg (Pet-Ritz)	⅙ of 24-oz. pie	200	28.0
Lemon cream:			
(Banquet)	⅙ of 14-oz. pie	173	23.0
(Pet-Ritz)	⅙ of 14-oz. pie	190	26.0
Lemon meringue (Mrs. Smith's)	⅛ of 8″ pie (3 oz.)	210	38.0
Mincemeat:			
(Banquet) Family size	⅙ of 20-oz. pie	260	38.0
(Mrs. Smith's):			
Small	⅛ of 26-oz. pie	220	30.0
Large	⅛ of 46-oz. pie	430	64.0
(Pet-Ritz)	⅙ of 26-oz. pie	280	48.0
Mud, Mississippi (Pepperidge Farm)	2¼-oz. serving	310	23.0
Neapolitan (Pet-Ritz)	⅙ of 14-oz. pie	180	17.0
Peach:			
(Banquet) Family size	⅙ of 20-oz. pie	245	35.0
(Mrs. Smith's):			
Regular:			
Small	⅛ of 26-oz. pie	200	28.0
Large	⅛ of 46-oz. pie	360	49.0
Natural juice	⅛ of 36.8-oz. pie	330	46.0
Pie In Minutes	⅛ of 25-oz. pie	210	29.0
(Pet-Ritz)	⅙ of 26-oz. pie	320	51.0
Pecan (Mrs. Smith's):			
Regular	⅛ of 24-oz. pie	330	51.0
Pie In Minutes	⅛ of 24-oz. pie	330	51.0
Pumpkin:			
(Banquet)	⅙ of 20-oz. pie	200	29.0
(Mrs. Smith's) *Pie In Minutes*	⅛ of 25-oz. pie	190	30.0
Pumpkin custard:			
(Mrs. Smith's):			
Small	⅛ of 26-oz. pie	180	28.0
Large	⅛ of 46-oz. pie	300	48.0
(Pet-Ritz)	⅙ of 26-oz. pie	250	39.0
Raspberry (Mrs. Smith's) red	⅛ of 26-oz. pie	220	32.0

(USDA) = United States Department of Agriculture
(HHS/FAO) = Health and Human Services/Food and Agriculture Organization
* = prepared as package directs

Food and Description	Measure or Quantity	Calories	Carbo-hydrates (grams)
Strawberry cream:			
(Banquet)	⅙ of 14-oz. pie	170	22.0
(Pet-Ritz)	⅙ of 14-oz. pie	170	20.0
Strawberry rhubarb			
(Mrs. Smith's)	⅛ of 26-oz. pie	230	33.0
PIECRUST:			
Home recipe (USDA), 9" pie, baked, made with vegetable shortening	1 crust	900	78.8
Frozen:			
(Empire Kosher)	7 oz.	1001	105.0
(Mrs. Smith's):			
8" shell	⅛ of 10-oz. shell	80	8.0
9" shell:			
Regular	⅛ of 12-oz. shell	90	10.0
Shallow	⅛ of 10-oz. shell	80	8.0
9⅝" shell	⅛ of 15-oz. shell	120	12.0
(Oronoque):			
Regular	⅙ of 7.4-oz. shell	170	14.0
Deep dish	⅙ of 8.5-oz. shell	200	16.0
(Pet-Ritz):			
Regular	⅙ of 5-oz. shell	110	11.0
Deep dish:			
Regular	⅙ of 6-oz. shell	130	12.0
Vegetable shortening	⅙ of 6-oz. shell	140	12.0
Graham cracker	⅙ of 5-oz. shell	110	8.0
Refrigerated (Pillsbury)	⅛ of 2-crust shell	240	24.0
*PIECRUST MIX:			
(Betty Crocker):			
Regular	1/16 of pkg.	120	10.0
Stick	⅛ of stick	120	10.0
(Flako)	⅙ of 9" pie shell	245	25.2
(Pillsbury) mix or stick	⅙ of 2-crust pie	270	25.0
PIE FILLING (See also **PUDDING OR PIE FILLING**):			
Regular:			
Apple:			
(Thank You Brand)	3½ oz.	91	23.0
(White House)	½ cup (4.8 oz.)	163	39.0

Food and Description	Measure or Quantity	Calories	Carbo-hydrates (grams)
Apple rings or slices (See **APPLE**, canned)			
Apricot (Comstock)	⅙ of 21-oz. can	110	24.0
Banana cream (Comstock)	⅙ of 21-oz. can	110	22.0
Blueberry (White House)	½ cup	159	38.0
Cherry:			
(Thank You Brand):			
Regular	3½ oz.	99	24.8
Sweet	3½ oz.	115	29.0
(White House)	½ cup (4.8 oz.)	190	45.0
Chocolate (Comstock)	⅙ of 21-oz. can	140	27.0
Coconut cream (Comstock)	⅙ of 21-oz. can	120	24.0
Coconut custard (USDA) home recipe, made with egg yolk & milk	5 oz. (inc. crust)	288	41.3
Lemon (Comstock)	⅙ of 21-oz. can	160	33.0
Mincemeat (Comstock)	⅙ of 21-oz. can	170	36.0
Peach (White House)	½ cup	158	39.0
Pineapple (Comstock)	⅙ of 21-oz. can	110	25.0
Pumpkin (See also **PUMPKIN**, canned):			
(Libby's)	1 cup	210	58.0
(Comstock)	⅙ of 27-oz. can	170	38.0
Raisin (Comstock)	⅙ of 21-oz. can	140	30.0
Strawberry (Comstock)	⅙ of 21-oz. can	130	28.0
Dietetic (Thank You Brand):			
Apple	3¼ oz.	60	.3
Cherry	3⅓ oz.	83	20.8
*PIE MIX:			
Boston cream (Betty Crocker)	⅛ of pie	270	50.0
Chocolate (Royal) No Bake	⅛ of pie	260	25.0
PIEROGIES, frozen (Empire Kosher):			
Cheese	1½-oz. serving	110	13.0
Onion	1½-oz. serving	90	13.0
PIGEON (See **SQUAB**)			

(USDA) = United States Department of Agriculture
(HHS/FAO) = Health and Human Services/Food and Agriculture Organization
* = prepared as package directs

Food and Description	Measure or Quantity	Calories	Carbo-hydrates (grams)
PIGEONPEA (USDA):			
Raw, immature seeds in pods	1 lb.	207	37.7
Dry seeds	1 lb.	1551	288.9
PIGNOLI (See **PINE NUT**)			
PIGS FEET, pickled (USDA)	4-oz. serving	226	0.
PIKE:			
Blue:			
Whole	1 lb. (weighed whole)	180	0.
Meat only	4 oz.	102	0.
Northern:			
Whole	1 lb. (weighed whole)	104	0.
Meat only	4 oz.	100	0.
Walleye:			
Whole	1 lb. (weighed whole)	140	0.
Meat only	4 oz.	105	0.
PIMIENTO, canned:			
(Dromedary) drained	1-oz. serving	10	2.0
(Sunshine) diced or sliced, solids & liq.	1 T.	4	.9
PIÑA COLADA COCKTAIL:			
Canned (Mr. Boston) 12½% alcohol	3 fl. oz.	249	34.2
*Mix (Bar-Tender's)	5 fl. oz.	254	24.0
PIÑA COLADA COCKTAIL MIX:			
Dry (Holland House)	.56-oz. pkg.	82	12.0
*Frozen (Bacardi)	4 fl. oz.	110	14.0
Liquid:			
*(Bar-Tender's)	5 fl. oz.	254	24.0
(Holland House)	1 fl. oz.	33	8.0
PINEAPPLE:			
Fresh (USDA):			
Whole	1 lb. (weighed untrimmed)	123	32.3
Diced	½ cup (2.8 oz.)	41	10.7

Food and Description	Measure or Quantity	Calories	Carbo-hydrates (grams)
Sliced	⅜″ × 3½″ slice (3 oz.)	44	11.5
Canned, regular pack, solids & liq.: (USDA):			
Juice pack	4 oz.	66	17.1
Light syrup	5 oz.	76	17.5
Heavy syrup:			
Crushed	½ cup (5.6 oz.)	97	25.4
Slices	1 large slice & 2 T. syrup (4.3 oz.)	90	23.7
Tidbits	½ cup (4.6 oz.)	95	25.0
(Del Monte):			
Juice pack:			
Chunks, slices or tidbits	½ cup (4 oz.)	70	18.0
Spears	2 spears (3.1 oz.)	50	14.0
Syrup pack	½ cup (4 oz.)	90	23.0
(Dole) Juice pack, chunk, crushed or sliced	½ cup (4 oz.)	70	18.0
(Town House) juice pack	½ cup	70	18.0
Canned, unsweetened or dietetic, solids & liq.:			
(Diet Delight) juice pack	½ cup (4.4 oz.)	70	18.0
(Libby's) Lite	½ cup (4.4 oz.)	60	16.0
(S&W) *Nutradiet,* blue label	1 slice	30	7.5
PINEAPPLE, CANDIED (USDA)	1-oz. serving	90	22.7
PINEAPPLE & MANDARIN ORANGE, canned (Dole) in light syrup, solids & liq.	½ cup (4.4-oz.)	75	19.0
PINEAPPLE JUICE: Canned:			
(Ardmore Farms)	6 fl. oz.	102	25.2
(Dole) unsweetened (Minute Maid):	6 fl. oz.	100	25.0

(USDA) = United States Department of Agriculture
(HHS/FAO) = Health and Human Services/Food and Agriculture Organization
* = prepared as package directs

Food and Description	Measure or Quantity	Calories	Carbo-hydrates (grams)
Regular	8.45-fl.-oz. container	139	34.1
On the Go	10-fl.-oz. bottle	165	40.4
(Mott's)	9½-fl.-oz. can	169	42.0
(Town House)	6 fl.-oz.	100	25.0
(Tree Top)	6 fl.-oz.	100	24.0
Chilled (Minute Maid)	6 fl.-oz.	99	24.2
*Frozen:			
(Dole) unsweetened	6 fl.-oz.	90	22.0
(Minute Maid)	6 fl.-oz.	99	24.2
PINEAPPLE & GRAPEFRUIT JUICE DRINK, canned:			
(Del Monte) regular or pink	6 fl. oz.	90	24.0
(Dole) pink	6 fl. oz.	101	25.4
(Texsun)	6 fl. oz.	91	22.0
*PINEAPPLE-ORANGE JUICE:			
Canned:			
(Andmore Farms)	6 fl.-oz.	102	25.2
(Dole)	6 fl.-oz.	100	23.0
(Johanna Farms) *Tree Ripe*	8.45 fl.-oz. container	132	32.4
*Frozen:			
(Dole)	6 fl.-oz.	90	22.0
(Minute Maid)	6 fl.-oz.	98	23.9
*PINEAPPLE-ORANGE-BANANA JUICE, frozen (Dole)	6 fl.-oz.	90	23.0
*PINEAPPLE-ORANGE-GUAVA JUICE, frozen (Dole)	6 fl.-oz.	100	22.0
*PINEAPPLE-PASSION-BANANA JUICE, frozen (Dole)	6 fl.-oz.	100	21.0
PINEAPPLE PRESERVE OR JAM, sweetened (Smucker's)	1 T. (.7 oz.)	54	12.0
PINE NUT (USDA):			
Pignoli, shelled	4 oz.	626	13.2

Food and Description	Measure or Quantity	Calories	Carbo-hydrates (grams)
Pinon, whole	4 oz. (weighed in shell)	418	13.5
Pinon, shelled	4 oz.	720	23.2
PINOT CHARDONNAY WINE			
(Paul Masson) 12% alcohol	3 fl. oz.	71	2.4
PISTACHIO NUT:			
Raw (USDA):			
In shell	4 oz. (weighed in shell)	337	10.8
Shelled	½ cup (2.2 oz.)	368	11.8
Shelled	1 T. (8 grams)	46	1.5
Roasted:			
(Fisher) salted:			
In shell	1 oz.	84	2.7
Shelled	1 oz.	174	5.4
(Flavor House) dry roasted	1 oz.	168	5.4
(Planters) dry roasted	1 oz.	170	6.0
PITANGA, fresh (USDA)			
Whole	1 lb. (weighed whole)	187	45.9
Flesh only	4 oz.	58	14.2
PIZZA PIE (See also *SHAKEY'S*):			
Regular, non-frozen:			
Home recipe (USDA) with cheese topping	⅛ of 14″ pie	177	21.2
(*Domino's*):			
Cheese:			
Plain:			
Small	⅛ of 12″ pizza	157	24.3
Large	1/12 of 16″ pizza	239	28.4
Double:			
Small	⅛ of 12″ pizza	240	24.7
Large	1/12 of 16″ pizza	350	29.1
Double, with pepperoni:			
Small	⅛ of 12″ pizza	227	24.8
Large	1/12 of 16″ pizza	389	29.1

(USDA) = United States Department of Agriculture
(HHS/FAO) = Health and Human Services/Food and Agriculture Organization
* = prepared as package directs

Food and Description	Measure or Quantity	Calories	Carbo-hydrates (grams)
Mushroom & sausage:			
Small	⅛ of 12" pizza	183	24.6
Large	1/12 of 16" pizza	266	28.9
Pepperoni:			
Plain:			
Small	⅛ of 12" pizza	192	24.3
Large	1/12 of 16" pizza	278	28.5
With sausage:			
Small	⅛ of 12" pizza	215	48.9
Large	1/12 of 16" pizza	303	57.3
Sausage:			
Small	⅛ of 12" pizza	180	24.4
Large	1/12 of 16" pizza	264	28.6
(Godfather's):			
Cheese:			
Original:			
Mini	¼ of pizza (2.8 oz.)	190	31.0
Small	⅙ of pizza (3.6 oz.)	240	32.0
Medium	⅛ of pizza (4 oz.)	270	36.0
Large:			
Regular	1/10 of pizza (4.4 oz.)	297	39.0
Hot slice	⅛ of pizza (5½ oz.)	370	48.0
Stuffed:			
Small	⅙ of pizza (4.4 oz.)	310	38.0
Medium	⅛ of pizza (4.8 oz.)	350	42.0
Large	1/10 of pizza (5.2 oz.)	381	44.0
Thin crust:			
Small	⅙ of pizza (2.6 oz.)	180	21.0
Medium	⅛ of pizza (3 oz.)	310	26.0
Large	1/10 of pizza (3.4 oz.)	228	28.0
Combo:			
Original:			
Mini	¼ of pizza (3.8 oz.)	240	32.0

Food and Description	Measure or Quantity	Calories	Carbo-hydrates (grams)
Small	⅙ of pizza (5.6 oz.)	360	35.0
Medium	⅛ of pizza (6.2 oz.)	400	39.0
Large:			
Regular	⅒ of pizza (6.8 oz.)	437	42.0
Hot Slice	⅛ of pizza (8.5 oz.)	550	52.0
Stuffed:			
Small	⅙ of pizza (6.3 oz.)	430	41.0
Medium	⅛ of pizza (7 oz.)	480	45.0
Large	⅒ of pizza (7.6 oz.)	521	47.0
Thin crust:			
Small	⅙ of pizza (4.3 oz.)	270	23.0
Medium	⅛ of pizza (4.9 oz.)	310	29.0
Large	⅒ of pizza (5.4 oz.)	336	31.0
Frozen:			
Bacon (Totino's)	½ of 10-oz. pizza	370	35.0
Bagel (Empire Kosher)	2-oz. serving	140	17.0
Canadian style bacon:			
(Jeno's) Crisp 'N Tasty	½ of 7.7-oz. pizza	250	27.0
(Stouffer's) french bread	½ of 11⅝-oz. pkg.	360	41.0
(Totino's)	½ of 10.2-oz. pizza	310	35.0
Cheese:			
(Banquet) Zap, french bread	4½-oz. serving	310	41.0
(Celentano):			
Nine-slice	2.7-oz. piece	150	22.0
Thick crust	⅓ of 13-oz. pizza	290	35.0

(USDA) = United States Department of Agriculture
(HHS/FAO) = Health and Human Services/Food and Agriculture Organization
* = prepared as package directs

Food and Description	Measure or Quantity	Calories	Carbohydrates (grams)
(Empire Kosher):			
Regular	⅓ of 10-oz. pie	195	27.0
Family size	⅕ of 15-oz. pie	215	30.0
3-pack	⅑ of 27-oz. pie	215	30.0
(Jeno's):			
Crisp 'N Tasty	½ of 7.4-oz. pizza	270	28.0
4-pack	¼ of 8.9-oz. pkg.	160	17.0
(Kid Cuisine)	6½-oz. serving	240	41.0
(Pappalo's) french bread	5.7-oz. piece	360	40.0
(Pepperidge Farm) croissant crust	1 pizza	430	41.0
(Pillsbury) microwave:			
Regular	½ of 7.1-oz. pizza	240	28.0
French bread	5.7-oz. piece	370	41.0
(Stouffer's) french bread:			
Regular:			
Plain	½ of 10⅜-oz. pkg.	340	41.0
Double cheese	½ of 11⅜-oz. pkg.	410	43.0
Lean Cuisine:			
Plain	5⅛-oz. serving	310	40.0
Extra Cheese	5½-oz. serving	350	39.0
(Totino's):			
Microwave	3.9-oz. pizza	250	34.0
My Classic, deluxe	⅙ of 18.6-oz. pizza	210	23.0
Pan, three cheese	⅙ of pizza (3.9 oz.)	290	33.0
Party	½ of 9.8-oz. pizza	340	34.0
Slices	2½-oz. slice	170	20.0
(Weight Watchers):			
Regular	5¾-oz. serving	310	39.0
French bread	5.1-oz. serving	310	31.0
Combination:			
(Jeno's):			
Crisp 'N Tasty	½ of 7.8-oz. pizza	300	27.0
4-pack	¼ of 9.6-oz. pkg.	180	17.0
(Pappalo's):			
French bread	6½-oz. serving	430	41.0

Food and Description	Measure or Quantity	Calories	Carbo-hydrates (grams)
Pan	⅙ of 26.5-oz. pizza	340	34.0
Thin crust	⅙ of 22-oz. pizza	260	29.0
(Pillsbury) microwave	½ of 9-oz. pizza	310	29.0
(Totino's):			
My Classic, deluxe	1⅙ of 22½-oz. pizza	270	23.0
Party	½ of 10½-oz. pizza	380	35.0
Slices	2.7-oz. piece	200	20.0
(Weight Watchers) deluxe	6¾-oz. serving	300	37.0
Deluxe:			
(Banquet) Zap	4.8-oz. serving	330	39.0
(Pepperidge Farm) croissant crust	1 pizza	440	43.0
(Stouffer's) french bread:			
Regular	6.2-oz. serving	430	41.0
Lean Cuisine	6 ⅛-oz. serving	350	40.0
(Weight Watchers) french bread	6.12-oz. serving	310	31.0
English muffin (Empire Kosher)	2-oz. serving	140	17.0
Golden topping (Fox Deluxe)	½ of 6.8-oz. pizza	240	25.0
Hamburger:			
(Fox Deluxe)	½ of 7.6-oz. pizza	260	26.0
(Jeno's):			
Crisp 'N Tasty	½ of 8.1-oz. pizza	290	28.0
4-pack	¼ of 10-oz. pkg.	180	17.0
(Pappalo's):			
Pan	⅙ of 26.3-oz. pizza	310	34.0
Thin crust	⅙ of 222-oz. pizza	240	28.0
(Stouffer's) french bread	½ of 12¼-oz. pkg.	410	40.0
(Totino's) party	½ of 10.6-oz. pizza	370	35.0

(USDA) = United States Department of Agriculture
(HHS/FAO) = Health and Human Services/Food and Agriculture Organization
* = prepared as package directs

Food and Description	Measure or Quantity	Calories	Carbo-hydrates (grams)
Mexican style (Totino's)	½ of 10.2-oz. pizza	380	35.0
Pepperoni:			
(Banquet) Zap, french bread	4½-oz. serving	350	36.0
(Fox Deluxe)	½ of 7-oz. pizza	250	26.0
(Jeno's):			
Crisp 'N Tasty	½ of 7.6-oz. pizza	280	27.0
4-pack	¼ of 9.2-oz. pkg.	170	17.0
(Pappalo's):			
French bread	6-oz. serving	410	41.0
Pan	⅙ of 25.2-oz. pizza	330	34.0
Thin crust	⅙ of 22-oz. pizza	270	28.0
(Pepperidge Farm) crois-sant crust	1 pizza	420	43.0
(Pillsbury) microwave:			
Regular	½ of 8½-oz. pizza	300	29.0
French bread	6-oz. serving	430	46.0
(Stouffer's) french bread:			
Regular	½ of 11¼-oz pkg.	410	41.0
Lean Cuisine	5½-oz. serving	340	40.0
(Totino's):			
Microwave, small	4-oz. pizza	280	34.0
My Classic	⅙ of 21.1-oz. pizza	260	23.0
Pan	⅙ of 25.2-oz. pizza	330	34.0
Party	½ of 10.2-oz. pizza	370	35.0
Slices	2.6-oz. slice	190	20.0
(Weight Watchers):			
Regular	5.87-oz. serving	320	38.0
French bread	5¼-oz. serving	310	28.0
Sausage:			
(Fox Deluxe)	½ of 7.2-oz. pizza	260	26.0
(Jeno's):			
Crisp 'N Tasty	½ of 7.8-oz. pizza	300	28.0
4-pack	¼ of 9.6-oz. pkg.	180	17.0
(Pappalo's):			
French bread	6.3-oz. piece	410	41.0

Food and Description	Measure or Quantity	Calories	Carbo- hydrates (grams)
Pan	⅙ of 26.3-oz. pizza	360	34.0
Thin crust	⅙ of 22-oz. pizza	250	28.0
(Pillsbury) microwave:			
Regular	½ of 8¾-oz. pizza	280	29.0
French bread	6.3-oz. piece	410	48.0
(Stouffer's) french bread:			
Regular	½ of 12-oz. pkg.	420	41.0
Lean Cuisine	6-oz. serving	350	40.0
(Totino's):			
Microwave, small	4.2-oz. pizza	320	33.0
Pan	⅙ of 26.3-oz. pizza	320	34.0
Party	½ of 10.6-oz. pizza	390	35.0
Slices	2.7-oz. slice	200	20.0
(Weight Watchers)	6¼-oz. serving	310	37.0
Sausage & pepperoni (Stouffer's) french bread	½ of 12½-oz. pkg.	450	40.0
Vegetable (Stouffer's) french bread	½ of 12¾-oz. pkg.	420	41.0
*Mix (Ragu) *Pizza Quick*	¼ of pie	300	37.0
PIZZA PIE CRUST:			
*Mix, *Gold Medal*	⅙ of mix	110	22.0
Refrigerated (Pillsbury)	⅛ of crust	90	16.0
PIZZA ROLL, frozen (Jeno's):			
Cheese	½ of 6-oz. pkg.	240	23.0
Hamburger	½ of 6-oz. pkg.	240	21.0
Pepperoni & cheese:			
Regular	½ of 6-oz. pkg.	230	22.0
Microwave	⅓ of 9-oz. pkg.	240	23.0
Sausage & pepperoni:			
Regular	½ of 6-oz. pkg.	230	22.0
Microwave	⅓ of 9-oz. pkg.	250	24.0

(USDA) = United States Department of Agriculture
(HHS/FAO) = Health and Human Services/Food and Agriculture Organization
* = prepared as package directs

Food and Description	Measure or Quantity	Calories	Carbo-hydrates (grams)
PIZZA SAUCE:			
(Contadina):			
Regular or with cheese	½ cup (4.2 oz.)	80	10.0
With pepperoni	½ cup (4.2 oz.)	90	10.0
With tomato chunks	½ cup (4.2 oz.)	50	10.0
(Ragu):			
Regular	15½-oz. jar	250	30.0
Pizza Quick:			
Chunky	14-oz. jar	332	44.2
Mushroom, sausage or traditional	14-oz. jar	329	32.9
Pepperoni	14-oz. jar	412	32.9
PIZZA SEASONING SPICE			
(French's)	1 tsp. (.1 oz.)	5	1.0
PLANTAIN, raw (USDA):			
Whole	1 lb. (weighed with skin)	389	101.9
Flesh only	4 oz.	135	35.4
PLUM:			
Fresh (USDA):			
Damson:			
Whole	1 lb. (weighed with pits)	272	73.5
Flesh only	4 oz.	75	20.2
Japanese & hybrid:			
Whole	1 lb. (weighed with pits)	205	52.5
	2.1-oz. plum (2″ dia.)	27	6.9
Diced	½ cup (2.9 oz.)	39	10.1
Halves	½ cup (3.1 oz.)	42	10.8
Slices	½ cup (3 oz.)	40	10.3
Prune type:			
Whole	1 lb. (weighed with pits)	320	84.0
Halves	½ cup (2.8 oz.)	60	52.8
Canned, purple, regular pack solids & liq.: (USDA):			
Extra heavy syrup	4 oz.	116	30.3
Heavy syrup, with pits	½ cup (4.5 oz.)	106	27.6
Heavy syrup, without pits	½ cup (4.2 oz.)	100	25.9
Light syrup	4 oz.	71	18.8

Food and Description	Measure or Quantity	Calories	Carbo-hydrates (grams)
(Stokely-Van Camp) (Thank You Brand):	½ cup	120	30.0
Heavy syrup	½ cup (4.8 oz.)	109	27.2
Light syrup	½ cup (4.7 oz.)	80	20.0
Canned, unsweetened or low calorie, solids & liq.: (Diet Delight) purple:			
Juice pack	½ cup (4.4 oz.)	70	19.0
Water pack	½ cup (4.4 oz.)	50	13.0
(S&W) *Nutradiet*, purple, juice pack	½ cup	80	20.0
(Thank You Brand)	½ cup (4.8 oz.)	49	12.2
PLUM JELLY:			
Sweetened (Bama)	1 T. (.7 oz.)	45	12.0
Dietetic or low calorie (Featherweight)	1 T.	16	4.0
PLUM PRESERVE OR JAM, sweetened (Smucker's)	1 T. (.7 oz.)	53	13.5
PLUM PUDDING (Richardson & Robbins)	2″ wedge (3.6 oz.)	270	61.0
POLISH-STYLE SAUSAGE (See **SAUSAGE**)			
POMEGRANATE, raw (USDA):			
Whole	1 lb. (weighed whole)	160	41.7
Pulp only	4 oz.	71	18.6
***PONDEROSA* RESTAURANT:**			
A-1 Sauce	1 tsp.	4	1.0
Beef, chopped, patty only			

(USDA) = United States Department of Agriculture
(HHS/FAO) = Health and Human Services/Food and Agriculture
Organization
* = prepared as package directs

Food and Description	Measure or Quantity	Calories	Carbohydrates (grams)
(see also Bun):			
Regular	3½ oz.	209	0.
Big	4.8 oz.	295	0.
Double Deluxe	5.9 oz.	362	0.
Junior (*Square Shooter*)	1.6 oz.	98	0.
Steakhouse Deluxe	2.96 oz.	181	0.
Beverages:			
Coca-Cola	8 fl. oz.	96	24.0
Coffee	6 fl. oz.	2	.5
Dr Pepper	8 fl. oz.	96	24.8
Lemon	8 fl. oz.	110	28.5
Milk:			
Regular	8 fl. oz.	159	12.0
Chocolate	8 fl. oz.	208	25.9
Orange drink	8 fl. oz.	110	30.0
Root beer	8 fl. oz.	104	25.6
Sprite	8 fl. oz.	95	24.0
Bun:			
Regular	2.4-oz. bun	190	35.0
Hot dog	1 bun	108	18.9
Junior	1.4-oz. bun	118	21.0
Steakhouse deluxe	2.4-oz. bun	190	35.0
Chicken strips:			
Adult portion	2⅜ oz.	282	15.8
Children's portion	1.4 oz.	141	7.9
Cocktail sauce	1½ oz.	57	.2
Filet mignon	3.8 oz. (edible portion)	152	.2
Filet of sole, fish only (See also Bun)	3-oz. piece	125	4.4
Fish, baked	4.9-oz. serving	268	11.6
Gelatin dessert	½ cup	97	23.5
Gravy, au jus	1 oz.	3	Tr.
Ham & cheese:			
Bun (See Bun)			
Cheese, Swiss	2 slices (.8 oz.)	76	.5
Ham	2½ oz.	184	1.4
Hot dog, child's, meat only (See also Bun)	1.6-oz. hot dog	140	2.0
Margarine:			
Pat	1 pat	36	Tr.
On potato, as served	½ oz.	100	.1
Mustard sauce, sweet & sour	1 oz.	50	9.5
New York strip steak	6.1 oz. (edible portion)	362	0.

Food and Description	Measure or Quantity	Calories	Carbo-hydrates (grams)
Onion, chopped	1 T. (.4 oz.)	4	.9
Pickle, dill	3 slices (.7 oz.)	2	.2
Potato:			
Baked	7.2-oz. potato	145	32.8
French fries	3-oz. serving	230	30.2
Prime ribs:	4.2 oz. (edible		
Regular	portion)	286	0.
Imperial	8.4 oz. (edible		
	portion)	572	0.
King	6 oz. (edible		
	portion)	409	0.
Pudding:			
Butterscotch	4½ oz.	200	27.4
Chocolate	4½ oz.	213	27.1
Vanilla	4½ oz.	195	27.5
Ribeye	3.2 oz. (edible		
	portion)	197	0.
Ribeye & shrimp:			
Ribeye	3.2 oz.	197	0.
Shrimp	2.2 oz.	139	0.
Roll, kaiser	2.2-oz. roll	184	33.0
Salad bar:			
Bean sprouts	1 oz.	13	1.5
Beets	1 oz.	5	.9
Broccoli	1 oz.	9	1.7
Cabbage, red	1 oz.	9	2.0
Carrots	1 oz.	12	2.8
Cauliflower	1 oz.	8	1.5
Celery	1 oz.	4	1.1
Chickpeas (Garbanzos)	1 oz.	102	17.3
Cucumber	1 oz.	4	.7
Mushrooms	1 oz.	8	1.2
Onion, white	1 oz.	11	2.6
Pepper, green	1 oz.	6	1.4
Radish	1 oz.	5	1.0
Tomato	1 oz.	6	1.3
Salad dressing:			
Blue cheese	1 oz.	129	2.1
Italian, creamy	1 oz.	138	2.8
Low calorie	1 oz.	14	.8
Oil & vinegar	1 oz.	124	.9

(USDA) = United States Department of Agriculture
(HHS/FAO) = Health and Human Services/Food and Agriculture Organization
* = prepared as package directs

Food and Description	Measure or Quantity	Calories	Carbo-hydrates (grams)
Sweet'n Tart	1 oz.	129	9.2
1000 Island	1 oz.	117	6.7
Shrimp dinner	7 pieces (3½ oz.)	220	9.8
Sirloin:			
Regular	3.3 oz. (edible portion)	197	0.
Super	6½ oz. (edible portion)	383	0.
Tips	4 oz. (edible portion)	192	0.
Steak sauce	1 oz.	23	4.0
Tartar sauce	1.5 oz.	285	4.5
T-bone	4.3 oz. (edible portion)	240	0.
Tomato (See also Salad Bar):			
Slices	2 slices (.9 oz.)	5	1.2
Whole, small	3.5 oz.	22	4.7
Topping, whipped	¼ oz.	19	1.2
Worcestershire sauce	1 tsp.	4	.9
POPCORN:			
*Plain, popped fresh:			
(General Mills) Top Secret		33	3.7
(Jiffy Pop)	½ of 5-oz. pkg.	244	29.8
(Jolly Time):			
Regular, no added butter or salt:			
White	1 cup	19	4.0
Yellow	1 cup	22	4.7
Microwave:			
Natural	1 cup	53	5.0
Butter flavor	1 cup	53	5.3
Cheese flavor	1 cup	60	5.7
(Orville Redenbacher's)			
Original:			
Plain	1 cup (.2 oz.)	22	4.5
With oil & salt	1 cup (.3 oz.)	40	5.3
Caramel crunch	1 cup	140	19.0
Hot air corn	1 cup	25	4.5
Microwave:			
Regular, butter flavored	1 cup	27	2.5
Regular, natural	1 cup	27	2.7

Food and Description	Measure or Quantity	Calories	Carbo-hydrates (grams)
Flavored:			
Caramel	1 cup	96	11.6
Cheese	1 cup	50	4.0
Sour cream & onions	1 cup	50	4.3
(Pillsbury) microwave:			
Regular	1 cup	70	6.5
Butter flavor, regular or			
frozen	1 cup	70	6.7
Salt free, frozen	1 cup	57	7.7
Butter flavor	1 cup	65	6.0
Dry popped	1 oz.	100	20.0
Oil popped	1 oz.	220	20.0
Packaged:			
Plain:			
Cape Cod	1 oz.	160	12.0
(Eagle)	1 oz.	160	12.0
(Wise) butter flavored	1 oz.	140	16.0
Caramel-coated:			
(Bachman)	1-oz. serving	110	25.0
(Old Dutch)	1 oz.	109	DNA
(Old London) without			
peanuts	1⅜-oz. serving	195	43.6
Cheese flavored (Snyder's)	1-oz. serving	180	14.0
Cracker Jack	1-oz. serving	120	22.0

POPCORN POPPING OIL
(Orville Redenbacher's)			
Gourmet, buttery flavor	1 T.	120	0.

POPOVER:
Home recipe (USDA)	1 average popover (2 oz.)	128	14.7
*Mix (Flako)	1 popover	170	25.0

POPPY SEED (French's)
	1 tsp.	13	.8

POPSICLE, twin
	3-fl.-oz. pop	70	17.0

(USDA) = United States Department of Agriculture
(HHS/FAO) = Health and Human Services/Food and Agriculture Organization
* = prepared as package directs

Food and Description	Measure or Quantity	Calories	Carbo-hydrates (grams)
PORGY, raw (USDA):			
Whole	1 lb. (weighed whole)	208	0.
Meat only	4 oz.	127	0.
PORK, medium-fat:			
Fat, separable, cooked	1 oz.	219	0.
Fresh (USDA):			
Boston butt:			
Raw:	1 lb. (weighed with bone & skin)	1220	0.
Roasted, lean & fat	4 oz.	400	0.
Roasted, lean only	4 oz.	277	0.
Chop:			
Broiled, lean & fat	1 chop (4 oz., weighed with bone)	295	0.
Broiled, lean & fat	1 chop (3 oz., weighed without bone)	332	0.
Broiled, lean only	1 chop (3 oz., weighed without bone)	230	0.
Ham:			
Raw	1 lb. (weighed with bone & skin)	1188	0.
Roasted, lean & fat	4 oz.	424	0.
Roasted, lean only	4 oz.	246	0.
Loin:			
Raw	1 lb. (weighed with bone)	1065	0.
Roasted, lean & fat	4 oz.	411	0.
Roasted, lean only	4 oz.	288	0.
Picnic:			
Raw	1 lb. (weighed with bone & skin)	1083	0.
Simmered, lean & fat	4 oz.	424	0.
Simmered, lean only	4 oz.	240	0.
Spareribs:			
Raw, with bone	1 lb. (weighed with bone)	976	0.
Braised, lean & fat	4 oz.	499	0.

Food and Description	Measure or Quantity	Calories	Carbohydrates (grams)
Cured, light commercial cure:			
Bacon (See **BACON**)			
Boston butt (USDA):			
Raw	1 lb. (weighed with bone & skin)	1227	0.
Roasted, lean & fat	4 oz.	374	0.
Roasted, lean only	4 oz.	276	0.
PORK, CANNED, chopped luncheon meat (USDA):			
Regular	1 oz.	83	.4
Chopped	1 cup (4.8 oz.)	400	1.8
Diced	1 cup	415	1.8
PORK DINNER OR ENTREE:			
*Canned:			
(Hunt's) *Minute Gourmet*	6.6-oz. serving	500	46.0
(La Choy) sweet & sour	¾ cup	250	48.0
Frozen (Swanson) loin of	10¾-oz. dinner	280	27.0
PORK, PACKAGED (Eckrich)	1-oz. serving	45	1.0
PORK, SALT (See **SALT PORK**)			
PORK, SWEET & SOUR, frozen:			
(Chun King)	13-oz. entree	400	78.0
(La Choy)	12-oz. entree	360	64.0
PORK & BEANS (See **BEAN, BAKED**)			
PORK RINDS (Old Dutch)	1-oz. serving	154	1.0

(USDA) = United States Department of Agriculture
(HHS/FAO) = Health and Human Services/Food and Agriculture Organization
* = prepared as package directs

Food and Description	Measure or Quantity	Calories	Carbo- hydrates (grams)
PORT WINE:			
(Gallo) 16% alcohol	3 fl. oz.	94	7.8
(Louis M. Martini) 19½% alcohol	3 fl. oz.	165	2.0
*POSTUM, instant, regular or coffee flavored	6 fl. oz.	11	2.6
POTATO (See also SWEET POTATO):			
Cooked (USDA)			
Au gratin, with cheese	½ cup (4.3 oz.)	177	16.6
Baked, peeled	2½" dia. potato (3.5 oz.)	92	20.9
Boiled, peeled before boiling, no salt	4.3-oz. potato	79	17.7
French-fried in deep fat, no salt	10 pieces (2 oz.)	156	20.5
Hash-browned, home recipe, after holding overnight	½ cup (3.4 oz.)	223	28.4
Mashed, milk & butter added	½ cup (3.5 oz.)	92	12.1
Canned, solids & liq.:			
(Allen's) Butterfield	½ cup	45	10.0
(Hunt's)	4 oz.	55	12.0
(Larsen) *Freshlike*	½ cup	60	13.0
(Town House)	½ cup	55	12.0
Frozen:			
(Bel-Air):			
With cheese	5-oz. serving	220	31.0
French fries:			
Regular	3-oz. serving	120	40.0
Crinkle cut	3-oz. serving	120	20.0
Hash brown	4-oz. serving	80	19.0
Shoestring	3-oz. serving	140	20.0
Sour cream & chives	5-oz. serving	230	31.0
(Birds Eye):			
Cottage fries	2.8-oz. serving	119	17.3
Crinkle cuts:			
Regular	3-oz. serving	115	18.4
Deep Gold	3-oz. serving	138	25.5
French fries:			
Regular	3-oz. serving	113	16.8
Deep Gold	3-oz. serving	161	24.4
Hash browns:			

Food and Description	Measure or Quantity	Calories	Carbo-hydrates (grams)
Regular	4-oz. serving	74	16.5
Shredded	¼ of 12-oz. pkg.	61	13.1
Steak fries	3-oz. serving	109	17.9
Tasti Fries	2½-oz. serving	136	16.5
Tasti Puffs	¼ of 10-oz. pkg.	192	19.4
Tiny Taters	⅕ of 16.oz. pkg.	204	22.0
Whole, peeled	3.2-oz. serving	59	12.8
(Empire Kosher) french fries	3-oz. serving	110	18.0
(Green Giant) One Serving:			
Au gratin	5½-oz. serving	200	20.0
& broccoli in cheese sauce	5½-oz. serving	130	14.0
(Larsen) diced	4-oz. serving	80	19.0
(McKenzie) whole, white, boiled	3-oz. serving	70	15.0
(Ore-Ida):			
Cheddar Browns	3-oz. serving	80	14.0
Cottage fries	3-oz. serving	120	19.0
Country Style Dinner Fries or *Home Style Potato Wedges*	3-oz. serving	110	19.0
Crispers!	3-oz. serving	230	25.0
Crispy Crowns	3-oz. serving	170	20.0
Golden Crinkles or *Golden Fries*	3-oz. serving	120	20.0
Golden Patties	2½-oz. serving	140	15.0
Golden Twirls	3-oz. serving	160	21.0
Hash browns:			
Microwave	2-oz. serving	120	13.0
Shredded or Southern style	3-oz. serving	70	15.0
Toaster	1¾-oz. serving	100	12.0
Lite Crinkle Cuts	3-oz. serving	90	16.0
Pixie Crinkles	3-oz. serving	140	21.0
Potatoes O'Brien	3-oz. serving	60	14.0
Shoestring	3-oz. serving	150	22.0
Tater Tots:			
Plain:			
Regular	3-oz. serving	150	20.0

(USDA) = United States Department of Agriculture
(HHS/FAO) = Health and Human Services/Food and Agriculture Organization
* = prepared as package directs

Food and Description	Measure or Quantity	Calories	Carbo-hydrates (grams)
Microwave	4-oz. serving	200	29.0
With onions	3-oz. serving	150	20.0
Whole, small, peeled (Stouffer's):	3-oz. serving	70	16.0
Au gratin	⅓ of 11½-oz. pkg.	110	10.0
Scalloped	⅓ of 11½-oz. pkg.	90	11.0
POTATO, STUFFED, BAKED, frozen (Green Giant):			
With cheese flavored topping	½ of 10-oz. pkg.	200	33.0
With sour cream & chives	½ of 10-oz. pkg.	230	31.0
POTATO CHIPS:			
(Cape Cod) any style	1 oz.	150	16.0
(Cottage Fries) unsalted	1 oz.	160	14.0
Delta Gold	1 oz.	160	14.0
(Frito-Lay):			
All flavors except sour cream & onion	1 oz.	150	15.0
Sour cream & onion	1 oz.	160	15.0
Ruffles:			
Regular:			
All flavors	1 oz.	150	15.0
Light	1 oz.	130	19.0
Cottage fries:			
BBQ	1 oz.	150	14.0
Sour cream & chive or unsalted	1 oz.	160	14.0
(Laura Scudder's):			
Barbecue	1 oz.	150	15.0
Sour cream & onion	1 oz.	150	14.0
(New York Deli)	1 oz.	160	14.0
(Old Dutch) O'Grady's:	1 oz.	150	16.0
All flavors except BBQ	1 oz.	150	16.0
BBQ	1 oz.	140	16.0
(Snyder's)	1 oz.	150	15.0
(Tom's):			
Regular, BBQ, rippled or sour cream & onion	1 oz.	160	14.0
Hot or vinegar and salt	1 oz.	160	15.0

Food and Description	Measure or Quantity	Calories	Carbo-hydrates (grams)
(Wise):			
Regular:			
Barbecue, garlic & onion	1 oz.	150	14.0
Lightly salted, natural or salt & vinegar	1 oz.	160	14.0
Cottage Fries:			
BBQ	1 oz.	150	14.0
No salt added or sour cream & chives	1 oz.	160	14.0
Ridgies	1 oz.	160	14.0
*POTATO MIX:			
Au gratin:			
(Betty Crocker)	½ cup	150	21.0
(French's) tangy	½ cup	130	20.0
(Lipton) & sauce	¼ of pkg.	108	22.4
(Town House)	½ cup	150	21.0
Beef & mushroom (Lipton)	½ cup	95	20.4
Casserole (French's) cheddar cheese & bacon	½ cup	130	18.0
Cheddar bacon (Lipton) & sauce	½ cup	106	20.5
Cheddar broccoli (Lipton)	½ cup	104	20.5
Chicken flavored mushroom (Lipton) & sauce	½ cup	90	19.2
Hash browns (Betty Crocker) with onion	½ cup	160	24.0
Italian (Lipton)	½ cup	107	20.8
Julienne (Betty Crocker)	½ cup	130	18.0
Mashed:			
(Betty Crocker) *Buds*	½ cup	130	17.0
(French's):			
Big Tate	½ cup	140	16.0
Idaho	½ cup	120	16.0
(Pillsbury) *Hungry Jack*, flakes	½ cup	140	17.0
(Town House)	½ cup	120	16.0
Nacho (Lipton) & sauce	½ cup	103	20.9

(USDA) = United States Department of Agriculture
(HHS/FAO) = Health and Human Services/Food and Agriculture Organization
* = prepared as package directs

Food and Description	Measure or Quantity	Calories	Carbo- hydrates (grams)
Scalloped:			
(Betty Crocker) plain	½ cup	140	19.0
(French's):			
Creamy Italian	½ cup	120	19.0
Crispy top or real cheese	½ cup	140	19.0
(Lipton) & sauce	½ cup	102	19.5
Sour cream & chive:			
(Betty Crocker)	½ cup	160	21.0
(French's)	½ cup	150	19.0
(Lipton)	¼ pkg.	113	21.0
*POTATO PANCAKE MIX			
(French's)	3" pancake	30	5.3
POTATO SALAD: home recipe (USDA):			
With cooked salad dressing seasonings	4 oz.	112	18.5
With mayonnaise & French dressing, hard-cooked eggs, seasonings	4 oz.	164	15.2
POTATO TOPPERS (Libby's)	1 T.	30	4.0
POT ROAST, frozen:			
(Armour) *Dinner Classics*	10-oz. meal	310	26.0
(Healthy Choice)	11-oz. meal	260	36.0
(Le Menu)	10-oz. meal	330	27.0
(Stouffer's) *Right Course*	9¼-oz. meal	220	22.0
POUND CAKE (See **CAKE,** Pound)			
PRESERVE OR JAM (See indi-- vidual flavors)			
PRETZELS:			
(Eagle) *A & Eagle*	1 oz.	110	22.0
(Estee) unsalted	1 piece (1.3 grams)	7	1.6

Food and Description	Measure or Quantity	Calories	Carbo-hydrates (grams)
(Nabisco) *Mister Salty:*			
Regular:			
Dutch	1 piece	55	11.0
Logs	1 piece	12	2.3
Mini	1 piece	7	1.3
Mini mix or nuggets	1 piece	5	1.0
Rings	1 piece	5	.9
Rods	1 piece	55	10.5
Sticks	1 piece	1	.2
Twists	1 piece	22	4.2
Juniors	1 piece	4	.7
(Old Dutch)	1-oz. serving	120	23.0
(Rokeach) Dutch style:			
Regular	1 oz.	110	24.0
Unsalted	1 oz.	110	20.0
Rold Gold	1 oz.	110	22.0
(Seyfert's) rods, butter	1 oz.	110	21.0
(Snyder's)			
Hard	1 oz.	102	22.7
Sticks or thins	1 oz.	110	22.0
(Tom's) twists	1 oz.	100	22.0
(Wise) nuggets	1 oz.	110	21.0
PRICKLY PEAR, fresh (USDA):			
Whole	1 lb. (weighed with rind & seeds)	84	21.8
Flesh only	4 oz.	48	12.4
PRODUCT 19, cereal (Kellogg's)	1 cup (1 oz.)	100	24.0
PROSCIUTTO (Hormel) boneless	1 oz.	90	0.

(USDA) = United States Department of Agriculture
(HHS/FAO) = Health and Human Services/Food and Agriculture
                        Organization
* = prepared as package directs

Food and Description	Measure or Quantity	Calories	Carbo-hydrates (grams)
PRUNE:			
Canned:			
(Featherweight) stewed, water pack	½ cup	130	35.0
(Sunsweet) stewed	½ cup (4.6 oz.)	120	32.0
Dried:			
(Sunsweet):			
Whole	2 oz.	120	31.0
Pitted	2 oz.	140	36.0
*(Town House)	2 oz.	140	36.0
PRUNE JUICE:			
(Algood) *Lady Betty*	6 fl. oz.	130	30.0
(Ardmore Farms)	6 fl. oz.	148	36.6
(Mott's) regular	6 fl. oz.	130	32.0
(Town House)	6 fl. oz.	120	31.0
PRUNE WHIP (USDA) home recipe	1 cup (4.8 oz.)	211	49.8
PUDDING OR PIE FILLING (See also **CUSTARD**):			
Home recipe (USDA):			
Bread (See **BREAD PUDDING**)			
Rice, made with raisins	½ cup (4.7 oz.)	1983	35.2
Tapioca:			
Apple	½ cup (4.4 oz.)	146	36.8
Cream	½ cup (2.9 oz.)	110	14.0
Canned, regular pack:			
Banana:			
(Hunt's) *Snack Pack*	4¼-oz. container	180	22.0
(Thank You Brand)	½ cup	150	33.8
(Town House)	5-oz. container	160	28.0
Butterscotch:			
(Hunt's) *Snack Pack*	4¼-oz. container	180	26.0
(Swiss Miss)	4-oz. container	160	23.0
(Town House)	5-oz. container	160	28.0
Chocolate:			
(Hunt's) *Snack Pack:*			
Regular	4¼-oz. container	160	28.0

Food and Description	Measure or Quantity	Calories	Carbo-hydrates (grams)
Fudge	4¼-oz. container	170	24.0
German	4¼-oz. container	190	30.0
Marshmallow	4¼-oz. container	170	26.0
(Swiss Miss):			
Regular	4-oz. container	180	27.0
Fudge:			
Regular	4-oz. container	170	26.0
Fruit on bottom:			
Black cherries	4-oz. container	170	30.0
Strawberries	4-oz. container	170	29.0
(Town House)	5-oz. container	160	28.0
Lemon (Thank You Brand)	½ cup	174	37.7
Rice (Hunt's) *Snack Pack*	4¼-oz. container	190	23.0
Tapioca:			
(Hunt's) *Snack Pack*	4¼-oz. container	160	28.0
(Swiss Miss)	4-oz. container	150	26.0
(Thank You Brand)	½ cup	144	24.7
(Town House)	5-oz. container	160	26.0
Vanilla:			
(Hunt's) *Snack Pack*	4¼-oz. container	170	28.0
(Swiss Miss)	4-oz. container	160	26.0
(Thank You Brand)	½ cup	150	26.0
(Town House)	5-oz. container	160	25.0
Canned, dietetic pack (Estee)	½ cup	70	13.0
Chilled (Swiss Miss):			
Butterscotch, chocolate malt or vanilla	4-oz. container	150	24.0
Chocolate or double rich	4-oz. container	160	24.0
Chocolate malt	4-oz. container	150	22.0
Chocolate sundae	4-oz. container	170	26.0
Rice	4-oz. container	150	24.0
Tapioca	4-oz. container	130	22.0
Vanilla sundae	4-oz. container	170	25.0
Frozen (Rich's):			
Butterscotch	4½-oz. container	198	27.2
Chocolate	4½-oz. container	212	27.0
Vanilla	4½-oz. container	194	27.4

(USDA) = United States Department of Agriculture
(HHS/FAO) = Health and Human Services/Food and Agriculture Organization
* = prepared as package directs

Food and Description	Measure or Quantity	Calories	Carbo-hydrates (grams)
*Mix, sweetened, regular & instant:			
Banana:			
(Jell-O) cream:			
Regular	½ cup	161	26.7
Instant	½ cup	174	30.0
(Jell-Well) cream	½ cup	180	31.0
(Royal) regular	½ cup	160	27.0
Butter pecan (Jell-O) instant	½ cup	175	29.1
Butterscotch:			
(Jell-O):			
Regular	½ cup	172	29.7
Instant	½ cup	175	30.0
(Jell-Well)	½ cup	180	31.0
(Royal) regular	½ cup	160	27.0
Chocolate:			
(Jell-O):			
Plain:			
Regular	½ cup	174	28.8
Instant	½ cup	181	30.6
Fudge:			
Regular	½ cup	169	27.8
Instant	½ cup	182	30.9
Milk:			
Regular	½ cup	171	28.2
Instant	½ cup	184	34.0
(Jell-Well)	½ cup	180	31.0
(Royal)	½ cup	190	35.0
Coconut:			
(Jell-O) cream:			
Regular	½ cup	176	24.4
Instant	½ cup	182	26.1
(Royal) instant	½ cup	170	30.0
*Flan (Knorr):			
Without sauce	½ cup	130	19.0
With sauce	½ cup	190	34.0
Lemon:			
(Jell-O):			
Regular	½ cup	181	38.8
Instant	½ cup	179	31.1
(Jell-Well)	½ cup	180	31.0
Lime (Royal) Key Lime, regular	½ cup	160	30.0

Food and Description	Measure or Quantity	Calories	Carbo- hydrates (grams)
Pineapple (Jell-O) cream, instant	½ cup	176	30.4
Pistachio (Jell-O) instant	½ cup	174	28.4
Raspberry (Salada) *Danish Dessert*	½ cup	130	32.0
Rice (Jell-O) *Americana*	½ cup	176	29.9
Strawberry (Salada) *Danish Dessert*	½ cup	130	32.0
Tapioca (Jell-O) *Americana:*			
Chocolate	½ cup	173	27.8
Vanilla	½ cup	162	27.4
Vanilla:			
(Jell-O):			
Plain, instant	½ cup	179	31.0
French, regular	½ cup	172	29.7
(Royal)	½ cup	180	29.0
*Mix, dietetic:			
Butterscotch:			
(D-Zerta)	½ cup	68	12.0
(Weight Watchers)	½ cup	90	16.0
Chocolate:			
(D-Zerta)	½ cup (4.6 oz.)	68	11.5
(Estee)	½ cup	70	13.0
(Louis Sherry)	½ cup (4.2 oz.)	50	9.0
(Weight Watchers)	½ cup	90	18.0
Vanilla:			
(D-Zerta)	½ cup	70	13.0
(Estee) instant	½ cup	70	13.0
(Royal)	½ cup	100	16.0
(Weight Watchers)	½ cup	90	17.0
PUDDING POPS (See *JELL-O PUDDING POPS*)			
PUDDING ROLL-UPS, *Fruit Corners* (General Mills):			
Butterscotch	.5-oz. piece	60	11.0

(USDA) = United States Department of Agriculture
(HHS/FAO) = Health and Human Services/Food and Agriculture Organization
* = prepared as package directs

Food and Description	Measure or Quantity	Calories	Carbo-hydrates (grams)
Chocolate fudge or milk chocolate	.5-oz. piece	60	10.0
PUDDING SUNDAE (Swiss Miss):			
Caramel or mint	4-oz. container	170	25.0
Chocolate	4-oz. container	190	29.0
Peanut butter	4-oz. container	200	23.0
Vanilla	4-oz. container	180	28.0
PUFF PASTRY (See PASTRY SHEET, PUFF)			
PUFFED RICE:			
(Malt-O-Meal)	1 cup (.5 oz.)	54	12.2
(Quaker)	1 cup	55	12.7
PUFFED WHEAT:			
(Malt-O-Meal)	1 cup (.5 oz.)	53	10.4
(Quaker)	1 cup (.5 oz.)	54	10.8
PUMPKIN:			
Fresh (USDA):			
Whole	1 lb. (weighed with rind & seeds	83	20.6
Flesh only	4 oz.	29	7.4
Canned:			
(Libby's) solid pack	½ of 16-oz. can	40	10.0
(Stokely-Van Camp)	½ cup (4.3 oz.)	45	9.5
PUMPKIN BUTTER (Smucker's) *Autumn Harvest*	1 T.	36	9.0
PUMPKIN SEED, dry (USDA):			
Whole	4 oz. (weighed in hull)	464	12.6
Hulled	4 oz.	627	17.0

Food and Description	Measure or Quantity	Calories	Carbohydrates (grams)
PUNCH DRINK (Minute Maid):			
Canned:			
Regular	8.45-fl. oz. container	131	32.7
On the Go	10-fl. oz. bottle	155	38.7
Tropical	8.45-fl. oz. container	130	32.0
Chilled, citrus	6 fl. oz.	93	23.1
*Frozen, citrus	6 fl. oz.	93	23.1
PURE & LIGHT, fruit juice, canned (Dole):			
Country raspberry or orchard peach	6 fl. oz.	90	24.0
Mandarin tangerine	6 fl. oz.	100	24.0
Mountain cherry	6 fl. oz.	90	20.0

Food and Description	Measure or Quantity	Calories	Carbo-hydrates (grams)

Q

QUAIL, raw (USDA) meat & skin	4 oz.	195	0.
QUIK (Nestlé):			
Chocolate	1 tsp. (.4 oz.)	45	9.5
Strawberry	1 tsp. (.4 oz.)	45	11.0
Sugar free	1 tsp. (.2 oz.)	18	3.0et
QUINCE JELLY, sweetened (Smucker's)	1 T.	54	12.0

Food and Description	Measure or Quantity	Calories	Carbo-hydrates (grams)

R

RABBIT (USDA)
Domesticated:
Raw, ready-to-cook	1 lb. (weighed with bones)	581	0.
Stewed, flesh only	4 oz.	245	0.
Wild, ready-to-cook	1 lb. (weighed with bones)	490	0.

| **RACCOON**, roasted, meat only | 4 oz. | 289 | 0. |

RADISH (USDA):
Common, raw:
Without tops	½ lb. (weighed untrimmed)	34	7.4
Trimmed, whole	4 small radishes (1.4 oz.)	7	1.4
Trimmed sliced	½ cup (2 oz.)	10	2.1
Oriental, raw, without tops	½ lb. (weighed unpared)	34	7.4
Oriental, raw, trimmed & pared	4 oz.	22	4.8

RAISIN:
Dried:
(USDA):
Whole, pressed down	½ cup (2.9 oz.)	237	63.5
Chopped	½ cup (2.9 oz.)	234	62.7
Ground	½ cup (4.7 oz.)	387	103.7
(Dole) regular or golden	¼ cup (1½-oz.)	125	33.0
(Sun-Maid) seedless, natural Thompson	1 oz.	96	23.0

(USDA) = United States Department of Agriculture
(HHS/FAO) = Health and Human Services/Food and Agriculture Organization
* = prepared as package directs

Food and Description	Measure or Quantity	Calories	Carbo-hydrates (grams)
(Town House)	¼ cup	130	33.0
Cooked (USDA) added sugar, solids & liq.	½ cup (4.3 oz.)	260	68.8
RAISIN BRAN (See BRAN BREAKFAST CEREAL)			
RAISIN SQUARES, cereal (Kellogg's)	½ cup (1 oz.)	90	22.0
RASPBERRY:			
Black (USDA):			
Fresh:			
Whole	1 lb. (weighed with caps & stems)	160	34.6
Without caps & stems	½ cup (2.4 oz.)	49	10.5
Canned, water pack unsweetened, solids & liq.	4 oz.	58	12.1
Red:			
Fresh (USDA):			
Whole	1 lb. (weighed with caps & stems)	126	29.9
Without caps & stems	½ cup (2.5 oz.)	41	9.8
Canned, water pack, unsweetened or low calorie, solids & liq. (USDA)	4 oz.	40	10.0
Frozen (Birds Eye) quick thaw:			
Regular	5-oz. serving	155	37.0
In lite syrup	5-oz. serving	110	25.7
RASPBERRY DRINK, mix (Funny Face)	8 fl. oz.	88	22.0
RASPBERRY PRESERVE OR JAM:			
Sweetened (Smucker's)	1 T. (.7 oz.)	53	13.5
Dietetic:			
(Estee; Louis Sherry)	1 T. (.6 oz.)	6	0.
(Featherweight) red	1 T.	16	4.0
(S&W) *Nutradiet*, red label	1 T.	12	3.0

Food and Description	Measure or Quantity	Calories	Carbo-hydrates (grams)
RAVIOLI:			
Canned, regular pack (Franco-American)			
beef, *RavioliOs*	7½-oz. serving	250	35.0
Canned, dietetic (Estee)			
beef	7½-oz. can	230	25.0
Frozen:			
(Buitoni):			
Regular, square:			
Cheese	4.8-oz. serving	331	45.2
Meat	4.8-oz. serving	318	44.9
Ravioletti:			
Cheese	2.6-oz. serving	221	36.9
Meat	2.6-oz. serving	233	37.1
(Celentano) cheese:			
Regular	½ of 13-oz. box	380	50.0
Mini	½ of 8-oz. box	250	39.0
(Kid Cuisine)	8¾-oz. meal	250	52.0
(Weight Watchers) baked	9-oz. meal	290	30.0
RED & GRAY SNAPPER, raw (USDA):			
Whole	1 lb. (weighed whole)	219	0.
Meat only	4 oz.	105	0.
RED LOBSTER			
RESTAURANT			
("Lunch portion" refers to a cooked serving weighing 5 oz. raw, unless otherwise noted):			
Calamari, breaded & fried	Lunch portion	360	30.0
Catfish	Lunch portion	170	0.
Chicken breast, skinless	4-oz. serving	140	0.
Cod, Atlantic	Lunch portion	100	0.
Crab legs:			
King	16-oz. serving	170	6.0
Snow	16-oz. serving	150	1.0
Flounder	Lunch portion	100	1.0

(USDA) = United States Department of Agriculture
(HHS/FAO) = Health and Human Services/Food and Agriculture Organization
* = prepared as package directs

Food and Description	Measure or Quantity	Calories	Carbo-hydrates (grams)
Grouper	Lunch portion	110	0.
Haddock	Lunch portion	100	2.0
Halibut	Lunch portion	110	1.0
Hamburger, without bun	5.3 oz.	410	0.
Langostino	Lunch portion	120	2.0
Lobster:			
Maine	1 lobster (edible portion)	240	5.0
Rock	1 tail	230	2.0
Mackerel	Lunch portion	190	1.0
Monkfish	Lunch portion	110	0.
Perch, Atlantic Ocean	Lunch portion	130	1.0
Pollock	Lunch portion	120	1.0
Rockfish, red	Lunch portion	90	0.
Salmon:			
Norwegian	Lunch portion	230	3.0
Sockeye	Lunch portion	160	3.0
Scallop:			
Calico	Lunch portion	180	8.0
Deep sea	Lunch portion	130	2.0
Shark:			
Blacktip	Lunch portion	150	0.
Mako	Lunch portion	140	0.
Shrimp	8-12 pieces	120	0.
Snapper, red	Lunch portion	110	0.
Sole, lemon	Lunch portion	120	1.0
Steak:			
Filet mignon	8-oz. serving	350	0.
Porterhouse	18-oz. serving	1140	0.
Rib eye	12-oz. serving	980	0.
Sirloin	8-oz. serving	350	0.
Strip	9-oz. serving	560	0.
Swordfish	Lunch portion	100	0.
Tilefish	Lunch portion	100	0.
Trout, rainbow	Lunch portion	170	0.
Tuna, yellowfin	Lunch portion	180	0.
RELISH:			
Dill (Vlasic)	1 oz.	2	1.0
Hamburger:			
(Heinz)	1 T.	30	8.0
(Vlasic)	1 oz.	40	9.0
Hot dog:			
(Heinz)	1 oz.	35	8.0
(Vlasic)	1 oz.	40	8.0

Food and Description	Measure or Quantity	Calories	Carbo-hydrates (grams)
India (Heinz)	1 oz.	35	9.0
Sour (USDA)	1 T. (.5 oz.)	3	.4
Sweet:			
(Heinz)	1 oz.	25	6.6
(Vlasic)	1 oz.	30	8.0
RHINE WINE:			
(Great Western) 12% alcohol	3 fl. oz.	73	2.9
(Taylor) 12½% alcohol	3 fl. oz.	75	.3
RHUBARB (USDA)			
Cooked, sweetened, solids & liq.	½ cup (4.2 oz.)	169	43.2
Fresh:			
Partly trimmed	1 lb. (weighed with part leaves, fends & trimmings)	54	12.6
Trimmed	4 oz.	18	4.2
Diced	½ cup (2.2 oz.)	10	2.3
***RICE:**			
Brown (Uncle Ben's) parboiled, with added butter & salt	⅔ cup	152	26.4
White:			
(USDA) instant or pre-cooked	⅔ cup (3.3 oz.)	101	22.5
(Minute Rice) instant, no added butter	⅔ cup (4.3 oz.)	120	27.4
(River)	½ cup	100	22.0
(Success) long grain	½ cup	110	23.0
*(Uncle Ben's):			
Cooked without butter or salt	⅔ cup	129	28.9
Cooked with butter and salt	⅔ cup	148	28.9
White & wild (Carolina)	½ cup	90	20.0
RICE, FRIED (See also **RICE MIX**):			
*Canned (La Choy)	⅓ of 11-oz. can	190	40.0

(USDA) = United States Department of Agriculture
(HHS/FAO) = Health and Human Services/Food and Agriculture Organization
* = prepared as package directs

Food and Description	Measure or Quantity	Calories	Carbo- hydrates (grams)
Frozen:			
(Birds Eye)	3.7-oz. serving	104	22.8
(Chun King):			
Chicken	8 oz.	254	40.0
Pork	8 oz.	263	43.0
(La Choy) & meat	8-oz. serving	280	52.0
RICE & VEGETABLE, frozen:			
(Birds Eye):			
For One:			
& broccoli, au gratin	5-oz. pkg.	229	25.0
with green beans & almonds	5½-oz. pkg.	200	23.6
Mexican, with corn	5½-oz. pkg.	158	29.9
Pilaf	5½-oz. pkg.	215	27.6
International:			
Country style	⅓ of 10-oz. pkg.	87	19.0
French style	⅓ of 10-oz. pkg.	106	23.0
Spanish style	⅓ of 10-oz. pkg.	111	24.0
(Green Giant):			
One Serving Vegetable:			
& broccoli in cheese sauce	4½-oz. pkg.	180	25.0
with peas & mushrooms with sauce	5½-oz. pkg.	130	27.0
Rice Originals:			
& broccoli in cheese sauce	4 oz.	120	18.0
Medley	4 oz.	100	19.0
& wild rice	4 oz.	130	24.0
***RICE & VEGETABLE MIX:**			
(Knorr) risotto:			
With mushroom or onions	½ cup	130	24.0
With peas & corn	½ cup	130	23.0
(Lipton) & sauce:			
Asparagus with hollandaise sauce	½ cup	123	24.9
& broccoli, with cheddar cheese sauce	½ cup	131	26.1
RICE BRAN (USDA)	1 oz.	78	14.4
RICE CAKE:			
(Hain):			
Regular, any type	1 piece	40	8.0

Food and Description	Measure or Quantity	Calories	Carbo-hydrates (grams)
Mini:			
Plain, apple cinnamon or teriyaki	½-oz. serving	50	12.0
Barbecue or nacho cheese	½-oz. serving	70	10.0
Cheese	½-oz. serving	60	10.0
Honeynut	½-oz. serving	60	12.0
Ranch	½-oz. serving	40	4.0
Heart Lovers (TKI Foods)	.3-oz. piece	35	6.0
(Pritikin)	1 piece	35	6.0
RICE MIX:			
Beef:			
(Lipton) & sauce	¼ of pkg.	120	25.9
*(Minute Rice) rib roast	½ cup (4.1 oz.)	149	25.1
Rice-A-Roni	⅙ of 8-oz. pkg.	130	26.0
*Cajun (Lipton) & sauce	¼ of pkg.	123	26.0
Chicken:			
*(Lipton) & sauce	½ cup	125	25.4
*(Minute Rice) drumstick	½ cup (3.8 oz.)	153	25.4
Rice-A-Roni	⅙ of 8-oz. pkg.	130	27.0
*Fried (Minute Rice)	½ cup (3.4 oz.)	156	25.2
*Herb & butter (Lipton) & sauce	½ cup	124	24.1
*Long grain & wild (Lipton) & sauce:			
Original	½ cup	121	26.1
Mushroom & herb	½ cup	125	26.4
(Minute Rice)	½ cup (4.1 oz.)	148	25.0
(Uncle Ben's):			
Without butter	½ cup	97	20.6
With butter	½ cup	112	20.6
*Medley (Lipton) & sauce	½ cup	150	26.0
*Milanese (Knorr)	½ cup	130	24.0
*Mushroom (Lipton) & sauce	½ cup	123	26.1
*Pilaf (Lipton) & sauce	½ cup	117	24.7

(USDA) = United States Department of Agriculture
(HHS/FAO) = Health and Human Services/Food and Agriculture Organization
* = prepared as package directs

Food and Description	Measure or Quantity	Calories	Carbo-hydrates (grams)
Spanish (See also **RICE, SPANISH**):			
*(Carolina) *Bake-It-Easy*	¼ of pkg.	110	23.0
*(Lipton) & sauce	½ cup	120	25.7
*(Minute Rice)	½ cup (5.2 oz.)	150	25.6
Rice-A-Roni	⅐ of 7½-oz. pkg.	110	22.0
*Tomato (Knorr)	½ cup	130	23.0
RICE PUDDING (See **PUDDING OR PIE FILLING**)			
***RICE SEASONING MIX:**			
Fried:			
*(Durkee)	1 cup	213	46.5
(Kikkoman)	1-oz. pkg.	91	15.6
Spice Your Rice (French's):			
Beef flavor & onion, cheese & chives or chicken flavor & parmesan	½ cup	160	27.0
Buttery herb	½ cup	170	27.0
Chicken flavor & herb	½ cup	160	26.0
RICE WINE (HEW/FAO):			
Chinese, 20.7% alcohol	1 fl. oz.	38	1.1
Japanese, 10.6% alcohol	1 fl. oz.	72	13.1
RIGATONI, frozen (Healthy Choice) & meat sauce	9½-oz. meal	240	36.0
ROCK & RYE (Mr. Boston) 27% alcohol	1 fl. oz.	75	6.8
ROCKY ROAD, cereal (General Mills)	⅔ cup (1 oz.)	120	23.0
ROE (USDA):			
Raw:			
Carp, cod haddock, herring, pike or shad	4 oz.	147	1.7
Salmon, sturgeon or turbot	4 oz.	235	1.6

Food and Description	Measure or Quantity	Calories	Carbohydrates (grams)
Baked or broiled, cod & shad	4 oz.	143	2.2
Canned, cod, haddock or herring, solids & liq.	4 oz.	134	.3

ROLL OR BUN:
Commercial type, non-frozen:

Food and Description	Measure or Quantity	Calories	Carbohydrates (grams)
Apple (Dolly Madison)	2-oz. piece	180	33.0
Banquet (Mrs. Wright's)	1-oz. roll	90	17.0
Biscuit (Mrs. Wright's)	1-oz. piece	90	15.0
Blunt (Mrs. Wright's)	2-oz. piece	150	28.0
Brown & serve:			
(Interstate Brands) *Merita*	1-oz. roll	70	14.0
(Mrs. Wright's):			
Buttermilk, cloverleaf, gem or twin	1 piece	90	13.0
Half & half	1 piece	100	15.0
Sesame	1 piece	80	15.0
Sesame seed	1 piece	90	15.0
(Pepperidge Farm):			
Club	1 piece	100	19.0
French	1 piece	240	48.0
Hearth	1 piece	50	10.0
(Roman Meal)	1-oz. piece	72	12.6
Cherry (Dolly Madison)	2-oz. piece	180	33.0
Cinnamon (Dolly Madison)	1¾-oz. piece	180	28.0
Country (Pepperidge Farm)	1 piece	50	9.0
Crescent (Pepperidge Farm) butter	1-oz. piece	110	13.0
Croissant (Pepperidge Farm)	1 piece	170	22.0
Danish (Dolly Madison) *Danish Twirls:*			
Apple	2-oz. piece	240	28.0
Cheese, cream	3½-oz. piece	380	43.0
Cherry	2-oz. piece	230	28.0
Cinnamon raisin	2-oz. piece	250	28.0
Deli krisp (Mrs. Wright's)	1.3-oz. roll	120	20.0

(USDA) = United States Department of Agriculture
(HHS/FAO) = Health and Human Services/Food and Agriculture Organization
* = prepared as package directs

Food and Description	Measure or Quantity	Calories	Carbohydrates (grams)
Dinner:			
Butternut	1-oz. roll	90	15.0
Eddy's	1-oz. roll	75	14.0
Holsum	1-oz. roll	90	15.0
(Mrs. Wright's) split top	1.1-oz. roll	80	14.0
(Roman Meal)	1-oz. roll	75	12.7
Egg, *Weber's*	1-oz. bun	70	12.0
Farmstyle (Mrs. Wright's)	1-oz. piece	90	15.0
Finger (Pepperidge Farm) poppy seed	1 piece	50	8.0
Frankfurter:			
(Mrs. Wright's):			
Regular	1 piece	110	19.0
Sesame	1 piece	120	21.0
Wheat, crushed	1.5-oz. piece	110	22.0
(Pepperidge Farm):			
Regular	1 piece	140	24.0
Dijon	1 piece	160	23.0
(Roman Meal)	1.5-oz. roll	114	19.3
French (Arnold) *Francisco:*			
Regular	2-oz. roll	160	31.0
Sourdough	1.1-oz. piece	90	16.0
Golden Twist (Pepperidge Farm)	1-oz. piece	110	14.0
Hamburger:			
(Mrs. Wright's):			
Regular	2.3-oz. piece	190	35.0
Giant, plain	2½-oz. piece	200	37.0
Lite	1 piece	80	15.0
Multi-meal or onion	1 piece	130	24.0
Sesame	1.7-oz. piece	140	25.0
Sesame	2.3-oz. piece	200	34.0
Wheat, crushed:			
Regular	1.6-oz. piece	120	24.0
Giant	2.3-oz. piece	170	34.0
(Pepperidge Farm)	1.5-oz. piece	130	22.0
(Roman Meal)	1.6-oz. piece	122	20.6
Hard (USDA)	1.8-oz. piece	156	29.8
Hoagie (Pepperidge Farms)	1 piece	210	34.0
Honey (Dolly Madison)	3½-oz. piece	420	47.0
Lemon (Dolly Madison)	2-oz. piece	180	31.0
Old fashioned (Pepperidge Farm)	.6-oz. piece	50	7.0

Food and Description	Measure or Quantity	Calories	Carbo-hydrates (grams)
Parkerhouse (Pepperidge Farm)	.6-oz. piece	50	9.0
Party (Pepperidge Farm)	.4-oz. piece	30	5.0
Potato:			
(Mrs. Wright's)	1 piece	100	18.0
(Pepperidge Farm):			
Hearty, classic	1 piece	90	14.0
Sandwich bun	1 piece	160	28.0
Pull-apart (Mrs. Wright's)	2-oz. piece	170	23.0
Raspberry (Dolly Madison)	2-oz. piece	190	31.0
Soft (Pepperidge Farm)	1¼-oz. piece	100	18.0
Steak, *Butternut*	1-oz. roll	80	14.0
Sub (Mrs. Wright's):			
Regular	5-oz. piece	310	70.0
Jr.	3-oz. piece	220	45.0
Tea (Mrs. Wright's)	1 piece	70	4.0
Frozen (Pepperidge Farm):			
Cinnamon	2¼-oz. piece	280	34.0
Danish:			
Apple	1 piece	220	35.0
Cheese	1 piece	240	25.0
Cinnamon raisin	1 piece	250	35.0
Raspberry	1 piece	220	31.0
*ROLL OR BUN DOUGH:			
Frozen (Rich's) home style	1 roll	75	14.0
Refrigerated (Pillsbury):			
Butterflake	1 piece	140	20.0
Caramel danish, with nuts	1 piece	160	19.0
Cinnamon:			
Regular	1 piece	210	29.0
With icing:			
Regular	1 piece	110	17.0
& raisin	1 piece	140	19.5
Crescent	1 piece	100	11.0
*ROLL MIX, HOT (Pillsbury)	1 piece	100	17.0

(USDA) = United States Department of Agriculture
(HHS/FAO) = Health and Human Services/Food and Agriculture Organization
* = prepared as package directs

Food and Description	Measure or Quantity	Calories	Carbo-hydrates (grams)
ROMAN MEAL CEREAL, HOT			
Regular:			
Cream of rye	⅓ cup (1.3 oz.)	112	27.3
Multi bran with cinnamon apples	⅓ cup (1.2 oz.)	112	23.8
Oat bran	¼ cup (1 oz.)	93	17.4
Oats, wheat, dates, raisins & almonds	⅓ cup (1.3 oz.)	136	25.6
Original:			
Plain	⅓ cup (1 oz.)	82	20.3
With oats	⅓ cup (1.2 oz.)	106	23.3
Instant, oats, wheat, honey, coconut & almond	⅓ cup (1.3 oz.)	154	23.9
ROSEMARY LEAVES			
(French's)	1 tsp	5	.8
ROSÉ WINE:			
Corbett Canyon (Glenmore)	3 fl. oz.	63	1.0
(Great Western) 12% alcohol	3 fl. oz.	80	2.4
(Paul Masson):			
Regular, 11.8% alcohol	3 fl. oz.	76	4.2
Light, 7.1% alcohol	3 fl. oz.	49	3.9
ROY ROGERS:			
Bar Burger, R.R.	1 burger	593	38.0
Biscuit	1 biscuit	231	26.2
Breakfast crescent sandwich:			
Regular	4.5-oz. sandwich	408	28.0
With bacon	4.7-oz. sandwich	446	28.0
With ham	5.8-oz. sandwich	456	29.0
With sausage	5.7-oz. sandwich	564	28.0
Cheeseburger:			
Regular	1 burger	525	37.0
With bacon	1 burger	552	31.0
Chicken:			
Breast	1 piece (5.1 oz.)	412	16.9
Breast & wing	6.9-oz. piece	604	25.4
Leg	1 piece (1.9 oz.)	140	5.5
Thigh	1 piece (3.5 oz.)	296	11.7
Thigh & leg	5.3-oz. piece	436	17.2
Wing	1 piece (1.8 oz.)	192	8.5
Chicken nugget	1 piece	48	3.5

Food and Description	Measure or Quantity	Calories	Carbohydrates (grams)
Cole slaw	3½-oz. serving	110	11.0
Drinks:			
Coffee, black	6 fl. oz.	Tr.	Tr.
Cola:			
Regular	12 fl. oz.	145	37.0
Diet	12 fl. oz.	1	0.
Hot chocolate	6 fl. oz.	123	22.0
Milk	8 fl.oz.	150	11.4
Orange juice:			
Regular	7 fl. oz.	99	22.8
Large	10 fl. oz.	136	31.2
Shake:			
Chocolate	1 shake	358	61.3
Strawberry	1 shake	306	45.0
Vanilla	1 shake	315	49.4
Tea, iced, plain	8 fl.oz.	0	0.
Egg & biscuit platter:			
Regular	1 meal	559	44.0
With bacon	1 meal	607	44.0
With ham	1 meal	607	44.0
With sausage	1 meal	713	44.0
Hamburger	1 burger	472	26.6
Pancake platter, with syrup & butter			
Plain	1 order	386	63.0
With bacon	1 order	436	63.0
With ham	1 order	434	64.0
With sausage	1 order	542	63.0
Potato, french fries:			
Small	3 oz.	238	29.0
Large	5.5 oz.	440	54.0
Potato salad	3½-oz. order	107	10.9
Roast beef sandwich:			
Plain:			
Regular	1 sandwich	350	37.0
Large	1 sandwich	373	35.0
With cheese:			
Regular	1 sandwich	403	29.0
Large	1 sandwich	427	30.3

(USDA) = United States Department of Agriculture
(HHS/FAO) = Health and Human Services/Food and Agriculture Organization
* = prepared as package directs

Food and Description	Measure or Quantity	Calories	Carbo-hydrates (grams)
Salad bar:			
Bacon bits	1 T.	33	2.2
Beets, sliced	¼ cup	18	2.0
Broccoli	½ cup	12	3.5
Carrot, shredded	¼ cup	12	9.7
Cheese, cheddar	¼ cup	112	.8
Croutons	1 T.	35	7.0
Cucumber	1 slice	Tr.	.2
Egg, chopped	1 T.	27	.3
Lettuce	1 cup	10	4.0
Macaroni salad	1 T.	30	3.1
Mushrooms	¼ cup	5	.7
Noodle, Chinese	¼ cup	55	6.5
Pea, green	¼ cup	7	1.2
Pepper, green	1 T.	2	.5
Potato salad	1 T.	25	2.8
Sunflower seeds	1 T.	78	2.5
Tomato	1 slice	7	1.6
Salad dressing:			
Regular:			
Bacon & tomato	1 T.	68	3.0
Bleu cheese	1 T.	75	1.0
Ranch	1 T.	77	2.0
1000 Island	1 T.	80	2.0
Low calorie, Italian	1 T.	35	1.0
Strawberry shortcake	7.2-oz. serving	447	59.3
Sundae:			
Caramel	1 sundae	293	51.5
Hot fudge	1 sundae	337	53.3
Strawberry	1 sundae	216	33.1

RUM (See **DISTILLED LIQUOR**)

RUTABAGA:

Raw (USDA):			
Without tops	1 lb. (weighed with skin)	177	42.4
Diced	½ cup (2.5 oz.)	32	7.7
Boiled (USDA) drained, diced	½ cup (3 oz.)	30	7.1
Canned (Sunshine) solids & liq.	½ cup (4.2 oz.)	32	6.9

Food and Description	Measure or Quantity	Calories	Carbo-hydrates (grams)
RYE, whole grain (USDA)	1 oz.	95	20.8

RYE FLOUR (See **FLOUR**)

RYE WHISKEY (See **DISTILLED LIQUOR**)

Food and Description	Measure or Quantity	Calories	Carbohydrates (grams)

S

SABLEFISH, raw (USDA):

Whole	1 lb. (weighed whole)	362	0.
Meat only	4 oz.	215	0.

SAFFLOWER SEED (USDA) in hull

	1 oz.	89	1.8

SAKE WINE (HEW/FAO)

19.8% alcohol	1 fl. oz.	39	1.4

*SALAD BAR PASTA (Buitoni):

Country buttermilk or homestyle	⅙ of pkg.	250	22.0
Italian:			
Creamy	⅙ of pkg.	290	20.0
Zesty	⅙ of pkg.	140	21.0

SALAD DRESSING:

Regular:			
Bacon & tomato (Henri's)	1 T.	70	4.0
Bleu or blue cheese:			
(USDA)	1 T. (.5 oz.)	76	1.1
(Henri's)	1 T.	60	3.0
(Nu Made)	1 T.	60	1.0
(Wish-Bone) chunky	1 T.	73	.8
Boiled (USDA) home recipe	1 T. (.6 oz.)	26	2.4
Buttermilk:			
(Hain)	1 T.	70	0.
(Nu Made)	1 T.	50	1.0
Caesar:			
(Hain) creamy	1 T.	60	1.0
(Wish-Bone)	1 T.	78	.9
Cheddar bacon (Wish-Bone)	1 T. (.5 oz.)	70	1.0

Food and Description	Measure or Quantity	Calories	Carbo-hydrates (grams)
Cucumber, creamy:			
(Nu Made)	1 T.	70	1.0
(Wish-Bone)	1 T. (.5 oz.)	80	1.0
Cucumber dill (Hain)	1 T.	80	0.
Dijon vinaigrette:			
(Hain)	1 T.	50	0.
(Wish-Bone)	1 T.	60	1.0
French:			
Home recipe (USDA)	1 T.	101	.6
(Hain) creamy	1 T.	60	1.0
(Henri's):			
Hearty	1 T.	70	4.0
Original	1 T.	60	3.0
Sweet 'n saucy	1 T.	70	5.0
(Nu Made) savory	1 T.	60	2.0
(Wish-Bone):			
Deluxe	1 T.	57	2.3
Red	1 T.	64	3.9
French mustard (Hain)	1 T.	50	1.0
Green tomato vinaigrette (Hain)	1 T.	60	1.0
Garlic & sour cream (Hain)	1 T.	70	0.
Green goddess (Nu Made)	1 T.	60	1.0
Honey & sesame (Hain)	1 T.	60	2.0
Italian:			
(Hain):			
Canola oil	1 T.	50	1.0
& cheese vinaigrette	1 T.	55	0.
Creamy or traditional	1 T.	80	0.
(Henri's):			
Authentic	1 T.	80	1.0
Creamy garlic	1 T.	50	3.0
(Wish-Bone):			
Creamy	1 T.	56	1.7
Herbal	1 T.	70	1.2
Robusto	1 T.	70	1.3
Mayonnaise (See **MAYONNAISE**)			
Mayonnaise-type:			
(Luzianne) Blue Plate	1 T.	70	3.0

(USDA) = United States Department of Agriculture
(HHS/FAO) = Health and Human Services/Food and Agriculture Organization
* = prepared as package directs

Food and Description	Measure or Quantity	Calories	Carbo-hydrates (grams)
Miracle Whip (Kraft)	1 T.	70	2.0
Ranch (Henri's) *Chef's Recipe*	1 T.	70	2.0
Red wine vinegar & oil (Wish-Bone)	1 T.	50	4.3
Roquefort (USDA)	1 T. (.5 oz.)	76	1.1
Russian:			
(USDA)	1 T.	74	1.6
(Henri's)	1 T.	60	4.0
(Wish-Bone)	1 T.	45	5.9
Swiss cheese vinaigrette (Hain)	1 T.	60	0.
Tangy citrus (Hain)	1 T.	50	1.0
Tas-Tee (Henri's)	1 T.	60	4.0
1000 Island:			
(USDA)	1 T.	80	2.5
(Hain)	1 T.	50	0.
(Henri's)	1 T.	50	2.0
(Nu Made)	1 T.	60	3.0
(Wish-Bone)	1 T.	61	32
Dietetic or low calorie:			
Bleu or blue cheese:			
(Estee)	1 T. (.5 oz.)	8	1.0
(Henri's)	1 T.	35	5.0
Herb Magic (Luzianne Blue Plate) creamy	1 T.	8	2.0
(Walden Farms) chunky	1 T.	27	1.7
(Wish-Bone) chunky	1 T.	40	1.0
Caesar:			
(Hain) low salt	1 T.	60	1.0
(Weight Watchers)	¾-oz. pouch	6	1.0
Catalina (Kraft)	1 T.	16	3.0
Chef's Recipe (Henri's) ranch	1 T.	40	6.0
Cucumber:			
(Kraft) creamy	1 T.	30	1.0
(Luzianne Blue Plate) *Herb Magic*, creamy	1 T. (.6 oz.)	8	2.0
Cucumber & onion (Henri's) creamy	1 T.	35	6.0
Dijon (Estee)	1 T.	8	1.0
French:			
(Estee)	1 T. (.5 oz.)	4	<1.0
(Henri's):			
Hearty	1 T.	30	5.0
Original	1 T.	40	6.0

Food and Description	Measure or Quantity	Calories	Carbo-hydrates (grams)
(Pritikin)	1 T.	10	2.0
(Walden Farms)	1 T.	33	2.6
(Wish-Bone):	1 T.	31	2.1
Regular	1 T.	30	1.9
Red	1 T.	17	3.2
Sweet & spicy	1 T.	18	3.2
Garlic (Estee)	1 T. (.5 oz.)	2	0.
Herb basket, *Herb Magic*			
(Luzianne Blue Plate)	1 T.	6	2.0
Italian:			
(Estee) creamy	1 T. (.5 oz.)	4	0.
(Estee) spicy	1 T.	4	1.0
(Hain) creamy	1 T.	80	1.0
(Henri's) authentic	1 T.	20	2.0
Herb Magic (Luzianne			
Blue Plate)	1 T.	4	1.0
(Kraft) zesty	1 T.	6	1.0
(Pritikin):			
Regular	1 T.	6	2.0
Creamy	1 T.	16	3.0
(Walden Farms):			
Regular or low sodium	1 T.	9	1.5
No sugar added	1 T.	6	Tr.
(Weight Watchers) regular	1 T.	50	2.0
(Wish-Bone)	1 T	7	.9
Ranch:			
Herb Magic (Luzianne			
Blue Plate)	1 T.	6	1.0
(Pritikin)	1 T.	18	4.0
(Weight Watchers)	¾-oz. pkg.	35	8.0
(Wish-Bone)	1 T.	46	2.3
Red wine/vinegar			
(Estee)	1 T.	2	0.
Russian:			
(Pritikin)	1 T.	12	3.0
(Weight Watchers)	1 T. (.5 oz.)	50	2.0
(Wish-Bone)	1 T. (.5 oz.)	22	3.9
Tas-Tee (Henri's)	1 T.	30	4.0

(USDA) = United States Department of Agriculture
(HHS/FAO) = Health and Human Services/Food and Agriculture Organization
* = prepared as package directs

Food and Description	Measure or Quantity	Calories	Carbo-hydrates (grams)
1000 Island:			
(Estee)	1 T.	8	2.0
(Henri's)	1 T.	30	4.0
Herb Magic (Luzianne Blue Plate)	1 T.	8	2.0
(Kraft)	1 T.	30	2.0
(Walden Farms)	1 T.	24	3.1
(Weight Watchers)	1 T.	50	2.0
(Wish-Bone)	1 T.	36	1.9
Vinaigrette (Pritikin)	1 T.	10	2.0
Whipped (Weight Watchers)	1 T. (.5 oz.)	45	2.0
*SALAD DRESSING MIX:			
Regular (Good Seasons):			
Blue cheese & herbs	1 T. (.6 oz.)	72	1.0
Buttermilk, farm style	1 T. (.6 oz.)	58	1.2
Classic dill	1 T.	70	.5
Garlic, cheese	1 T.	72	1.0
Garlic & herb	1 T.	71	1.0
Italian:			
Regular, cheese or zesty	1 T. (.6 oz.)	71	.6
Mild	1 T. (.6 oz.)	73	1.0
Ranch	1 T.	57	1.0
Dietetic:			
Blue cheese (Hain)	1 T.	14	1.0
Buttermilk (Hain)	1 T.	11	1.0
Caesar (Hain) no oil	1 T.	6	1.0
French (Hain) no oil	1 T.	12	3.0
Garlic & cheese (Hain)	1 T.	6	1.0
Herb (Hain)	1 T.	2	1.0
Italian:			
(Good Seasons):			
Regular	1 T.	8	1.8
Lite	1 T.	27	.8
(Hain) no oil	1 T.	2	1.0
Ranch (Good Seasons)	1 T.	29	2.0
Russian (Weight Watchers)	1 T.	4	1.0
1000 Island:			
Hain	1 T.	12	3.0
Weight Watchers	1 T.	12	1.0
SALAD SUPREME			
(McCormick)	1 tsp. (.1 oz.)	11	.5

Food and Description	Measure or Quantity	Calories	Carbo-hydrates (grams)
SALAMI:			
(USDA):			
Dry	1 oz.	128	.3
Cooked	1 oz.	88	.4
(Eckrich):			
Beer or cooked	1 oz.	70	1.0
Cotto:			
Beef	.7-oz. slice	50	1.0
Meat	1-oz. slice	70	1.0
Hard	1 oz.	130	1.0
Hebrew National	1 oz.	80	1.0
(Hormel):			
Beef	1 slice	25	0.
Cotto:			
Chub	1 oz.	100	0.
Sliced	1 slice	52	5.
Genoa:			
Regular or *Gran Value*	1 oz.	110	0.
Di Lusso	1 oz.	100	0.
Hard:			
Packaged, sliced	1 slice	40	0.
Whole:			
Regular	1 oz.	110	0.
National Brand	1 oz.	120	0.
Party slice	1 oz.	90	0.
Piccolo, stick	1 oz.	120	0.
(Ohse) cooked	1 oz.	65	1.0
(Oscar Mayer):			
Beer:			
Regular	.8-oz. slice	50	.4
Beef	.8-oz. slice	64	.4
Cotto:			
Regular	.8-oz. slice	53	.4
Beef	.5-oz. slice	29	.2
Beef	.8-oz. slice	46	.4
Genoa	.3-oz. slice	34	.1
Hard	.3-oz. slice	33	.1
(Smok-A-Roma):			
Beef or cotto	1-oz. slice	80	1.0
Turkey	1-oz. slice	45	1.0

(USDA) = United States Department of Agriculture
(HHS/FAO) = Health and Human Services/Food and Agriculture
                        Organization
* = prepared as package directs

Food and Description	Measure or Quantity	Calories	Carbo-hydrates (grams)
SALISBURY STEAK, frozen:			
(Armour):			
Classics Lite	11½-oz. meal	300	29.0
Dining Lite	9-oz. meal	200	14.0
Dinner Classics, regular	11¼-oz. meal	350	26.0
(Banquet):			
Regular	11-oz. dinner	500	26.0
Extra Helping	18-oz. dinner	910	49.0
(Healthy Choice)	11½-oz. meal	300	41.0
(Le Menu):			
Regular	10½-oz. meal	370	28.0
Healthy style	10-oz. meal	280	31.0
(Morton)	10-oz. dinner	300	23.0
(Stouffer's):			
Regular, with onion gravy	9⅞-oz. pkg.	250	9.0
Lean Cuisine, with Italian style sauce & vegetables	9½-oz. pkg.	280	12.0
(Swanson):			
Regular	10¾-oz. dinner	400	43.0
Homestyle Recipe	10-oz. entree	320	22.0
Hungry Man	16½-oz. dinner	680	37.0
(Weight Watchers) beef, Romana	8¾-oz. meal	310	26.0
SALMON:			
Atlantic (USDA):			
Raw:			
Whole	1 lb. (weighed whole)	640	0.
Meat only	4 oz.	246	0.
Canned, solids & liq., including bones	4 oz.	230	.9
Chinook or King (USDA)			
Raw:			
Steak	1 lb. (weighed whole)	886	0.
Meat only	4 oz.	252	0.
Canned, solids & liq., including bones	4 oz.	238	0.
Chum, canned (USDA), solids & liq., including bones	4 oz.	158	0.
Coho, canned (USDA) solids & liq., including bones	4 oz.	174	0.

Food and Description	Measure or Quantity	Calories	Carbohydrates (grams)
Keta, canned (Peter Pan) solids & liq., including bones	½ cup (3.9 oz.)	140	0.
Pink or Humpback (USDA):			
Raw:			
Steak	1 lb. (weighed whole)	475	0.
Meat only	4 oz.	135	0.
Canned, solids & liq.:			
(USDA) including bones	4 oz.	135	0.
(Bumble Bee) including bones	½ cup (4 oz.)	155	0.
(Del Monte)	7¾-oz. can	277	0.
Sockeye or Red or Blueback, canned, solids & liq.:			
(USDA)	4 oz.	194	0.
(Bumble Bee) including bones	½ cup (4 oz.)	155	0.
(Del Monte)	½ of 7¾-oz. can	165	0.
Unspecified kind of salmon (USDA) baked or broiled	4.2 oz. steak (approx. 4" × 3" × ½")	218	0.
SALMON, SMOKED (USDA)	4 oz.	200	0.
SALT:			
Regular:			
Butter-flavored (French's) imitation	1 tsp. (3.6 grams)	8	0.
Garlic (Lawry's)	1 tsp. (4 grams)	5	1.0
Hickory smoke (French's)	1 tsp. (4 grams)	2	Tr.
Onion (Lawry's)	1 tsp.	4	.9
Seasoned (Lawry's)	1 tsp.	3	.6
Table:			
(USDA)	1 tsp.	0	0.
(Morton) iodized	1 tsp. (7 grams)	0	0.
Lite Salt (Morton) iodized	1 tsp. (6 grams)	0	0.

(USDA) = United States Department of Agriculture
(HHS/FAO) = Health and Human Services/Food and Agriculture Organization
* = prepared as package directs

Food and Description	Measure or Quantity	Calories	Carbo-hydrates (grams)
Substitute:			
(Adolph's):			
Regular	1 tsp. (6 grams)	1	Tr.
Packet	8-gram packet	*1	Tr.
Seasoned	1 tsp.	6	1.1
(Estee) *Salt-It*	½ tsp.	0	0.
(Morton):			
Regular	1 tsp. (6 grams)	Tr.	Tr.
Seasoned	1 tsp. (6 grams)	3	.5
SALT PORK, raw (USDA):			
With skin	1 lb. (weighed with skin)	3410	0.
Without skin	1 oz.	222	0.
SANDWICH SPREAD:			
(USDA)	1 T. (.5 oz.)	57	2.4
(USDA)	½ cup (4.3 oz.)	466	19.5
(Hellmann's)	1 T. (.5 oz.)	55	2.4
(Nu Made)	1 T.	60	4.0
(Oscar Mayer)	1-oz. serving	67	3.6
SANGRIA (Taylor) 11.6% alcohol	3 fl. oz.	99	10.8
SARDINE:			
Raw (HEW/FAO):			
Whole	1 lb. (weighed whole)	321	0.
Meat only	4 oz.	146	0.
Canned:			
Atlantic:			
(USDA) in oil:			
Solids & liq.	3¾-oz. can	330	.6
(Drained solids, with skin & bones	3¾-oz. can	187	DNA
(Del Monte) in tomato sauce, solids & liq.	7½-oz. can	330	4.0
(Underwood):			
In mustard sauce	3¾-oz. can	220	2.0
In tomato sauce	3⅜-oz. can	220	2.0
Norwegian:			
(Granadaisa Brand) in tomato sauce	3¾-oz. can	195	0.

Food and Description	Measure or Quantity	Calories	Carbo-hydrates (grams)
(King David Brand) brisling, in olive oil	3¾-oz. can	293	0.
(King Oscar Brand):			
In mustard sauce, solids & liq.	3¾-oz. can	240	2.0
In oil, drained	3-oz. can	260	1.0
In tomato sauce, solids & liq.	3¾-oz. can	240	2.0
(Queen Helga Brand) sild, in sild oil	3¾-oz. can	310	0.
(Underwood) drained	3-oz. serving	230	1.0
Pacific (USDA) in brine or mustard, solids & liq.	4 oz.	222	1.9
SAUCE:			
Regular:			
A-1	1 T. (.6 oz.)	12	3.1
Barbecue:			
(USDA)	1 cup (8.8 oz.)	228	20.0
(French's) regular hot or smoky	1 T. (.6 oz.)	14	3.0
(Gold's)	1 T.	16	3.9
(Heinz):			
Regular	½ cup	160	27.0
Hickory smoked & hot	½ cup	160	31.0
(Hunt's) all natural:			
Any type except Texas	1 T. (.5 oz.)	20	5.0
Texas	1 T. (.5 oz.)	25	6.0
(Kraft):			
Plain or hot	½ cup	160	DNA
Onion bits	½ cup	200	DNA
(La Choy) oriental	1 T.	16	3.8
Caramel (Knorr)	1 T. (.7 oz.)	60	14.7
Cheese (Snow's) Welsh Rarebit	½ cup	170	10.0
Chicken Tonight, simmer sauce (Ragú):			
Cacciatore	4 oz.	70	12.0
Country french	4 oz.	140	6.0
Creamy, with mushrooms	4 oz.	110	5.0

(USDA) = United States Department of Agriculture
(HHS/FAO) = Health and Human Services/Food and Agriculture Organization
* = prepared as package directs

Food and Description	Measure or Quantity	Calories	Carbo-hydrates (grams)
Herb, with wine	4 oz.	100	13.0
Oriental	4 oz.	70	14.0
Salsa	4 oz.	35	7.0
Chili (See **CHILI SAUCE**)			
Cocktail (See also Seafood cocktail):			
(Gold's)	1 oz.	31	7.5
(Pfeiffer)	1-oz. serving	50	6.0
Grilling & broiling (Knorr):			
Chardonnay	⅛ of container	50	4.5
Spicy plum	⅛ of container	60	11.2
Tequila lime	⅛ of container	50	6.4
Tuscan herb	⅛ of container	55	4.6
Hollandaise (Knorr) microwave	1/12 of pkg. (1 oz.)	50	1.0
Hot dog, *Just Right*	2 oz.	60	6.0
Mandarin ginger (Knorr) microwave	⅛ of pkg.	55	5.3
Newberg (Snow's)	⅓ cup	120	10.0
Orange (La Choy)	1 T. (.6 oz.)	23	6.1
Parmesano (Knorr) microwave	⅛ of pkg.	50	3.3
Picante (Pace)	1 tsp.	2	.3
Plum (La Choy) tangy	1 oz.	44	10.8
Salsa Brava (La Victoria)	1 T.	6	1.0
Salsa Casera (La Victoria)	1 T.	4	1.0
Salsa Mexicana (Contadina)	4 fl. oz. (4.4 oz.)	38	6.8
Salsa Ranchera (La Victoria)	1 T.	6	1.0
Salsa verde (Old El Paso)	1 T.	5	1.0
Seafood cocktail (Del Monte)	1 T. (.6 oz.)	21	4.9
Soy:			
(USDA)	1 oz.	19	2.7
(Chun King)	1 tsp.	5	.7
(Gold's)	1 T.	10	1.0
(Kikkoman):			
Regular	1 T. (.6 oz.)	10	.9
Light, low sodium	1 T.	11	1.3
(La Choy)	1 T. (.5 oz.)	8	.9
Sparerib (Gold's)	1 oz.	60	14.0
Stir-fry (Kikkoman)	1 tsp.	6	2.3
Sweet & sour:			
(Chun King)	1.8-oz. serving	57	14.4

Food and Description	Measure or Quantity	Calories	Carbo-hydrates (grams)
(Contadina)	4 fl. oz. (4.4 oz.)	150	29.6
(Kikkoman)	1 T.	18	4.0
(La Choy)	1-oz. serving	30	7.0
Szechuan (La Choy)	1 oz.	48	12.0
Tabasco	¼ tsp.	Tr.	Tr.
Taco:			
(El Molino) red, mild	1 T.	5	1.0
(La Victoria):			
Green	1 T.	4	1.0
Red	1 T.	6	1.0
(Old El Paso), hot or mild	1 T.	5	1.2
(Ortega) hot or mild	1 oz.	13	3.1
Tartar:			
(USDA)	1 T. (.5 oz.)	74	.6
(Hellmann's)	1 T. (.5 oz.)	70	.1
Teriyaki (Kikkoman)	1 T. (.6 oz.)	15	2.7
Vera Cruz (Knorr) microwave	¼ of pkg. (3.4 oz.)	65	9.3
White (USDA) home recipe:			
Thin	¼ cup (2.2 oz.)	74	4.5
Medium	¼ cup (2.5 oz.)	103	5.6
Thick	¼ cup (2.2 oz.)	122	6.8
Worcestershire:			
(French's) regular or smoky	1 T. (.6 oz.)	10	2.0
(Gold's)	1 T.	42	3.3
(Lea & Perrins)	1 T. (.6 oz.)	12	3.0
Dietetic:			
Barbecue (Estee)	1 T. (.6 oz.)	18	3.0
Mexican (Pritikin)	1 oz.	12	2.0
Soy:			
(Kikkoman) lite	1 T.	9	.3
(La Choy)	1 T.	1	.8
Steak (Estee)	½ oz.	14	3.0
Tartar (USDA)	1 T. (.5 oz.)	31	.9

(USDA) = United States Department of Agriculture
(HHS/FAO) = Health and Human Services/Food and Agriculture Organization
* = prepared as package directs

Food and Description	Measure or Quantity	Calories	Carbohydrates (grams)
SAUCE MIX:			
Regular:			
*Au jus (Knorr)	2 fl. oz.	8	1.1
*Bearnaise (Knorr)	2 fl. oz.	170	5.0
*Demi-glace (Knorr)	2 fl. oz.	30	3.9
*Hollandaise (Knorr)	2 fl. oz.	170	5.0
*Hunter (Knorr)	2 fl. oz.	25	3.7
*Italian (Knorr) Napoli	4 fl. oz.	100	17.0
*Lyonnaise (Knorr)	2 fl. oz.	20	3.4
*Mushroom (Knorr)	2 fl. oz.	60	5.0
*Pepper (Knorr)	2 fl. oz.	20	3.0
*Sour cream:			
(Durkee)	⅔ cup	214	15.0
(French's)	2½ T.	60	5.0
*Stroganoff (French's)	⅓ cup	110	11.0
Sweet & sour:			
*(Durkee)	½ cup	115	22.5
*(French's)	½ cup	55	14.0
(Kikkoman)	1 T.	18	4.0
Teriyaki:			
*(French's)	1 T.	17	3.5
(Kikkoman)	1.5-oz. pkg.	125	22.3
*White (Durkee)	½ cup	119	20.5
SAUERKRAUT, canned:			
(USDA):			
Solids & liq.	½ cup (4.1 oz.)	21	4.7
Drained solids	½ cup (2.5 oz.)	15	3.1
(Claussen) drained	½ cup (2.7 oz.)	16	2.9
(Comstock) solids & liq.:			
Regular	½ cup (4.1 oz.)	30	4.0
Bavarian	½ cup (4.2 oz.)	35	7.0
(Frank's) solids & liq.:			
Regular	½ cup	28	4.0
Bavarian	½ cup	64	12.0
(Vlasic)	1 oz.	4	1.0
SAUERKRAUT JUICE, canned			
(USDA) 2% salt	½ cup (4.3 oz.)	12	2.8
SAUSAGE:			
*Brown & serve:			
(USDA)	1 oz.	120	.8
(Hormel)	1 sausage	70	0.
Country style (USDA) smoked	1 oz.	98	0.

Food and Description	Measure or Quantity	Calories	Carbohydrates (grams)
German (Smok-A-Roma)	4-oz. link	350	1.0
Italian style, hot or mild (Hillshire Farms)	3-oz. serving	263	*1.0
Knockwurst (*Hebrew National*) hot	1 oz.	79	.6
Links (Ohse) hot	1 oz.	80	4.0
Patty (Hormel) hot or mild	1 patty	150	0.
Polish-style:			
(Eckrich) meat:			
Regular	1 oz.	95	1.0
Skinless	1-oz. link	90	1.0
Skinless	1-oz. link	180	2.0
(Hormel):			
Regular	1 sausage	85	0.
Kielbasa, skinless	½ a link	180	1.0
Kolbase	3 oz.	220	1.0
(Ohse):			
Regular	1 oz.	80	1.0
Hot	1 oz.	70	3.0
Pork:			
*(USDA)	1 oz.	135	Tr.
(Eckrich):			
Links	1-oz. link	110	.5
Patty	2-oz. patty	240	1.0
Roll, hot	2-oz. serving	240	1.0
*(Hormel):			
Little Sizzlers	1 link	51	0.
Midget links	1 link	71	0.
Smoked	1 oz.	96	.3
(Jimmy Dean)	2-oz. serving	227	Tr.
*(Oscar Mayer) *Little Friers*	1 link	79	.3
Roll (Eckrich) minced	1-oz. slice	80	1.0
Smoked:			
(Eckrich):			
Beef:			
Regular	2 oz.	190	1.0
Smok-Y-Links	.8-oz. link	70	1.0
Cheese	2 oz.	180	2.0
Ham, *Smok-Y-Links*	.8-oz. link	75	1.0

(USDA) = United States Department of Agriculture
(HHS/FAO) = Health and Human Services/Food and Agriculture Organization
* = prepared as package directs

Food and Description	Measure or Quantity	Calories	Carbo-hydrates (grams)
Maple flavored, *Smok-Y-Links*	.8-oz. link	75	1.0
Meat:			
Regular	2 oz.	190	1.0
Hot	2.7-oz. link	240	3.0
Skinless:			
Regular	2-oz. link	180	2.0
Smok-Y-Links	.8-oz. link	75	1.0
(Hormel) Smokies:			
Regular	1 link	80	.5
Cheese	1 link	84	.5
(Ohse)	1 oz.	80	1.0
(Oscar Mayer):			
Beef	1½-oz. link	126	.7
Cheese	1½-oz. link	127	.8
Little Smokies	1 link	28	.1
Meat	1.5-oz. link	126	.7
Thuringer (See **THURINGER**)			
Turkey (Louis Rich) links or tube	1-oz. serving	45	Tr.
Vienna, canned:			
(USDA)	1 link (5-oz. can)	38	Tr.
(Hormel) drained:			
Regular	1 link	50	.3
Chicken	1 link	45	.3
(Libby's):			
In barbecue sauce	2½-oz. serving	180	2.0
In beef broth	1 link	46	.3
SAUTERNE:			
(Great Western)	3 fl. oz.	79	4.5
(Taylor)	3 fl. oz.	81	4.8
SCALLION (See **ONION, GREEN**)			
SCALLOP:			
Raw (USDA) muscle only	4-oz. serving	92	3.7
Steamed (USDA)	4-oz. serving	127	DNA
Frozen:			
(Captain's Choice) fried	1 piece	33	1.5
(Mrs. Paul's) fried, light	3 oz.	160	18.0

Food and Description	Measure or Quantity	Calories	Carbo-hydrates (grams)
SCHNAPPS:			
Apple (Mr. Boston) 27% alcohol	1 fl. oz.	78	8.0
Cinnamon (Mr. Boston) 27% alcohol	1 fl. oz.	76	8.0
Peppermint:			
(De Kuyper)	1 fl. oz.	79	7.5
(Mr. Boston) 50% alcohol	1 fl. oz.	115	8.0
Spearmint (Mr. Boston)	1 fl. oz.	78	7.8
Strawberry (Mr. Boston)	1 fl. oz.	68	6.2
SCOTCH WHISKY (See DISTILLED LIQUOR)			
SCREWDRIVER COCKTAIL (Mr. Boston) 12½% alcohol	3 fl. oz.	111	12.0
SCROD, frozen (Gorton's)	1 pkg.	320	17.0
SEA BASS, raw (USDA) meat only	4 oz.	109	0.
SEASON-ALL SEASONING (McCormick)	1 tsp.	4	.6
SEAFOOD CREOLE, frozen (Swanson) *Homestyle Recipe*	9-oz. entree	240	40.0
SEAFOOD NEWBERG, frozen (Healthy Choice)	8-oz. meal	200	30.0
SEAWEED, dried (HHS/FAO):			
Agar	1 oz.	88	23.7
Lavar	1 oz.	67	12.6
SEGO DIET FOOD, canned:			
Regular:			
Very chocolate, very chocolate malt or very Dutch chocolate	10 fl. oz.	225	43.0

(USDA) = United States Department of Agriculture
(HHS/FAO) = Health and Human Services/Food and Agriculture
          Organization
* = prepared as package directs

Food and Description	Measure or Quantity	Calories	Carbohydrates (grams)
Very strawberry or very vanilla	10 fl. oz.	225	34.0
Lite:			
Chocolate, chocolate jamocha almond, chocolate malt or Dutch chocolate	10-fl.-oz. can	150	20.0
Double chocolate	10-fl.-oz. can	150	21.0
French vanilla, strawberry or vanilla	10-fl.-oz. can	150	17.0

SELTZER (See **MINERAL WATER**)

SESAME NUT MIX, canned (Planters) roasted | 1 oz. | 160 | 8.0

SESAME SEEDS, dry (USDA):

| Whole | 1 oz. | 160 | 6.1 |
| Hulled | 1 oz. | 165 | 5.0 |

7 GRAIN CEREAL
(Loma Linda):

| Crunchy | 1 oz. | 110 | 21.0 |
| No sugar | 1 oz. | 110 | 20.0 |

SHAD (USDA):
Raw:

| Whole | 1 lb. (weighed whole) | 370 | 0. |
| Meat only | 4 oz. | 193 | 0. |

Cooked, home recipe:

Baked with butter or margarine & bacon slices	4 oz.	228	0.
Creole	4 oz.	172	1.8
Canned, solids & liq.	4 oz.	172	0.

SHAD, GIZZARD, raw (USDA):

| Whole | 1 lb. (weighed whole) | 229 | 0. |
| Meat only | 4 oz. | 227 | 0. |

SHAD ROE (*See* **ROE**)

Food and Description	Measure or Quantity	Calories	Carbohydrates (grams)
SHAKE 'N BAKE:			
Chicken:			
Original recipe	5½-oz. pkg.	617	108.9
Barbecue	7-oz. pkg.	741	146.9
Country mild	4¾-oz. pkg.	610	79.5
Italian herb	5¾-oz. pkg.	613	111.0
Fish, original recipe	5¼-oz. pkg.	582	111.1
Pork or ribs:			
Original recipe	6-oz. pkg.	652	131.4
Barbecue	5¾-oz. pkg.	609	118.1
Extra crispy, *Oven Fry*	4.2-oz. pkg.	482	83.1
SHAKEY'S:			
Chicken, fried, & potatoes:			
3-piece	1 order	947	51.0
5-piece	1 order	1700	130.0
Ham & cheese sandwich	1 sandwich	550	56.0
Pizza:			
Cheese:			
Homestyle pan crust	⅒ of 12″ pizza	303	31.0
Thick crust	⅒ of 12″ pizza	170	21.6
Thin crust	⅒ of 12″ pizza	133	13.2
Onion, green pepper, black olives & mushrooms:			
Homestyle pan crust	⅒ of 12″ pizza	320	32.1
Thick crust	⅒ of 12″ pizza	162	22.2
Thin crust	⅒ of 12″ pizza	125	13.8
Pepperoni:			
Homestyle pan crust	⅒ of 12″ pizza	343	31.1
Thick crust	⅒ of 12″ pizza	185	21.8
Thin crust	⅒ of 12″ pizza	148	13.2
Sausage & mushroom:			
Homestyle pan crust	⅒ of 12″ pizza	343	31.4
Thick crust	⅒ of 12″ pizza	178	21.8
Thin crust	⅒ of 12″ pizza	141	13.3
Sausage & pepperoni:			
Homestyle pan crust	⅒ of 12″ pizza	374	31.2
Thick crust	⅒ of 12″ pizza	177	21.7
Thin crust	⅒ of 12″ pizza	166	13.2

(USDA) = United States Department of Agriculture
(HHS/FAO) = Health and Human Services/Food and Agriculture Organization
* = prepared as package directs

Food and Description	Measure or Quantity	Calories	Carbo-hydrates (grams)
Special:			
Homestyle pan crust	1/10 of 12" pizza	384	31.6
Thick crust	1/10 of 12" pizza	208	22.3
Thin crust	1/10 of 12" pizza	171	13.5
Potatoes	15-piece order	950	120.0
Spaghetti with meat sauce & garlic bread	1 order	940	134.0
Super hot hero	1 sandwich	810	67.0
SHELLS, PASTA, STUFFED, frozen:			
(Buitoni) jumbo:			
Cheese stuffed	5½-oz. serving	288	25.1
Florentine	5½-oz. serving	264	23.1
(Celentano):			
Broccoli & cheese	13½-oz. pkg.	540	60.0
Cheese:			
Plain	½ of 12½-oz. pkg.	340	31.0
With sauce	½ of 16-oz. box	330	41.0
(Le Menu) healthy style, 3-cheese	10-oz. dinner	280	34.0
SHERBET OR SORBET:			
Lemon (Häagen-Dazs)	4 fl. oz.	140	32.0
Lime (Lucerne)	½ cup	120	26.0
Orange:			
(USDA)	½ cup	129	29.7
(Baskin-Robbins)	4 fl. oz.	158	33.4
(Borden)	½ cup	110	25.0
(Dole)	½ cup	110	28.0
(Häagen-Dazs)	4 fl. oz.	113	30.0
(Lucerne)	½ cup	120	26.0
Peach (Dole)	½ cup	130	28.0
Pineapple:			
(Dole)	½ cup	120	28.0
(Lucerne)	½ cup	120	26.0
Raspberry:			
(Baskin-Robbins)	4 fl. oz.	140	34.0
(Häagen-Dazs)	4 fl. oz.	96	24.4
(Sealtest)	½ cup	140	30.0

Food and Description	Measure or Quantity	Calories	Carbo- hydrates (grams)
SHERBET OR SORBET & ICE CREAM:			
(Häagen-Dazs):			
Bar, orange & cream	2.6 fl.-oz. bar	130	18.0
Bulk:			
Blueberry & cream	4 fl. oz.	190	25.0
Key lime & cream	4 fl. oz.	190	29.0
Orange & cream	4 fl. oz.	190	27.0
(Lucerne) vanilla ice cream & orange sherbet	½ cup	130	21.0
SHERBET SHAKE, mix (Weight Watchers)	1 envelope	70	11.0
SHREDDED WHEAT:			
(Nabisco):			
Regular	¾-oz. biscuit	90	19.0
& bran	1 oz.	110	23.0
Spoon Size	⅔ cup (1 oz.)	110	23.0
(Quaker)	1 biscuit (.6 oz.)	52	11.0
(Sunshine):			
Regular	1 biscuit	90	19.0
Bite size	⅔ cup (1 oz.)	110	22.0
Frosted:			
(Kellogg's) *Frosted Mini- Wheats*, regular & bite size	1 oz.	100	24
(Nabisco) *Frosted Wheat Squares*	1 oz.	100	24
SHRIMP:			
Raw (USDA):			
Whole	1 lb. (weighed in shell)	285	4.7
Meat only	4 oz.	103	1.7
Canned (Bumble Bee) solids & liq.	4½-oz. can	90	.9
Frozen:			
(Mrs. Paul's) fried	3-oz. serving	190	15.0
(Sau-Sea) cooked	5-oz. pkg.	90	0.

(USDA) = United States Department of Agriculture
(HHS/FAO) = Health and Human Services/Food and Agriculture Organization
* = prepared as package directs

Food and Description	Measure or Quantity	Calories	Carbohydrates (grams)
SHRIMP & CHICKEN CANTONESE, frozen (Stouffer's) with noodles	10⅛-oz. meal	270	25.0
SHRIMP COCKTAIL, canned or frozen (Sau-Sea)	4 oz.	113	19.0
SHRIMP DINNER OR ENTREE, frozen:			
(Armour) *Classics Lite:*			
Baby bay	9¾-oz. meal	220	31.0
Creole	11¼-oz. meal	260	53.0
(Captain's Choice):			
Breaded:			
Gourmet	1 piece	18	.7
Jumbo	3 oz.	206	10.0
Cooked plain	3 oz.	84	0.
(Gorton's):			
Crunchy, whole	5-oz. serving	380	35.0
Scampi	1 pkg.	470	33.0
(Healthy Choice):			
Creole	11¼-oz. meal	210	42.0
Marinara	10½-oz. meal	220	42.0
(La Choy) Fresh & Lite, with lobster sauce	10-oz. meal	240	36.4
(Stouffer's) *Right Course,* primavera	9⅝-oz. meal	240	32.0
SHRIMP PASTE, canned (USDA)	1 oz.	51	.4
SKATE, raw (USDA) meat only	4 oz.	111	0.
SLENDER (Carnation):			
Bar:			
Chocolate or chocolate chip	1 bar	135	13.0
Chocolate peanut butter or vanilla	1 bar	135	12.0
Dry	1 packet	110	21.0
Liquid	10-fl.-oz. can	220	34.0

Food and Description	Measure or Quantity	Calories	Carbo-hydrates (grams)
SLOPPY JOE:			
Canned:			
(Hormel) *Short Orders*	7½-oz. can	340	15.0
(Libby's):			
Beef	⅓ cup (2.5 oz.)	110	7.0
Pork	⅓ cup	120	6.0
*Manwich	1 sandwich	310	31.0
Frozen (Banquet) *Cookin' Bag*	5-oz. pkg.	210	12.0
SLOPPY JOE SAUCE, canned			
(Ragú) *Joe Sauce*	3½-oz.	50	11.0
SLOPPY JOE SEASONING MIX:			
*(Durkee)			
Regular	1¼ cup	128	32.0
Pizza flavor	1¼ cup	746	26.0
(French's)	1.5-oz. pkg.	128	32.0
*(Hunt's) *Manwich*	5.9-oz. serving	320	31.0
(McCormick)	1.3-oz. pkg.	103	23.4
SMELT, Atlantic, jack & bar (USDA):			
Raw:			
Whole	1 lb. (weighed whole)	244	0.
Meat only	4 oz.	111	0.
Canned, solids & liq.	4 oz.	227	0.
S'MORES CRUNCH, cereal			
(General Mills)	¾ cup (1 oz.)	120	24.0
SMOKED SAUSAGE (See SAUSAGE)			
SNACKS (See CRACKERS, PUFFS & CHIPS; *NATURE SNACKS*; POPCORN;			

(USDA) = United States Department of Agriculture
(HHS/FAO) = Health and Human Services/Food and Agriculture Organization
* = prepared as package directs

Food and Description	Measure or Quantity	Calories	Carbo-hydrates (grams)
POTATO CHIPS; PRETZELS; etc.)			
SNAIL, raw (USDA):			
Unspecified kind	4 oz.	102	2.3
Giant African	4 oz.	83	5.0
SNAPPER (See RED SNAPPER)			
SOAVE WINE (Antinori) 12% alcohol	3 fl. oz.	84	6.3
SOFT DRINK:			
Sweetened:			
Apple (Slice)	6 fl. oz.	98	24.0
Birch beer (Canada Dry)	6 fl. oz.	82	21.0
Bitter lemon:			
(Canada Dry)	6 fl. oz. (6.5 oz.)	75	19.5
(Schweppes)	6 fl. oz. (6.5 oz.)	82	20.0
Bubble Up	6 fl. oz.	73	18.5
Cactus Cooler (Canada Dry)	6 fl. oz. (6.5 oz.)	90	21.8
Cherry:			
(Canada Dry) wild	6 fl. oz. (6.5 oz.)	98	24.0
(Cragmont)	6 fl. oz.	91	23.0
(Shasta) black	6 fl. oz.	81	22.0
Cherry-lime (Spree) all natural	6 fl. oz.	79	21.5
Chocolate (Yoo-hoo)	6 fl. oz.	93	18.0
Citrus Mist (Shasta)	6 fl. oz.	85	23.0
Club	Any quantity	0	0.
Cola:			
Coca-Cola:			
Regular, caffeine-free or cherry coke	6 fl. oz.	77	20.0
Classic	6 fl. oz.	72	19.0
(Cragmont) regular	6 fl. oz.	82	20.0
Pepsi-Cola, regular or *Pepsi Free*	6 fl. oz.	80	19.8

Food and Description	Measure or Quantity	Calories	Carbohydrates (grams)
RC 100, caffeine-free	6 fl. oz.	86	21.4
(Royal Crown)	6 fl. oz.	86	21.4
(Shasta):			
Regular	6 fl. oz.	73	20.0
Cherry	6 fl. oz.	70	19.1
Shasta Free	6 fl. oz.	75	20.5
(Slice) cherry	6 fl. oz.	82	21.6
(Spree) all natural	6 fl. oz.	73	20.0
Collins mix (Canada Dry)	6 fl. oz. (6.5 oz.)	60	15.0
Cream:			
(Canada Dry) vanilla	6 fl. oz. (6.6 oz.)	97	24.0
(Cragmont) regular or red	6 fl. oz.	84	21.0
(Shasta)	6 fl. oz.	77	21.0
Dr. Diablo (Shasta)	6 fl. oz.	70	19.0
Dr. Nehi (Royal Crown)	6 fl. oz.	82	20.4
Dr Pepper	6 fl. oz. (6.5 oz.)	75	19.4
Fruit punch:			
(Nehi)	6 fl. oz.	107	26.7
(Shasta)	6 fl. oz.	87	23.5
Ginger ale:			
(Canada Dry):			
Regular	6 fl. oz.	68	15.8
Golden	6 fl. oz.	75	18.0
(Cragmont)	6 fl. oz.	63	16.0
(Fanta)	6 fl. oz.	63	16.0
(Nehi)	6 fl. oz.	76	19.0
(Schweppes)	6 fl. oz.	65	16.0
(Shasta)	6 fl. oz.	60	16.5
(Spree) all natural	6 fl. oz.	60	16.5
Ginger beer (Schweppes)	6 fl. oz.	70	17.0
Grape:			
(Canada Dry) concord	6 fl. oz. (6.6 oz.)	97	24.0
(Cragmont)	6 fl. oz.	96	24.0
(Fanta)	6 fl. oz.	86	22.0
(Hi-C)	6 fl. oz.	74	19.5
(Nehi)	6 fl. oz.	97	24.4
(Schweppes)	6 fl. oz.	95	23.0
(Shasta)	6 fl. oz.	88	24.0

(USDA) = United States Department of Agriculture
(HHS/FAO) = Health and Human Services/Food and Agriculture Organization
* = prepared as package directs

Food and Description	Measure or Quantity	Calories	Carbo-hydrates (grams)
Grapefruit:			
(Schweppes)	6 fl. oz.	80	20.0
(Spree) all natural	6 fl. oz.	77	21.0
Half & half (Canada Dry)	6 fl. oz. (6.5 oz.)	82	19.5
Hi-Spot (Canada Dry)	6 fl. oz. (6.5 oz.)	75	18.7
Island Lime (Canada Dry)	6 fl. oz. (6.6 oz.)	97	24.8
Kick (Royal Crown)	6 fl. oz.	99	24.8
Lemon (Hi-C)	6 fl. oz.	71	17.1
Lemon-lime:			
(Cragmont):			
Regular	6 fl. oz.	74	19.0
Cherry	6 fl. oz	82	20.0
(Minute Maid)	6 fl. oz.	71	18.0
(Shasta)	6 fl. oz.	73	19.5
(Spree) all natural	6 fl. oz.	77	21.0
Lemon sour (Schweppes)	6 fl. oz.	79	19.0
Lemon-tangerine (Spree) all natural	6 fl. oz.	82	22.0
Manderin-lime (Spree) all natural	6 fl. oz.	77	21.0
Mello Yello	6 fl. oz.	87	22.0
Mr. PiBB	6 fl. oz.	71	19.0
Mountain Dew	6 fl. oz.	89	22.2
Orange:			
(Canada Dry) *Sunripe*	6 fl. oz. (6.6 oz.)	97	24.7
(Cragmont)	6 fl. oz.	89	22.0
(Fanta)	6 fl. oz.	88	23.0
(Hi-C)	6 fl. oz.	74	19.5
(Minute Maid)	6 fl. oz.	87	22.0
(Nehi)	6 fl. oz.	104	26.0
(Schweppes) sparkling	6 fl. oz.	88	22.0
(Shasta)	6 fl. oz.	88	24.0
(Slice)	6 fl. oz.	97	25.2
Peach (Nehi)	6 fl. oz.	102	25.6
Punch (Hi-C)	6 fl. oz.	74	19.4
Quinine or tonic water:			
(Schweppes)	6 fl. oz.	64	16.0
(Shasta)	6 fl. oz.	60	16.5
Red berry (Shasta)	6 fl. oz.	79	22.5
Red pop (Shasta)	6 fl. oz.	79	22.5
Root beer:			
(Cragmont)	6 fl. oz.	84	21.0
(Fanta)	6 fl. oz.	78	20.0
(Nehi)	6 fl. oz.	97	24.4
(Ramblin')	6 fl. oz.	88	23.0
(Schweppes)	6 fl. oz.	76	19.0

Food and Description	Measure or Quantity	Calories	Carbo-hydrates (grams)
(Shasta)	6 fl. oz.	77	21.0
(Spree) all natural	6 fl. oz.	77	21.0
Seltzer	Any quantity	0	0.
7UP	6 fl. oz.	72	18.1
Slice	6 fl. oz.	76	19.8
Sprite	6 fl. oz.	71	18.0
Strawberry:			
(Cragmont)	6 fl. oz.	88	22.0
(Nehi)	6 fl. oz.	97	24.3
(Shasta)	6 fl. oz.	73	20.0
The Skipper (Cragmont)	6 fl. oz.	77	19.0
Tropical blend (Spree) all natural	6 fl. oz.	73	20.5
Upper 10 (Royal Crown)	6 fl. oz.	85	21.1
Dietetic:			
Apple (Slice)	6 fl. oz.	10	2.4
Birch beer (Shasta)	6 fl. oz.	2	.5
Blackberry (Schweppes) mid-calorie royal	6 fl. oz.	35	8.0
Cherry:			
(Cragmont) black	6 fl. oz.	0	0.
Diet Rite	6 fl. oz.	2	.4
(Shasta) black	6 fl. oz.	Tr.	Tr.
Chocolate (Shasta)	6 fl. oz. (6.2 oz.)	0	0.
Cola:			
Coca-Cola, regular, caffeine free or cherry	6 fl. oz.	Tr.	.1
(Cragmont) regular, lite or cherry	6 fl. oz.	0	0.
Diet Rite (Royal Crown)	6 fl. oz.	Tr.	.2
Pepsi, diet, light or caffeine free	6 fl. oz.	Tr.	Tr.
RC	6 fl. oz.	Tr.	.2
(Shasta)	6 fl. oz.	0	0.
(Slice) cherry	6 fl. oz.	10	2.4
Cream:			
(Cragmont)	6 fl. oz.	0	0.
Diet Rite, caramel	6 fl. oz.	<1	.2
(Shasta)	6 fl. oz.	0	0.
Fresca	6 fl. oz.	2	.1

(USDA) = United States Department of Agriculture
(HHS/FAO) = Health and Human Services/Food and Agriculture Organization
* = prepared as package directs

Food and Description	Measure or Quantity	Calories	Carbohydrates (grams)
Frolic (Shasta)	6 fl. oz.	0	0.
Ginger ale:			
(Schweppes)	6 fl. oz.	2	<1.0
(Shasta)	6 fl. oz.	0	0.
Grape (Shasta)	6 fl. oz.	0	0.
Grapefruit, *Diet Rite*	6 fl. oz.	2	.4
Kiwi-passion fruit (Schweppes) mid-calorie royal	6 fl. oz.	35	8.0
Lemon-lime:			
(Cragmont) any type	6 fl. oz.	0	0.
Diet Rite	6 fl. oz.	2	.6
(Minute Maid)	6 fl. oz.	10	2.0
(Shasta)	6 fl. oz.	0	0.
Orange:			
(Fanta)	6 fl. oz.	<1	.1
(Minute Maid)	6 fl. oz.	4	.4
(No-Cal)	6 fl. oz.	1	0.
(Shasta)	6 fl. oz.	0	0.
(Slice)	6 fl. oz.	10	2.1
Peach, *Diet Rite*, golden	6 fl. oz.	1	.3
Peaches 'n Cream (Schweppes) mid-calorie royal	6 fl. oz.	35	8.0
Quinine or tonic (Canada Dry: No-Cal)	6 fl. oz.	3	Tr.
Raspberry, *Diet Rite*	6 fl. oz.	2	.5
Root beer:			
(Cragmont)	6 fl. oz.	0	0.
(No-Cal)	6 fl. oz.	1	0.
(Shasta)	6 fl. oz.	0	0.
7UP	6 fl. oz.	2	0.
Slice	6 fl. oz.	13	3.0
Sprite	6 fl. oz.	2	Tr.
Strawberry (Shasta)	6 fl. oz.	0	0.
Strawberry-banana (Schweppes) mid-calorie royal	6 fl. oz.	35	8.0
Tangerine, *Diet Rite*	6 fl. oz.	2	.3
The Skipper (Cragmont)	6 fl. oz.	0	0.
Tropical citrus (Schweppes) mid-calorie royal	6 fl. oz.	35	8.0
Upper 10 (RC)	6 fl. oz.	2	.6

Food and Description	Measure or Quantity	Calories	Carbohydrates (grams)
SOLE, frozen:			
Raw, meat only (USDA)	4 oz.	90	0.
Frozen:			
(Captain's Choice)	3-oz. fillet	99	0.
(Frionor) *Norway Gourmet*	4-oz. fillet	60	0.
(Gorton's):			
Fishmarket Fresh	4 oz.	90	1.0
Light Recipe, fillet, with lemon butter sauce	1 pkg.	250	8.0
(Healthy Choice):			
Au gratin	11-oz. meal	270	40.0
Lemon butter sauce	8¼-oz. meal	230	33.0
(Mrs. Paul's) fillet, light	1 piece	240	20.0
(Weight Watchers) stuffed	10½-oz. meal	310	38.0
SOUFFLE:			
Cheese, home recipe (USDA)	1 cup (collapsed)	207	5.9
Corn, frozen (Stouffer's)	4-oz. serving	160	18.0
Spinach, frozen (Stouffer's)	4-oz. serving	140	8.0
SOUP:			
Canned, regular pack:			
*Asparagus (Campbell's), condensed, cream of	8-oz. serving	80	10.0
Bean:			
(Campbell's):			
Chunky, with ham, old fashioned:			
Small	11-oz. can	290	38.0
Large	19¼-oz. can	500	66.0
*Condensed, with bacon	8-oz. serving	140	21.0
Home Cookin', & ham	10¾-oz. can	210	29.0
(Grandma Brown's)	8-oz. serving	182	29.1
*(Town House) & bacon	8-oz. serving	140	20.0
Beef:			
(Campbell's):			
Chunky:			

(USDA) = United States Department of Agriculture
(HHS/FAO) = Health and Human Services/Food and Agriculture
                Organization
* = prepared as package directs

Food and Description	Measure or Quantity	Calories	Carbo-hydrates (grams)
Regular:			
Small	10¾-oz. can	200	24.0
Large	19-oz. can	340	42.0
Stroganoff style	10¾-oz. can	320	28.0
*Condensed:			
Regular	8-oz. serving	80	10.0
Broth	8-oz. serving	16	1.0
Consommé	8-oz. serving	25	2.0
Mushroom	8-oz. serving	60	5.0
Noodle:			
Regular	8-oz. serving	70	7.0
Homestyle	8-oz. serving	90	8.0
Home Cookin'	10¾-oz. can	140	18.0
(Progresso):			
Regular	10½-oz. can	180	14.0
Regular	½ of 19-oz. can	160	12.0
Hearty	½ of 19-oz. can	160	15.0
Noodle	½ of 19-oz. can	160	17.0
Tomato, with rotini	½ of 19-oz. can	170	19.0
Vegetable	10½-oz. can	160	20.0
(Swanson)	7¼-oz. can	18	1.0
Beef barley (Progresso)	10½-oz. can	170	17.0
Borscht (See **BORSCHT**)			
*Broccoli (Campbell's)			
condensed	8-oz. serving	140	14.0
Celery:			
*(Campbell's) condensed,			
cream of	8-oz. serving	100	8.0
*(Rokeach):			
Prepared with milk	10-oz. serving	190	19.0
Prepared with water	10-oz. serving	90	12.0
Chickarina (Progresso)	½ of 19-oz. can	130	13.0
Chicken:			
(Campbell's):			
Chunky:			
Noodle	10¾-oz. can	200	20.0
Nuggets	10¾-oz. can	190	24.0
Old fashioned:			
Small	10¾-oz. can	180	21.0
Large	19-oz. can	300	36.0
With rice	19-oz. can	280	32.0
Vegetable	19-oz. can	340	38.0
*Condensed:			
Alphabet	8-oz. serving	80	10.0

Food and Description	Measure or Quantity	Calories	Carbo-hydrates (grams)
Broth:			
Plain	8-oz. serving	30	2.0
Noodles	8-oz. serving	45	8.0
Cream of	8-oz. serving	110	9.0
& dumplings	8-oz. serving	80	9.0
Gumbo	8-oz. serving	60	8.0
Mushroom, creamy	8-oz. serving	120	8.0
Noodle	8-oz. serving	60	8.0
NoodleOs	8-oz. serving	70	8.0
& rice	8-oz. serving	60	7.0
& stars	8-oz. serving	60	7.0
Vegetable	8-oz. serving	70	8.0
Home Cookin':			
Gumbo, with sausage	10¾-oz. can	140	15.0
With noodles	19-oz. can	220	20.0
Rice	10¾-oz. can	150	10.0
(College Inn) broth	1 cup (8.3 oz.)	35	0.
(Hain):			
Broth	8¾-oz. can	70	0.
Noodle	9½-oz. serving	120	12.0
(Manischewitz):			
Clear	1 cup	46	DNA
Barley or rice	1 cup	83	DNA
Vegetable	1 cup	55	DNA
(Progresso):			
Barley	½ of 18½-oz. can	100	12.0
Broth	8 oz.	16	0.
Cream of	½ of 19-oz. can	180	13.0
Hearty	10½-oz. can	130	9.0
Homestyle	½ of 19-oz. can	110	12.0
Noodle	10½-oz. can	120	8.0
Rice	10½-oz. can	120	12.0
Vegetable	½ of 19-oz. can	130	16.0
(Swanson):			
Regular	7¼-oz. can	30	2.0
Natural Goodness	7¼-oz. can	20	1.0
Chili beef (Campbell's):			
Chunky:			
Small	11-oz. can	290	37.0
Large	19½-oz. can	520	66.0
*Condensed	8-oz. serving	140	20.0

(USDA) = United States Department of Agriculture
(HHS/FAO) = Health and Human Services/Food and Agriculture
              Organization
* = prepared as package directs

Food and Description	Measure or Quantity	Calories	Carbo-hydrates (grams)
Chowder:			
Beef'n vegetable (Hormel)			
Short Orders	7½-oz. can	120	15.0
Clam:			
Manhattan style:			
(Campbell's):			
Chunky:			
Small	10¾-oz. can	160	24.0
Large	19-oz. can	300	42.0
*Condensed	8-oz. serving	70	10.0
(Progresso)	½ of 19-oz. can	120	17.0
*(Snow's) condensed	7½-oz. serving	70	9.0
New England style:			
*(Campbell's):			
Chunky:			
Small	10¾-oz. can	290	26.0
Large	19-oz. can	520	46.0
Condensed:			
Made with milk	8-oz. serving	150	17.0
Made with water	8-oz. serving	80	12.0
*(Gorton's)	1 can	560	68.0
(Hain)	9¼-oz. serving	180	26.0
(Progresso)	10½-oz. can	240	22.0
*(Snow's) condensed, made with milk	7½-oz. serving	140	13.0
*Corn (Snow's) New England, condensed, made with milk	7½-oz. serving	150	18.0
*Fish (Snow's) New England, condensed, made with milk	7½-oz. serving	130	11.0
*Seafood (Snow's) New England, condensed, made with milk	7½-oz. serving	130	11.0
Escarole (Progresso) in chicken broth	½ of 18½-oz. can	30	2.0
Ham'n butter bean (Campbell's) *Chunky*	10¾-oz. can	280	34.0
Italian vegetable pasta (Hain)	9½-oz. serving	160	25.0
Lentil:			
(Campbell's) *Home Cookin'*	10¾-oz. can	170	28.0
(Hain) vegetarian	9½-oz. serving	160	25.0

Food and Description	Measure or Quantity	Calories	Carbo-hydrates (grams)
(Progresso):			
Regular	½ of 19-oz. can	140	25.0
With sausage	½ of 19-oz. can	180	20.0
Macaroni & bean (Progresso)	½ of 19-oz. can	170	25.0
Minestrone:			
(Campbell's):			
Chunky	19-oz. can	320	48.0
*Condensed	8-oz. serving	80	13.0
Home Cookin':			
Regular	10¾-oz. can	140	22.0
Chicken	½ of 19-oz. can	180	15.0
(Hain)	9½-oz. serving	170	27.0
(Progresso):			
Beef	10½-oz. can	190	16.0
Chicken	½ of 19-oz. can	130	12.0
Hearty	½ of 18½-oz. can	110	16.0
Zesty	½ of 19-oz. can	150	19.0
*(Town House) condensed	8-oz. serving	80	12.0
Mushroom:			
*(Campbell's) condensed:			
Cream of	8-oz. serving	100	8.0
Golden	8-oz. serving	70	9.0
(Hain) creamy	9¼-oz. serving	110	16.0
(Progresso) cream of	½ of 18½-oz. can	160	14.0
*(Rokeach) cream of, prepared with water	10-oz. serving	150	3.0
Mushroom barley (Hain)	9½-oz. serving	100	17.0
*Noodle (Campbell's):			
Curly, & chicken	8-oz. serving	80	11.0
& ground beef	8-oz. serving	90	10.0
*Onion (Campbell's):			
Regular	8-oz. serving	60	9.0
Cream of:			
Made with water	8-oz. serving	100	12.0
Made with water & milk	8-oz. serving	140	15.0
*Oyster stew (Campbell's):			
Made with milk	8-oz. serving	140	10.0
Made with water	8-oz. serving	70	5.0
*Pea, green (Campbell's) condensed	8-oz. serving	160	25.0

(USDA) = United States Department of Agriculture
(HHS/FAO) = Health and Human Services/Food and Agriculture Organization
* = prepared as package directs

Food and Description	Measure or Quantity	Calories	Carbo-hydrates (grams)
Pea, split:			
(Campbell's):			
Chunky, with ham:			
Small	10¾-oz. can	230	33.0
Large	19-oz. can	420	60.0
*Condensed, with ham & bacon	8-oz. serving	160	24.0
Home Cookin', with ham	10¾-oz. can	230	38.0
(Grandma Brown's)	8-oz. serving	184	28.2
(Hain)	9½-oz. serving	170	28.0
(Progresso):			
Regular	½ of 19-oz. can	160	27.0
With ham	10½-oz. can	190	27.0
*Pepper pot (Campbell's)	8-oz. serving	90	9.0
*Potato (Campbell's):			
Cream of, made with water	8-oz. serving	80	12.0
Cream of, made with water & milk	8-oz. serving	120	15.0
*Scotch broth (Campbell's) condensed	8-oz. serving	80	9.0
Shav (Gold's)	8-oz. serving	25	4.0
Shrimp:			
*(Campbell's) condensed, cream of:			
Made with milk	8-oz. serving	160	13.0
Made with water	8-oz. serving	90	8.0
(Crosse & Blackwell)	6½-oz. serving	90	7.0
Sirloin burger (Campbell's) Chunky:			
Small	10¾-oz. can	220	23.0
Large	19-oz. can	400	40.0
Steak & potato (Campbell's) Chunky:			
Small	10¾-oz. can	200	24.0
Large	19-oz. can	340	42.0
*Teddy bear (Campbell's) condensed	8-oz. serving	70	11.0
Tomato:			
(Campbell):			
Condensed:			
Regular:			
Made with milk	8-oz. serving	150	22.0
Made with water	8-oz. serving	90	17.0
Bisque	8-oz. serving	120	22.0

Food and Description	Measure or Quantity	Calories	Carbo-hydrates (grams)
Homestyle, cream of:			
Made with milk	8-oz. serving	180	25.0
Made with water	8-oz. serving	110	20.0
& rice, old fashioned	8-oz. serving	110	22.0
Home Cookin', garden	10¾-oz. can	150	29.0
*(Rokeach):			
Plain, made with water	10-oz. serving	90	20.0
& rice	10-oz. serving	160	25.0
Tortellini (Progresso):			
Regular	½ of 19-oz. can	90	12.0
Creamy	½ of 18½-oz. can	240	17.0
Tomato	½ of 18½-oz. can	130	16.0
Turkey (Campbell's):			
Chunky	18¾-oz. can	300	32.0
*Condensed:			
Noodle	8-oz. serving	70	9.0
Vegetable	8-oz. serving	70	8.0
Vegetable:			
(Campbell's):			
Chunky:			
Regular:			
Small	10¾-oz. can	160	28.0
Large	19-oz. can	300	50.0
Beef, old fashioned:			
Small	10¾-oz. can	190	20.0
Large	19-oz. can	320	34.0
Mediterranean	19-oz. can	320	48.0
*Condensed:			
Regular	8-oz. serving	90	14.0
Beef	8-oz. serving	70	10.0
Old fashioned	8-oz. serving	60	9.0
Vegetarian	8-oz. serving	80	13.0
Home Cookin':			
Beef	10¾-oz. can	140	17.0
Country	10¾-oz. can	120	20.0
(Hain):			
Broth	9½-oz. serving	45	10.0
Chicken	9½-oz. serving	120	14.0
Vegetarian	9½-oz. serving	140	22.0
(Progresso)	½ of 19-oz. can	80	15.0
*(Rokeach) vegetarian	10-oz. serving	90	15.0

(USDA) = United States Department of Agriculture
(HHS/FAO) = Health and Human Services/Food and Agriculture
Organization
* = prepared as package directs

Food and Description	Measure or Quantity	Calories	Carbo-hydrates (grams)
Vichyssoise (Crosse & Blackwell) cream of	6½-oz. serving	70	5.0
*Won ton (Campbell's)	8-oz. serving	40	5.0
Canned, dietetic pack:			
Bean:			
*(Campbell's) condensed, *Special Request*, with bacon, less salt	8-oz. serving	140	21.0
(Pritikin) navy	½ of 14¾-oz. can	130	22.0
Beef (Pritikin) broth	½ of 13¾-oz. can	20	3.0
Chicken:			
(Campbell's):			
Regular:			
Broth	10½-oz. can	30	2.0
& noodles	10¾-oz. can	170	17.0
Special Request:			
Cream of	8-oz. serving	110	9.0
Noodle	8-oz. serving	60	8.0
Rice	8-oz. serving	60	7.0
(Estee) & vegetable	7¼-oz. can	130	10.0
(Hain):			
Broth	8¾-oz. can	60	0.
Noodle	9½-oz. serving	110	10.0
(Pritikin):			
Broth, defatted	½ of 13¾-oz. can	14	0.
Gumbo or ribbon pasta	7¼-oz. serving	60	8.0
Vegetable	½ of 14½-oz. can	70	12.0
(Weight Watchers) noodle	10½-oz. can	80	9.0
Chowder, clam (Pritikin):			
Manhattan	½ of 14¾-oz. can	70	14.0
New England	½ of 14¾-oz. can	118	20.0
Lentil (Pritikin)	½ of 14¾-oz. can	100	17.0
Minestrone:			
(Estee)	7½-oz. can	165	19.0
(Hain)	9½-oz. serving	160	28.0
(Pritikin)	½ of 14¾-oz. can	110	19.0
Mushroom:			
(Campbell's) cream of, low sodium:			
Regular	10½-oz. can	210	18.0
Special Request	8-oz. serving	100	8.0

Food and Description	Measure or Quantity	Calories	Carbo-hydrates (grams)
(Pritikin)	½ of 14¾-oz. can	60	11.0
(Weight Watchers) cream of	10½-oz. can	90	14.0
Pea, split:			
(Campbell's) low sodium	10¾-oz. can	230	37.0
(Pritikin)	½ of 15-oz. can	130	23.0
Tomato (Campbell's) low sodium, with tomato pieces	10½-oz. can	190	30.0
Turkey (Pritikin) vegetable, with ribbon pasta	½ of 14¾-oz. can	50	7.0
Vegetable:			
(Campbell's) low sodium:			
Chunky	10¾-oz. can	180	19.0
Special Request:			
Regular	8-oz. serving	90	14.0
Beef	8-oz. serving	70	10.0
(Estee) & beef	7½-oz. serving	140	9.0
(Pritikin)	½ of 14¾-oz. can	70	14.0
(Weight Watchers):			
With beef stock	10½-oz. can	90	13.0
Vegetarian, chunky	10½-oz. can	100	18.0
Frozen:			
Asparagus (Kettle Ready) cream of	6 fl. oz.	62	5.1
*Barley & mushroom:			
(Empire Kosher)	½ of 15-oz. polybag	69	12.0
(Tabatchnick)	8 oz.	92	16.0
Bean & barley (Tabatchnick)	8 oz.	63	22.0
Bean & ham (Kettle Ready):			
Black	6 fl. oz.	154	23.0
Savory	6 fl. oz.	113	20.2
Beef (Kettle Ready) vegetable	6 fl. oz.	85	10.7
Broccoli, cream of:			
(Kettle Ready):			
Regular	6 fl. oz.	94	6.4
Cheddar	6 fl. oz.	137	4.7
(Tabatchnick)	7½ oz.	90	10.0

(USDA) = United States Department of Agriculture
(HHS/FAO) = Health and Human Services/Food and Agriculture Organization
* = prepared as package directs

Food and Description	Measure or Quantity	Calories	Carbo-hydrates (grams)
Cauliflower (Kettle Ready) cream of	6 fl. oz.	93	5.5
Cheese (Kettle Ready) cheddar, cream of	6 fl. oz.	158	7.3
Chicken:			
(Empire Kosher):			
Corn	½ of 15-oz. polybag	71	7.0
Noodle	½ of 15-oz. polybag	267	13.0
(Kettle Ready):			
Cream of	6 fl. oz.	98	5.0
Gumbo	6 fl. oz.	93	12.1
Noodle	6 fl. oz.	94	12.0
Chili (Kettle Ready):			
Jalapeño	6 fl. oz.	173	14.7
Traditional	6 fl. oz.	161	13.8
Chowder:			
Clam:			
Boston (Kettle Ready)	6 fl. oz.	131	12.8
Manhattan:			
(Kettle Ready)	6 fl. oz.	69	7.9
(Tabatchnick)	7½ oz.	94	15.0
New England:			
(Kettle Ready)	6 fl. oz.	116	11.4
(Stouffer's)	8 oz.	180	16.0
(Tabatchnick)	7½-oz.	97	16.0
Corn & broccoli (Kettle Ready)	6 fl. oz.	101	12.8
Lentil (Tabatchnick)	8 oz.	173	27.0
Minestrone:			
(Kettle Ready)	6 fl. oz.	104	15.2
(Tabatchnick)	8 oz.	147	24.0
Mushroom (Kettle Ready) cream of	6 fl. oz.	85	6.2
Northern bean (Tabatchnick)	8 oz.	80	29.0
Onion (Kettle Ready) french	6 fl. oz.	42	4.9
Pea:			
(Empire Kosher)	7½ oz.	56	6.0
(Kettle Ready) split	6 fl. oz.	155	25.3
(Tabatchnick)	8 oz.	186	31.0
Potato (Tabatchnick)	8 oz.	95	19.0

Food and Description	Measure or Quantity	Calories	Carbo-hydrates (grams)
Spinach, cream of:			
(Stouffer's)	8 oz.	210	12.0
(Tabatchnick)	7½ oz.	90	12.0
Tomato (Empire Kosher) with rice	7½ oz.	227	50.0
Tortellini (Kettle Ready)	6 fl. oz.	122	14.9
Turkey chili (Empire Kosher)	7½ oz.	200	DNA
Vegetable:			
(Empire Kosher)	7½ oz.	111	22.0
(Kettle Ready)	6 fl. oz.	85	12.3
(Tabatchnick)	8 oz.	97	18.0
Won ton (La Choy)	7½ oz.	50	6.0
*Mix, regular:			
Asparagus (Knorr)	8 fl. oz.	80	11.0
Barley (Knorr) country	10 fl. oz.	120	22.5
*Beef:			
(Campbell's) *Cup-a-Ramen*, with vegetables	8 fl. oz.	270	38.0
(Lipton) & noodles, hearty	7 fl. oz.	107	20.2
Broccoli (Lipton) *Cup-a-Soup*, & cheese	6 fl. oz.	69	9.8
Cauliflower (Knorr)	8 fl. oz.	100	13.0
Cheese (Hain) savory	¾ cup	250	20.0
Cheese & broccoli (Hain)	¾ cup	310	19.0
Chicken:			
(Campbell's):			
Campbell's Cup, creamy	6 fl. oz.	90	12.0
Cup-a-Ramen, & vegetables	8 fl. oz.	270	38.0
(Knorr):			
Noodle	8 fl. oz.	100	17.9
'N pasta	8 fl. oz.	90	16.2
(Lipton):			
Regular:			
Plain	8 fl. oz.	82	12.1
With diced white meat	8 fl. oz.	81	12.1
Hearty	8 fl. oz.	83	13.3
Cup-a-Soup:			

(USDA) = United States Department of Agriculture
(HHS/FAO) = Health and Human Services/Food and Agriculture Organization
* = prepared as package directs

Food and Description	Measure or Quantity	Calories	Carbo- hydrates (grams)
Regular:			
Broth	6 fl. oz.	19	3.3
Country style	6 fl. oz.	107	11.8
Cream of	6 fl. oz.	84	9.7
Noodle	6 fl. oz.	48	8.0
& rice	6 fl. oz.	47	7.7
Vegetable	6 fl. oz.	47	7.8
Hearty:			
Country style	6 fl. oz.	69	11.1
& noodles	6 fl. oz.	110	20.0
Lots-a-Noodles, creamy, hearty	7 fl. oz.	179	21.4
Chowder, New England (Gorton's)	¼ of can	140	17.0
Herb (Knorr) fine	8 fl. oz.	130	15.0
Hot & Sour (Knorr) oriental	8 fl. oz.	80	9.0
Leek (Knorr)	8 fl. oz.	110	14.0
Lentil (Hain) savory	¾ cup	130	20.0
Minestrone:			
(Hain) savory	¾ cup	110	20.0
(Knorr) hearty	10 fl.-oz.	130	22.7
(Manischewitz)	6 fl.-oz.	50	9.0
Mushroom:			
(Hain)	¾ cup	210	11.0
(Knorr)	8 fl. oz.	100	12.0
(Lipton):			
Regular:			
Beef	8 fl. oz.	38	6.7
Onion	8 fl. oz.	41	6.8
Cup-a-Noodles, cream of	6 fl. oz.	70	9.1
Noodle:			
(Campbell's):			
Campbell's Cup:			
Regular:			
With broth	6 fl. oz.	90	15.0
Chicken, with white meat	6 fl. oz.	90	12.0
Microwavable:			
Beef flavor	1 cup	130	23.0
Chicken broth	1 cup	130	23.0
Chicken flavor	1 cup	140	22.0
Hearty	1 cup	180	32.0
Quality soup recipe:			
Regular	8 fl. oz.	110	19.0
Chicken	8 fl. oz.	100	16.0

Food and Description	Measure or Quantity	Calories	Carbo-hydrates (grams)
Hearty	8 fl. oz.	90	15.0
Raman:			
Beef, chicken or oriental	8 fl. oz.	190	26.0
Pork	8 fl. oz	200	26.0
(4C)	8 fl. oz.	50	7.0
Onion:			
(Campbell's) Quality Soup	8 fl. oz.	30	7.0
(Hain) Savory	¾ cup	50	6.0
(Knorr) french	8 fl. oz.	50	9.1
(Lipton):			
Regular:			
Plain	8 fl. oz.	20	4.3
Beefy	8 fl. oz.	24	4.1
Cup-a-Soup	6 fl. oz.	27	4.7
Oxtail (Knorr) hearty beef	8 fl. oz.	70	10.2
Pea, green (Lipton)			
Cup-a-Soup	6 fl.oz.	113	14.4
Pea, split (Manischewitz)	6 fl. oz.	45	8.0
Potato Leek (Hain)	¾ cup	260	20.0
Shrimp (Campbell's)			
Cup-a-Ramen, with vegetables	8 fl. oz.	280	40.0
Tomato:			
(Hain) savory	¾ cup	220	19.0
(Knorr) basil	8 fl. oz.	85	14.3
(Lipton) *Cup-A-Soup*	6 fl. oz.	103	21.2
Tortellini (Knorr) in brodo	8 fl. oz.	60	10.9
Vegetable:			
(Campbell's) quality soup	8 fl. oz.	40	8.0
(Hain) savory	¾ cup	80	13.0
(Knorr):			
Plain	8 fl. oz.	35	6.5
Spring, with herbs	8 fl. oz.	30	6.0
(Lipton):			
Regular:			
Plain	8 fl. oz.	39	6.9
Country	8 fl. oz.	80	15.7

(USDA) = United States Department of Agriculture
(HHS/FAO) = Health and Human Services/Food and Agriculture Organization
* = prepared as package directs

Food and Description	Measure or Quantity	Calories	Carbo-hydrates (grams)
Cup-a-Soup:			
Regular:			
Harvest	6 fl. oz.	91	18.8
Spring	6 fl. oz.	41	6.6
Lots-a-Noodles,			
garden	7 fl. oz.	123	23.1
(Manischewitz)	6 fl. oz.	50	9.0
*Mix, dietetic:			
Beef:			
(Campbell's) *Cup-a-Ramen,* with vegetables, low fat	8 fl. oz.	220	44.0
(Estee) noodle	6 fl. .oz.	20	3.0
Broccoli (Lipton) *Cup-a-Soup),* golden	6 fl. oz.	42	6.3
Chicken:			
(Campbell's) *Cup-a-Ramen,* with vegetables, low fat	8 fl. oz.	220	44.0
(Estee) noodle	2 fl. oz.	25	4.0
(Lipton) *Cup-a-Soup,* lite:			
Florentine	6 fl. oz.	42	7.6
Lemon	6 fl. oz.	48	9.1
(Weight Watchers) broth	1 packet	8	1.0
Mushroom (Hain) savory	¾ cup	250	15.0
Noodle (Campbell's) ramen, low fat block:			
Beef or chicken flavor	8 fl. oz.	160	32.0
Oriental or pork flavor	8 fl. oz.	150	31.0
Onion:			
(Estee)	6 fl. oz.	25	4.0
(4C)	8 fl. oz.	30	5.0
(Hain) savory	¾ cup	50	9.0
Oriental:			
(Campbell's) *Cup-a-Ramen,* with vegetables	8 fl. oz.	220	44.0
(Lipton) *Cup-a-Soup*	6 fl. oz.	45	5.8
Shrimp (Campbell's) *Cup-a-Ramen,* with vegetables, low fat	8 fl. oz.	230	45.0
Tomato:			
(Estee)	6 fl. oz	40	5.0
(Lipton) *Cup-a-Soup,* herb, creamy	6 fl. oz.	65	14.1

Food and Description	Measure or Quantity	Calories	Carbo-hydrates (grams)
SOUR CREAM (See **CREAM,** Sour)			
SOURSOP, raw (USDA):			
Whole	1 lb. (weighed with skin & seeds)	200	50.3
Flesh only	4 oz.	74	18.5
SOUSE (USDA)	1 oz.	51	.3
SOUTHERN COMFORT:			
80 proof	1 fl. oz.	79	3.4
100 proof	1 fl. oz.	95	3.5
SOYBEAN:			
(USDA):			
Young seeds:			
Raw	1 lb. (weighed in pod)	322	31.7
Boiled, drained	4 oz.	134	11.5
Canned:			
Solids & liq.	4 oz.	85	7.1
Drained solids	4 oz.	117	8.4
Mature seeds:			
Raw	1 lb.	1828	152.0
Raw	1 cup (7.4 oz.)	846	70.4
Cooked	4 oz.	147	12.2
Oil roasted:			
(Soy Ahoy) regular, or garlic	1 oz.	152	4.8
(Soytown)	1 oz.	152	4.8
SOYBEAN CURD OR TOFU (USDA):			
Regular	4 oz.	82	2.7
Cake	4.2-oz. cake	86	2.9
SOYBEAN FLOUR (See **FLOUR**)			

(USDA) = United States Department of Agriculture
(HHS/FAO) = Health and Human Services/Food and Agriculture Organization
* = prepared as package directs

Food and Description	Measure or Quantity	Calories	Carbo-hydrates (grams)
SOYBEAN GRITS, high fat (USDA)	1 cup (4.9 oz.)	524	46.0
SOYBEAN MILK (USDA):			
Fluid	4 oz.	37	1.5
Powder	1 oz.	122	7.9
SOYBEAN PROTEIN (USDA)	1 oz.	91	4.3
SOYBEAN PROTEINATE (USDA)	1 oz.	88	2.2
SOYBEAN SPROUT (See **BEAN SPROUT**)			
SOY SAUCE (See **SAUCE,** Soy)			
SPAGHETTI (See also **NOODLE**). Plain spaghetti products are essentially the same in calorie value and carbohydrate content on the same weight basis. The longer the cooking, the more water is absorbed and this affects the nutritive and caloric value:			
Dry (Pritikin) whole wheat	1 oz.	110	18.0
Cooked (USDA):			
8—10 minutes, "Al Dente"	1 cup (5.1 oz.)	216	43.9
14—20 minutes, tender	1 cup (4.9 oz.)	155	32.2
Canned, regular pack:			
(Franco-American):			
With meatballs in tomato sauce, *SpaghettiOs*	7⅜-oz. can	220	25.0
With meatballs, in tomato sauce	7⅜-oz. can	220	28.0
With sliced franks in tomato sauce, *SpaghettiOs*	7⅜-oz. can	220	26.0
In tomato & cheese sauce, *SpaghettiOs*	7⅜-oz. can	170	33.0
In tomato sauce with cheese	7⅜-oz. can	180	36.0

Food and Description	Measure or Quantity	Calories	Carbo-hydrates (grams)
(Hormel) *Short Orders:*			
& beef	7½-oz. can	260	25.0
& meatballs	7½-oz. can	210	26.0
Canned, dietetic:			
(Estee) & meatballs	7½-oz. serving	240	19.0
(Featherweight) & meatballs	7½-oz. serving	200	28.0
Frozen:			
(Armour) *Dining Lite,* with beef	9-oz. meal	220	25.0
(Banquet):			
Casserole, with meat sauce	8-oz. meal	270	35.0
Dinner, & meatballs	10-oz. meal	290	44.0
(Healthy Choice) with meat sauce	10-oz. meal	280	42.0
(Kid Cuisine)	9¼-oz. meal	310	43.0
(Le Menu) healthy style, with beef sauce & mushroom	9-oz. meal	280	45.0
(Morton) & meatballs	10-oz. dinner	200	39.0
(Stouffer's):			
Regular:			
With meatballs	12⅝-oz. meal	380	42.0
With meat sauce	12⅞-oz. meal	370	49.0
Lean Cuisine, with beef & mushroom sauce	11½-oz. meal	280	38.0
(Swanson):			
Regular, & meatballs	12½-oz. meal	390	46.0
Homestyle Recipe, with Italian style meatballs	13-oz. meal	490	60.0
(Weight Watchers) with meat sauce	10½-oz. meal	280	34.0
SPAGHETTI SAUCE, canned:			
Regular pack:			
Alfredo (Progresso):			
Regular	½ cup	340	6.0
Seafood	½ cup	220	5.0
Beef (Prego Plus) ground sirloin, with onion	4-oz. serving	160	20.0

(USDA) = United States Department of Agriculture
(HHS/FAO) = Health and Human Services/Food and Agriculture Organization
* = prepared as package directs

Food and Description	Measure or Quantity	Calories	Carbo-hydrates (grams)
Bolognese (Progresso)	½ cup	150	2.0
Cheese, three (Prego)	4 oz.	100	17.0
Chunky (Hunt's)	4 oz.	50	12.0
Chunk style (Town House)	4 oz.	80	14.0
Clam (Progresso):			
Red	½ cup	70	7.0
White:			
Regular	½ cup	110	1.0
Authentic pasta sauce	½ cup	130	4.0
Garden combinations (Prego) extra chunky	4 oz.	80	14.0
Garden Style (Ragú) chunky:			
Extra tomato, garlic & onion, green pepper & mushroom or mushroom & onion	¼ of 15½-oz. jar	80	14.0
Italian garden combination or sweet green & red bell pepper	¼ of 15½-oz. jar	80	12.0
Home style (Ragú):			
Plain or mushroom	4-oz. serving	70	12.0
Meat flavored	4-oz. serving	80	12.0
Lobster (Progresso) rock	½ cup	120	11.0
Marinara:			
(Prince)	4-oz. serving	80	12.4
(Progresso):			
Regular	½ cup	90	9.0
Authentic pasta sauce	½ cup	110	10.0
(Ragú)	4-oz. serving	120	12.0
Meat or meat flavored:			
(Hunt's)	4-oz. serving	70	12.0
(Prego)	4-oz. serving	140	20.0
(Progresso)	½ cup	110	13.0
(Town House)	4 oz.	80	11.0
Meatless or plain:			
(Prego)	4-oz. serving	130	20.0
(Progresso)	½ cup	110	13.0
(Town House)	4 oz.	80	11.0
Mushroom:			
(Hunt's)	4-oz. serving	70	12.0
(Prego):			
Regular	4-oz. serving	130	20.0
Extra chunky:			
Extra spice	4 oz.	100	17.0
& green pepper	4 oz.	100	14.0

Food and Description	Measure or Quantity	Calories	Carbo-hydrates (grams)
& onion	4 oz.	100	13.0
& tomato	4 oz.	110	14.0
(Progresso)	½ cup	110	13.0
(Ragú):			
Regular	4-oz. serving	90	9.0
Extra Thick & Zesty	4-oz. serving	110	13.0
Onion & garlic (Prego)	4 oz.	110	16.0
Primavera (Progresso)			
creamy	½ cup	190	8.0
Romano (Progresso)	½ cup	220	7.0
Sausage & green pepper			
(Prego)	4-oz. serving	160	19.0
Seafood (Progresso):			
Regular	½ cup	110	12.0
Authentic pasta sauce	½ cup	190	5.0
Sicilian (Progresso)	½ cup	30	2.0
Tomato & basil (Prego)	4 oz.	100	18.0
Tomato & onion (Prego)			
extra chunky	4 oz.	110	14.0
Traditional (Hunt's)	4 oz.	70	12.0
Dietetic pack:			
(Estee)	4-oz. serving	60	13.0
(Furman's) low sodium	½ cup	83	12.7
(Prego) plain, no salt added	4 oz.	110	11.0
(Pritikin) plain or mushroom	4-oz. serving	60	12.0
(Weight Watchers):			
Meat flavored	⅓ cup	50	9.0
Mushroom flavored	⅓ cup	40	9.0
SPAGHETTI SAUCE MIX:			
(Lawry's):			
With imported mushrooms	1½-oz. pkg.	143	26.0
Rich & thick	1½-oz. pkg.	147	28.1
*(Spatini)	½ cup	84	8.4
SPAM, luncheon meat (Hormel):			
Regular, smoke flavored or			
with cheese chunks	1-oz. serving	85	0.
Deviled	1 T.	35	0.

(USDA) = United States Department of Agriculture
(HHS/FAO) = Health and Human Services/Food and Agriculture
Organization
* = prepared as package directs

Food and Description	Measure or Quantity	Calories	Carbo-hydrates (grams)
SPANISH MACKEREL (See also **MACKEREL**, raw (USDA):			
Whole	1 lb. (weighed whole)	490	0.
Meat only	4 oz.	201	0.
SPARKLING COOLER, CITRUS, *La Croix,* 3½% alcohol	12 fl. oz.	215	30.0
SPECIAL K, cereal (Kellogg's)	1 cup (1 oz.)	110	20.0
SPICES (See individual spice names)			
SPINACH:			
Raw (USDA):			
Untrimmed	1 lb. (weighed with large stems & roots)	85	14.0
Trimmed or packaged	1 lb.	118	19.5
Trimmed, whole leaves	1 cup (1.2 oz.)	9	1.4
Trimmed, chopped	1 cup (1.8 oz.)	14	2.2
Boiled (USDA) whole leaves, drained	1 cup (5.5 oz.)	36	5.6
Canned, regular pack:			
(USDA):			
Solids & liq.	½ cup (4.1 oz.)	21	3.5
Drained solids	½ cup	27	4.0
(Allen's) chopped, solids & liq.	½ cup	25	4.0
(Larsen) *Freshlike,* cut	½ cup (4.3 oz.)	25	4.0
(Town House) whole leaf	½ cup	28	3.0
Canned, dietetic or low calorie:			
(USDA) low sodium:			
Solids & liq.	4 oz.	24	3.9
Drained solids	4 oz.	29	4.5
(Allen's) low sodium, solids & liq.	½ cup	25	4.0
(Del Monte) no salt added, solids & liq.	½ cup	25	4.0
(Larsen) *Fresh-Lite,* cut, no salt added	½ cup (4.3 oz.)	20	4.0
Frozen:			
(Bel-Air)	3.3 oz.	20	3.0

Food and Description	Measure or Quantity	Calories	Carbo-hydrates (grams)
(Birds Eye):			
Chopped or leaf	⅓ of pkg. (3.3 oz.)	28	3.4
Creamed	⅓ of pkg. (3 oz.)	60	4.9
& water chestnuts with selected seasonings	⅓ of 10-oz. pkg.	32	5.0
(Green Giant):			
Creamed	3.3 oz.	70	8.0
Cut or leaf, in butter sauce	5 oz.	40	6.0
Harvest Fresh	4½ oz.	25	4.0
(McKenzie) chopped or cut	⅓ of pkg.	25	3.0
(Stouffer's) creamed	½ of 9-oz. pkg.	170	7.0
SPINACH, NEW ZEALAND (USDA):			
Raw	1 lb.	86	14.1
Boiled, drained	4 oz.	15	2.4
SPINACH PUREE, canned			
(Larsen) no salt added	½ cup (4.3 oz.)	22	3.5
SPLEEN, raw (USDA):			
Beef & calf	4 oz.	118	0.
Hog	4 oz.	121	0.
Lamb	4 oz.	130	0.
SPLIT PEA (See **PEA, MATURE SEED**, dry)			
SQUAB, pigeon, raw (USDA):			
Dressed	1 lb. (weighed with feet, inedible viscera & bones)	569	0.
Meat & skin	4 oz.	333	0.
Meat only	4 oz.	161	0.
Light meat only, without skin	4 oz.	142	0.
Giblets	1 oz.	44	.3

(USDA) = United States Department of Agriculture
(HHS/FAO) = Health and Human Services/Food and Agriculture Organization
* = prepared as package directs

Food and Description	Measure or Quantity	Calories	Carbo-hydrates (grams)
SQUASH, SUMMER:			
Fresh (USDA):			
Crookneck & straightneck, yellow:			
Whole	1 lb. (weighed untrimmed)	89	19.1
Boiled, drained:			
Diced	½ cup (3.6 oz.)	15	3.2
Slices	½ cup (3.1 oz.)	13	2.7
Scallop, white & pale green:			
Whole	1 lb. (weighed untrimmed)	93	22.7
Boiled, drained, mashed	½ cup (4.2 oz.)	19	4.5
Zucchini & cocazelle, green:			
Whole	1 lb. (weighed untrimmed)	73	15.5
Boiled, drained slices	½ cup (2.7 oz.)	9	1.9
Canned (Progresso) zucchini, Italian style	½ cup	50	8.0
Frozen:			
(Birds Eye):			
Regular	⅓ of 10-oz. pkg.	22	3.9
Zucchini	⅓ of 10-oz. pkg.	19	3.3
(Larsen):			
Yellow crookneck	3.3-oz.	18	4.0
Zucchini	3.3-oz.	16	3.0
(McKenzie):			
Crookneck	⅓ of pkg. (3.3 oz.)	20	4.0
Zucchini	3.3 oz.	18	3.0
(Ore-Ida) zucchini, breaded	3 oz.	150	15.0
(Southland):			
Crookneck	⅕ of 16-oz. pkg.	15	4.0
Zucchini	⅕ of 16-oz. pkg.	15	3.0
SQUASH, WINTER:			
Fresh (USDA):			
Acorn:			
Whole	1 lb. (weighed with skin & seeds)	152	38.6
Baked, flesh only, mashed	½ cup (3.6 oz.)	56	14.3
Boiled, mashed	½ cup (4.1 oz.)	39	9.7

Food and Description	Measure or Quantity	Calories	Carbo-hydrates (grams)
Butternut:			
Whole	1 lb. (weighed with skin & seeds)	171	44.4
Baked, flesh only	4 oz.	77	19.8
Boiled, flesh only	4 oz.	46	11.8
Hubbard:			
Whole	1 lb. (weighed with skin & seeds)	117	28.1
Baked, flesh only	4 oz.	57	13.3
Boiled, flesh only, diced	½ cup (4.2 oz.)	35	8.1
Boiled, flesh only, mashed	½ cup (4.3 oz.)	37	8.4
Frozen:			
(USDA) heated	½ cup (4.2 oz.)	46	11.0
(Birds Eye)	⅓ of pkg. (3.3 oz.)	43	9.2
(Southland) butternut	⅓ of 20-oz. pkg.	45	11.0
SQUASH PUREE, canned			
(Larsen) no salt added	½ cup (4.5 oz.)	35	7.5
SQUASH SEEDS, dry (USDA):			
In hull	4 oz.	464	12.6
Hulled	1 oz.	157	4.3
SQUID, raw (USDA) meat only	4 oz.	95	1.7
STARCH (See **CORNSTARCH**)			
STEAK UMM	2-oz. serving	180	0.
STEW (See individual listings such as **BEEF STEW**)			
STOMACH, PORK, scalded (USDA)	4 oz.	172	0.
STRAINED FOOD (See **BABY FOOD**)			

(USDA) = United States Department of Agriculture
(HHS/FAO) = Health and Human Services/Food and Agriculture Organization
* = prepared as package directs

Food and Description	Measure or Quantity	Calories	Carbo-hydrates (grams)
STRAWBERRY:			
Fresh (USDA):			
Whole	1 lb. (weighed with caps & stems)	161	36.6
Whole, capped	1 cup (5.1 oz.)	53	2.1
Canned (USDA) unsweetened or low calorie, water pack, solids & liq.	4 oz.	25	6.4
Frozen (Birds Eye):			
Halves:			
Regular	1/3 of 16-oz. pkg.	164	34.9
Quick thaw in lite syrup	1/2 of 10-oz. pkg.	68	15.8
Whole:			
Regular	1/4 of 16-oz. pkg.	89	21.4
In lite syrup	1/4 of 16-oz. pkg.	61	14.4
Quick thaw	1.2 of 10-oz. pkg.	125	30.1
*STRAWBERRY DRINK,			
mix (Funny Face)	8 fl. oz.	88	22.0
STRAWBERRY FRUIT JUICE,			
canned (Smucker's)	8 fl. oz.	120	30.0
STRAWBERRY JELLY:			
Sweetened (Smucker's)	1 T. (.7 oz.)	53	13.5
Dietetic:			
(Diet Delight)	1 T. (.6 oz.)	12	3.0
(Estee)	1 T.	18	4.8
(Featherweight)	1 T.	16	4.0
STRAWBERRY NECTAR,			
canned (Libby's)	6 fl. oz.	60	14.0
STRAWBERRY PRESERVE OR JAM:			
Sweetened:			
(Smucker's)	1 T. (.7 oz.)	53	13.5
(Welch's)	1 T.	52	13.5
Dietetic or low calorie:			
(Estee)	1 T. (.6 oz.)	6	0.
(Featherweight) calorie reduced	1 T.	16	4.0

Food and Description	Measure or Quantity	Calories	Carbohydrates (grams)
(Louis Sherry) wild	1 T. (.6 oz.)	6	0.
(S&W) *Nutradiet*, red label	1 T.	12	3.0

STUFFING MIX:
Apple & raisin (Pepperidge Farm)	1 oz.	110	21.0
*Beef, *Stove Top*	½ cup	181	21.5
*Chicken:			
(Bell's)	½ cup	224	25.0
(Betty Crocker)	⅕ of pkg.	180	21.0
(Pepperidge Farm)	1 oz.	110	20.0
Stove Top	½ cup	178	20.2
*(Town House)	½ cup	180	20.0
Cornbread:			
(Pepperidge Farm)	1 oz.	110	22.0
Stove Top	½ cup	174	21.6
(Town House)	½ cup	170	20.0
Cube (Pepperidge Farm)	1 oz.	110	22.0
*Herb (Betty Crocker) seasoned	⅙ of pkg.	190	22.0
*New England style, *Stove Top*	½ cup	180	20.8
*Pork, *Stove Top*	½ cup	176	20.3
*Premium blend (Bell's)	½ cup	180	24.0
*Ready mix (Bell's)	½ cup	224	25.0
*San Francisco style, *Stove Top*	½ cup	175	19.9
Turkey, *Stove Top*	½ cup	177	20.7
White bread (Mrs. Cubbison's)	1 oz.	101	20.5
Wild rice & mushroom (Pepperidge Farm)	1 oz.	130	17.0

STURGEON (USDA)
Raw:			
Section	1 lb. (weighed with skin & bones)	362	0.
Meat only	4 oz.	107	0.
Smoked	4 oz.	169	0.

(USDA) = United States Department of Agriculture
(HHS/FAO) = Health and Human Services/Food and Agriculture Organization
* = prepared as package directs

Food and Description	Measure or Quantity	Calories	Carbo-hydrates (grams)
Steamed	4 oz.	181	0.
SUCCOTASH:			
Canned, solids & liq.:			
(Comstock):			
Cream style	½ cup (4.4 oz.)	110	20.0
Whole kernel	½ cup (4.4 oz.)	80	15.0
(Larsen) *Freshlike*	½ cup (4.5 oz.)	80	18.0
Frozen (Bel-Air)	⅓ of 10-oz. pkg.	100	19.0
SUCKER, CARP (USDA) raw:			
Whole	1 lb. (weighed whole)	196	0.
Meat only	4 oz.	126	0.
SUCKER, including **WHITE MULLET** (USDA) raw:			
Whole	1 lb. (weighed whole)	203	0.
Meat only	4 oz.	118	0.
SUDDENLY SALAD (Betty Crocker):			
Caesar	⅙ of pkg.	170	20.0
Classic pasta	⅙ of pkg.	160	23.0
Creamy macaroni	⅙ of pkg.	200	21.0
Italian pasta	⅙ of pkg.	150	20.0
Pasta primavera	⅙ of pkg.	190	20.0
Tortellini Italiano	⅕ of pkg.	160	21.0
SUET, raw (USDA)	1 oz.	242	0.
SUGAR, beet or cane (there are no differences in calories and carbohydrates among brands) (USDA):			
Brown:			
Regular	1 lb.	1692	437.3
Brownulated	1 cup (5.4 oz.)	567	146.5
Firm-packed	1 cup (7.5 oz.)	791	204.4
Firm-packed	1 T. (.5 oz.)	48	12.5

Food and Description	Measure or Quantity	Calories	Carbo-hydrates (grams)
Confectioner's:			
Unsifted	1 cup (4.3 oz.)	474	122.4
Unsifted	1 T. (8 grams)	30	7.7
Sifted	1 cup (3.4 oz.)	366	94.5
Sifted	1 T. (6 grams)	23	5.9
Stirred	1 cup (4.2 oz.)	462	119.4
Stirred	1 T. (8 grams)	29	7.5
Granulated	1 lb.	1746	451.3
Granulated	1 cup (6.9 oz.)	751	194.0
Granulated	1 T. (.4 oz.)	46	11.9
Granulated	1 lump (1⅛″ × ¾″ × ⅜″, 6 grams)	23	6.0
Maple	1 lb.	1579	408.0
Maple	1¾″ × 1¼″ × ½″ piece (1.2 oz.)	104	27.0
SUGAR APPLE, raw (USDA):			
Whole	1 lb. (weighed with skin & seeds)	192	48.4
Flesh only	4 oz.	107	26.9
SUGAR PUFFS, cereal (Malt-O-Meal)	⅞ cup (1 oz.)	109	24.7
SUGAR SUBSTITUTE:			
(Estee) fructose	1 tsp.	12	3.0
Spoon for Spoon	1 tsp.	2	1.0
Sprinkle Sweet (Pillsbury)	1 tsp.	2	.5
Sweet 'N Low:			
Brown	1 tsp.	20	10.0
Granulated	1-gram packet	14	.9
Liquid	1 drop	0	0.
Sweet'n It (Estee) liquid	6 drops	0	0.
*Sweet *10* (Pillsbury)	⅛ tsp.	0	0.
(Weight Watchers)	1-gram packet	4	1.0
*****SUKIYAKI DINNER,** canned:			
(Chun King) stir fry	6-oz. serving	257	9.6
(La Choy)	⅜ cup	210	9.0

(USDA) = United States Department of Agriculture
(HHS/FAO) = Health and Human Services/Food and Agriculture Organization
* = prepared as package directs

Food and Description	Measure or Quantity	Calories	Carbo-hydrates (grams)
SUNFLAKES MULTI-GRAIN, cereal (Ralston Purina)	1 cup (1 oz.)	100	24.0
SUNFLOWER SEED:			
(USDA):			
In hulls	4 oz. (weighed in hull)	343	12.2
Hulled	1 oz.	159	5.6
(Fisher):			
In hull, roasted, salted	1 oz.	86	3.0
Hulled, roasted:			
Dry, salted	1 oz.	164	5.6
Oil, salted	1 oz.	167	5.6
(Party Pride) dry roasted	1 oz.	190	3.0
(Planters):			
Dry roasted	1 oz.	160	5.0
Unsalted	1 oz.	170	5.0
SUNFLOWER SEED FLOUR, (See **FLOUR**)			
SUNSHINE PUNCH DRINK, canned (Johanna Farms) *Ssips*	8.45-fl.-oz. container	130	32.0
SUNTOPS (Dole)	1 bar	40	9.0
SURIMI (See **CRAB, IMITATION**)			
SWAMP CABBAGE (USDA):			
Raw, whole	1 lb. (weighed untrimmed)	107	19.8
Boiled, trimmed, drained	4 oz.	24	4.4
SWEETBREADS (USDA):			
Beef:			
Raw	1 lb.	939	0.
Braised	4 oz.	363	0.
Calf:			
Raw	1 lb.	426	0.
Braised	4 oz.	363	0.
Hog (See **PANCREAS**)			

Food and Description	Measure or Quantity	Calories	Carbo-hydrates (grams)
Lamb:			
Raw	1 lb.	426	0.
Braised	4 oz.	198	0.
SWEET POTATO (See also **YAM**):			
Baked (USDA) peeled after baking	5″ × 2″ potato (3.9 oz.)	155	35.8
Candied, home recipe (USDA)	3½″ × 2¼″ piece (6.2 oz.)	294	59.8
Canned:			
(USDA):			
In syrup	4-oz. serving	129	31.2
Vacuum or solid pack	½ cup (3.8 oz.)	118	27.1
(Joan of Arc):			
Mashed	½ cup (4 oz.)	90	24.0
Whole:			
Candied	½ cup (5.2 oz.)	240	60.0
Heavy syrup	½ cup (4.5 oz.)	130	34.0
Light syrup	½ cup (4 oz.)	110	28.0
In pineapple-orange sauce	½ cup (5 oz.)	210	54.0
(Trappey's) *Sugary Sam:*			
Cut, in light syrup	½ cup (4.3 oz.)	110	25.0
Mashed	½ cup (4.3 oz.)	100	25.0
Whole, in heavy syrup	½ cup (4.3 oz.)	130	30.0
Frozen (Mrs. Paul's) candied:			
Regular	4-oz. serving	170	42.0
N' apples	4-oz. serving	160	38.0
SWEET POTATO PIE (USDA) home recipe	⅙ of 9″ pie (5.4 oz.)	324	36.0
SWEET N' SOUR COCKTAIL MIX, liquid (Holland House)	1 fl. oz.	34	8.0

(USDA) = United States Department of Agriculture
(HHS/FAO) = Health and Human Services/Food and Agriculture Organization
* = prepared as package directs

Food and Description	Measure or Quantity	Calories	Carbo-hydrates (grams)
SWEET & SOUR PORK (See **PORK**)			
SWISS STEAK, frozen, (Swanson) 4-compartment dinner	10-oz. dinner	350	37.0
SWORDFISH (USDA):			
Raw, meat only	1 lb.	535	0.
Broiled, with butter or margarine	3″ × 3″ × ½″ steak (4.4 oz.)	218	0.
Canned, solids & liq.	4 oz.	116	0.
Frozen (Captain's Choice)	3-oz. steak	132	0.
SYRUP (See also **TOPPING**):			
Regular:			
Apricot (Smucker's)	1 T. (.6 oz.)	50	13.0
Blackberry (Smucker's)	1 T. (.6 oz.)	50	13.0
Blueberry (Smucker's)	1 T.	50	13.0
Boysenberry	1 T.	50	13.0
Chocolate or chocolate-flavored:			
(Hershey's)	1 T. (.7 oz.)	40	8.5
(Nestlé) *Quik*	1 oz.	80	18.0
Cane (USDA)	1 T. (.7 oz.)	55	14.0
Corn, *Karo*, dark or light	1 T. (.7 oz.)	58	14.5
Maple:			
(USDA)	1 T. (.7 oz.)	50	13.0
(Home Brands)	1 T. (.7 oz.)	55	13.0
Karo, imitation	1 T.	57	14.2
Pancake or waffle:			
(Aunt Jemima)	1 T. (.7 oz.)	53	13.1
Golden Griddle	1 T. (.7 oz.)	55	14.2
Karo	1 T. (.7 oz.)	60	14.9
Mrs. Butterworth's	1 T. (.7 oz.)	55	7.5
Strawberry (Smucker's)	1 T.	50	13.0
Dietetic or low calorie:			
Blueberry:			
(Estee)	1 T. (.5 oz.)	8	1.0
(Featherweight)	1 T.	14	3.0
Chocolate or chocolate-flavored:			
(Estee) *Choco-Syp*	1 T.	20	5.0
(Diet Delight)	1 T. (.6 oz.)	8	2.0
(No-Cal)	1 T.	6	0.

Food and Description	Measure or Quantity	Calories	Carbo-hydrates (grams)
Coffee (No-Cal)	1 T.	6	1.2
Cola (No-Cal)	1 T.	0	Tr.
Maple:			
(Cary's)	1 T.	6	2.0
(S&W) *Nutradiet*, imitation	1 T.	12	3.0
Pancake or waffle:			
(Aunt Jemima)	1 T. (.6 oz.)	29	7.3
(Diet Delight)	1 T. (.6 oz.)	6	4.0
(Estee)	1 T.	8	1.0
Log Cabin	1 T. (.7 oz.)	34	9.1
(Mrs. Butterworth's)	1 T.	30	7.5
(Weight Watchers)	1 T. (.6 oz.)	25	6.0

Food and Description	Measure or Quantity	Calories	Carbohydrates (grams)

T

TACO:
  *(Ortega) | 1 oz. | 54 | .9

*Mix:			
*(Durkee)	½ cup	321	3.7
(French's)	1¼-oz. pkg.	120	24.0
(McCormick)	1¼-oz. pkg.	123	23.7
(Old El Paso)	1 pkg.	100	20.7
Shell:			
(Gebhardt)	1 shell (.4 oz.)	30	4.0
(Lawry's)	1 shell	50	8.0
(Old El Paso):			
Regular	1 shell	55	6.0
Mini	1 shell	23	2.3
Super	1 shell	100	11.0
(Rosarita)	1 shell (.4 oz.)	45	6.0

TACO BELL RESTAURANTS:

Burrito:			
Bean:			
Green sauce	6¾-oz. serving	351	52.9
Red sauce	6¾-oz. serving	357	54.5
Beef:			
Green sauce	6¾-oz. serving	398	37.7
Red sauce	6¾-oz. serving	403	39.1
Supreme:			
Regular:			
Green sauce	8½-oz. serving	407	45.2
Red sauce	8½-oz. serving	413	46.6
Double beef:			
Green sauce	9-oz. serving	451	40.3
Red sauce	9-oz. serving	456	41.7
Cinnamon crispas	1.7-oz. serving	259	27.5
Enchirito:			
Green sauce	7½-oz. serving	371	28.0
Red sauce	7½-oz. serving	382	30.9
Fajita:			
Chicken	4¾-oz. serving	225	19.8
Steak	4¾-oz. serving	234	19.5

Food and Description	Measure or Quantity	Calories	Carbo-hydrates (grams)
Guacamole	¾-oz. serving	34	2.9
Meximelt	3¾-oz. serving	266	18.7
Nachos:			
Regular	3¾-oz. serving	345	37.5
Bellgrande	10.1-oz. serving	648	60.6
Pepper, jalapeño	3½-oz. serving	20	4.0
Pico De Gallo	1-oz. serving	8	1.1
Pintos & cheese:			
Green sauce	4½-oz. serving	184	17.5
Red sauce	4½-oz. serving	190	18.9
Pizza, Mexican	7.9-oz. serving	575	39.7
Ranch dressing	2.6-oz. serving	235	1.5
Salsa	.3-oz. serving	18	3.6
Sour cream	¾-oz. serving	46	.9
Taco:			
Regular	2¾-oz. serving	183	10.6
Bellgrande	5¾-oz. serving	355	17.6
Light	6-oz. serving	410	18.1
Soft:			
Regular	3¼-oz. serving	338	17.9
Supreme	4.4-oz. serving	275	19.1
Super combo	5-oz. serving	286	20.9
Taco salad:			
With shell	18.7-oz. serving	502	26.3
With salsa:			
Regular	21-oz. serving	941	63.1
Without shell	18.7-oz. serving	520	30.0
Taco sauce:			
Regular	.4-oz. packet	2	.4
Hot	.4-oz. packet	2	.3
Tostada:			
Green sauce	5½-oz. serving	237	25.1
Red sauce	5½-oz. serving	243	26.6

TACO JOHN'S:

Burrito:			
Bean	5-oz. serving	197	37.0
Beef	5-oz. serving	303	25.0

(USDA) = United States Department of Agriculture
(HHS/FAO) = Health and Human Services/Food and Agriculture Organization
* = prepared as package directs

Food and Description	Measure or Quantity	Calories	Carbo-hydrates (grams)
Chicken:			
— Regular	5-oz. serving	227	19.0
With green chili	12¼-oz. serving	344	29.0
Combo	5-oz. serving	250	31.0
Smothered:			
With green chili	12¼-oz. serving	367	40.0
With Texas chili	12¼-oz. serving	455	47.0
Super:			
Regular	8¼-oz. serving	389	51.0
With chicken	8¼-oz. serving	366	40.0
Chimichanga:			
Regular	12-oz. serving	464	67.0
With chicken	12-oz. serving	441	55.0
Mexican rice	8-oz. serving	340	59.0
Nachos:			
Regular	5-oz. serving	468	45.0
Super	11¼-oz. serving	669	60.0
Potato Ole, large	6-oz. serving	414	96.0
Taco:			
Regular	4¼-oz. serving	178	15.0
With chicken	4¼-oz. serving	140	12.0
Softshell:			
Regular	5-oz. serving	224	23.0
With chicken	5-oz. serving	180	20.0
Taco Bravo:			
Regular	6¾-oz. serving	319	42.0
Super	8-oz. serving	361	43.0
Taco burger	6-oz. serving	281	31.0
Taco salad:			
Regular:			
Without dressing	6-oz. serving	229	30.0
With dressing	8-oz. serving	359	35.0
Chicken:			
Without dressing	12¼-oz. serving	377	56.0
With dressing	14¼-oz. serving	507	61.0
Super:			
Without dressing	12¼-oz. serving	428	59.0
With dressing	14¼-oz. serving	558	65.0
TAMALE:			
Canned:			
(Hormel) beef:			
Regular	1 tamale	70	4.0

Food and Description	Measure or Quantity	Calories	Carbohydrates (grams)
Hot & Spicy	1 tamale	70	4.5
Short Orders	7½-oz. can	270	17.0
(Old El Paso), with chili gravy	1 tamale	95	8.0
(Pride of Mexico) beef	2-oz. tamale	115	7.5
Frozen (Patio)	13-oz. dinner	470	58.0
TAMARIND, fresh (USDA):			
Whole	1 lb. (weighed with peel, membrane & seeds) ½ cup (4.4 oz.)	104	24.6
Juice	½ cup (4.4 oz.)	51	12.0
TANG:			
Canned, *Fruit Box*:			
Cherry or strawberry	8.45-fl. oz. container	121	31.5
Grape	8.45-fl. oz. container	131	33.7
Mixed fruit	8.45-fl. oz. container	137	36.0
Orange, tropical	8.45-fl. oz. container	147	37.2
*Mix:			
Regular	6 fl. oz.	86	22.0
Dietetic	6 fl. oz.	5	Tr.
TANGELO, fresh (USDA):			
Whole	1 lb. (weighed with peel, membrane & seeds)	104	24.6
Juice	½ cup (4.4 oz.)	51	12.0

Food and Description	Measure or Quantity	Calories	Carbo-hydrates (grams)
TANGERINE OR MANDARIN ORANGE:			
Fresh (USDA):			
Whole	1 lb. (weighed with peel, membrane & seeds)	154	38.9
Whole	4.1-oz. tangerine (2⅜″ dia.)	39	10.0
Sections (without membranes)	1 cup (6.8 oz.)	89	22.4
Canned, regular pack:			
(Dole)	½ cup (4.4 oz.)	70	19.0
(Town House)	5½-oz.	100	25.0
Canned, dietetic or low calorie, solids & liq.:			
(Diet Delight) juice pack	½ cup (4.3 oz.)	50	13.0
(S&W) *Nutradiet*	½ cup	28	7.0
*TANGERINE JUICE, frozen (Minute Maid)	6 fl. oz.	91	21.9
TAPIOCA, dry, *Minute,* quick cooking	1 T. (.3 oz.)	32	7.9
TAQUITO, frozen, shredded (Van de Kamp's) beef	8-oz. serving	490	45.0
TARO, raw (USDA):			
Tubers, whole	1 lb. (weighed with skin)	373	90.3
Tubers, skin removed	4 oz.	111	26.9
Leaves & stems	1 lb.	181	33.6
TARRAGON (French's)	1 tsp. (1.4 grams)	5	.7
TAUTUG OR BLACKFISH, raw (USDA):			
Whole	1 lb. (weighed whole)	149	0.
Meat only	4 oz.	101	0.

Food and Description	Measure or Quantity	Calories	Carbo-hydrates (grams)
*TEA:			
Bag:			
(Celestial Seasonings):			
After dinner:			
Amaretto Nights or *Cinnamon Vienna*	1 cup	<3	.3
Bavarian Chocolate Orange	1 cup	7	1.6
Caffeine free	1 cup	4	.8
Fruit & tea	1 cup	<3	1.0
Herb:			
Almond Sunset, Cinnamon Rose or *Cranberry Cove*	1 cup	3	<2.0
Emperor's Choice, Lemon Zinger or *Raspberry Patch*	1 cup	4	<2.0
Mandarin Orange Spice or *Orange Zinger*	1 cup	5	<2.0
Roastaroma	1 cup	11	2.0
Premium black tea	1 cup	3	.4
(Lipton):			
Plain or flavored	1 cup	2	Tr.
Herbal:			
Almond pleasure, dessert mint, gentle orange or cinnamon apple	1 cup	2	0.
Quietly chamomile or toasty spice	1 cup	4	Tr.
(Sahadi):			
Herbal	6 fl. oz.	2	0.
Spearmint	6 fl. oz.	4	Tr.
Instant (Lipton) 100% tea or lemon flavored	8 fl. oz.	2	0.

(USDA) = United States Department of Agriculture
(HHS/FAO) = Health and Human Services/Food and Agriculture Organization
* = prepared as package directs

Food and Description	Measure or Quantity	Calories	Carbohydrates (grams)
TEA, ICED:			
Canned:			
Regular:			
(Johanna Farms) *Ssips* container	8.45 fl. oz.	100	26.0
(Lipton) lemon & sugar flavored	6 fl. oz.	70	18.0
(Shasta)	6 fl. oz.	61	16.5
Dietetic (Lipton) lemon flavored	6 fl. oz.	2	0.
*Mix:			
Regular:			
Country Time, sugar & lemon flavored	8 fl. oz.	121	30.2
(Lipton)	8 fl. oz.	60	16.0
(Nestea) lemon & sugar flavored	8 fl. oz.	93	12.0
Decaffeinated (Lipton) sugar & lemon flavored	8 fl. oz.	80	20
Dietetic:			
Crystal Light	8 fl. oz.	2	.2
(Lipton) lemon flavored	8 fl. oz.	2	0.
(Nestea) light	8 fl. oz.	5	1.3
TEAM, cereal (Nabisco)	1 cup (1 oz.)	110	24.0
TEENAGE MUTANT NINJA TURTLES, cereal (Ralston Purina)	1 cup (1-oz.)	110	26.0
TEQUILA SUNRISE COCKTAIL (Mr. Boston) 12% alcohol	3 fl. oz.	120	14.4
TERIYAKI, frozen:			
(Chun King) beef	13-oz. entree	379	68.0
(La Choy) Fresh & Light, with rice & vegetables	10-oz. meal	240	39.9
(Stouffer's) beef, with rice & vegetables	9¾-oz. meal	290	33.0
TERIYAKI BASTE & GLAZE (Kikkoman)	1 T. (.8 oz.)	28	6.0

Food and Description	Measure or Quantity	Calories	Carbo-hydrates (grams)
TERIYAKI MARINADE & SAUCE (La Choy)	1 oz.	30	5.0
***TEXTURED VEGETABLE PROTEIN,** Morningstar Farms:*			
Breakfast link	1 link	73	1.3
Breakfast patties	1 patty (1.3 oz.)	100	3.5
Breakfast strips	1 strip (.3 oz.)	37	.6
Grillers	1 patty (2.3 oz.)	190	6.0
THURINGER:			
(Eckrich):			
Sliced	1-oz. slice	90	1.0
Smoky Tangy	1-oz. serving	80	1.0
(Hormel):			
Packaged, sliced	1 slice	80	0.
Whole:			
Regular or tangy, chub	1 oz.	90	0.
Beefy	1-oz. serving	100	0.
Old Smokehouse	1-oz. serving	90	1.0
(Louis Rich) turkey	1-oz. slice	50	Tr.
(Ohse):			
Regular	1 oz.	75	2.0
Beef	1 oz.	80	1.0
(Oscar Mayer):			
Regular	.8-oz. slice	71	.3
Beef	.8-oz. slice	69	.1
THYME (French's)	1 tsp.	5	1.0
TOASTED WHEAT AND RAISINS, cereal (Nabisco)	1 oz.	100	23.0

TOASTER CAKE OR PASTRY:

(USDA) = United States Department of Agriculture
(HHS/FAO) = Health and Human Services/Food and Agriculture Organization
* = prepared as package directs

Food and Description	Measure or Quantity	Calories	Carbo-hydrates (grams)
Pop-Tarts (Kellogg's):			
Regular:			
Blueberry or cherry	1.8-oz. pastry	210	37.0
Brown sugar cinnamon	1¾-oz. pastry	210	33.0
Strawberry	1.8-oz. pastry	200	37.0
Frosted:			
Blueberry or strawberry	1 pastry	200	37.0
Brown sugar cinnamon	1 pastry	210	34.0
Cherry chocolate fudge	1 pastry	200	36.0
Chocolate-vanilla creme	1 pastry	210	37.0
Concord grape, dutch apple or raspberry	1 pastry	210	36.0
Toaster Tarts (Pepperidge Farm):			
Apple cinnamon	1 piece	170	25.0
Cheese	1 piece	190	22.0
Strawberry	1 piece	190	28.0
Toastettes (Nabisco):			
Regular, any flavor	1 pastry	200	36.0
Frosted:			
Brown sugar cinnamon or strawberry	1 pastry	200	36.0
Fudge	1 pastry	220	35.0
Toast-R-Cake (Thomas'):			
Blueberry	1 piece	108	18.0
Bran	1 piece	103	17.6
Corn	1 piece	120	19.2
TOASTY O's, cereal (Malt-O-Meal)	1¼ cups (1 oz.)	107	20.3
TOFU (See **SOYBEAN CURD**)			
TOFUTTI:			
Frozen:			
Regular:			
Chocolate supreme	4 fl. oz.	210	20.0
Maple walnut	4 fl. oz.	230	20.0
Vanilla	4 fl. oz.	200	21.0
Vanilla almond bark	4 fl. oz.	230	23.0
Wildberry supreme	4 fl. oz.	210	22.0

Food and Description	Measure or Quantity	Calories	Carbo- hydrates (grams)
Cuties:			
Chocolate	1 piece	140	21.0
Vanilla	1 piece	130	21.0
Lite Lite, chocolate-vanilla	4 fl. oz.	90	20.0
Love Drops	4 fl. oz.	230	26.0
Soft serve:			
Regular	4 fl. oz.	158	20.0
Hi-Lite:			
Chocolate	4 fl. oz.	100	18.0
Vanilla	4 fl. oz.	90	18.0
TOMATO:			
Fresh (USDA):			
Green:			
Whole, untrimmed	1 lb. (weighed with core & stem end)	99	21.1
Trimmed, unpeeled	4 oz.	27	5.8
Ripe:			
Whole:			
Eaten with skin	1 lb.	100	21.3
Peeled	1 lb. (weighed with skin, stem ends & hard core)	88	18.8
Peeled	1 med. (2″ × 2½″, 5.3 oz.)	33	7.0
Peeled	1 small (1¾″ × 2½″, 3.9 oz.)	24	5.2
Sliced, peeled	½ cup (3.2 oz.)	20	4.2
Boiled (USDA)	½ cup (4.3 oz.)	31	6.7
Canned, regular pack, solids & liq.:			
(Contadina):			
Sliced, baby	½ cup (4.2 oz.)	50	10.0
Pear shape	½ cup (4.2 oz.)	25	6.0
Stewed	½ cup (4.3 oz.)	35	9.0
Whole, peeled	½ cup (4.2 oz.)	25	5.0

(USDA) = United States Department of Agriculture
(HHS/FAO) = Health and Human Services/Food and Agriculture
Organization
* = prepared as package directs

Food and Description	Measure or Quantity	Calories	Carbo-hydrates (grams)
(Del Monte):			
Stewed	4 oz.	35	8.0
Wedges	½ cup (4 oz.)	30	8.0
Whole, peeled	½ cup (4 oz.)	25	5.0
(Hunt's):			
Crushed	½ cup	40	9.0
Cut, peeled	4-oz. serving	20	5.0
Pear shaped,			
Italian	4-oz. serving	20	5.0
Stewed, regular	4-oz. serving	35	8.0
Whole	4-oz. serving	20	5.0
(La Victoria) green, whole	1 T.	4	1.0
(Town House):			
Stewed	½ cup	35	9.0
Whole	½ cup	25	6.0
Canned, dietetic pack, solids & liq.:			
(Diet Delight) whole, peeled	½ cup (4.3 oz.)	25	5.0
(Furman's) crushed	½ cup	72	13.1
(Hunt's) no added salt:			
Stewed	4-oz. serving	35	8.0
Whole	4-oz. serving	20	5.0
TOMATO, PICKLED			
(Claussen) green	1 piece (1 oz.)	6	1.1
TOMATO & PEPPER, HOT CHILI:			
(Old El Paso), Jalapeño	¼ cup	13	2.5
(Ortega) Jalapeño	1 oz.	10	2.6
TOMATO JUICE, CANNED:			
Regular pack:			
(Ardmore Farms)	6 fl. oz.	36	7.8
(Campbell's)	6 fl. oz.	40	8.0
(Hunt's)	6 fl. oz.	30	7.0
(Town House)	6 fl. oz.	35	8.0
Dietetic pack:			
(Diet Delight)	6 fl. oz.	35	7.0
(Hunt's) no added salt	6 fl. oz.	30	8.0
TOMATO PASTE, canned:			
Regular pack:			
(Contadina):			
Regular	6 oz.	150	35.0

Food and Description	Measure or Quantity	Calories	Carbo-hydrates (grams)
Italian:			
Plain	6 oz.	210	36.0
With mushroom	6 oz.	180	36.0
(Hunt's):			
Regular	2 oz.	45	11.0
Garlic	2 oz.	60	11.0
Italian style	2 oz.	50	11.0
(Town House)	6 oz.	150	35.0
Dietetic (Hunt's) low sodium	2 oz.	45	11.0
TOMATO PUREE, canned:			
Regular (Hunt's)	½ cup (4.2 oz.)	45	10.0
Dietetic (Featherweight) low sodium	1 cup	90	20.0
TOMATO SAUCE, canned:			
(Contadina):			
Regular	½ cup (4.4 oz.)	45	9.0
Italian style	½ cup (4.4 oz.)	40	8.0
(Furman's)	½ cup	58	9.8
(Hunt's):			
Regular or with bits	4 oz.	30	7.0
With garlic	4 oz.	70	10.0
Herb	4 oz.	70	12.0
Italian	4 oz.	60	10.0
With mushrooms	4 oz.	25	6.0
With onions	4 oz.	40	9.0
Special	4 oz.	35	8.0
(Town House)	4 oz.	40	9.0
TOMCOD, ATLANTIC, raw (USDA):			
Whole	1 lb. (weighed whole)	136	0.
Meat only	4 oz.	87	0.
TOM COLLINS (Mr. Boston) 12½% alcohol	3 fl. oz.	111	10.8

(USDA) = United States Department of Agriculture
(HHS/FAO) = Health and Human Services/Food and Agriculture Organization
* = prepared as package directs

Food and Description	Measure or Quantity	Calories	Carbo-hydrates (grams)
*TOM COLLINS MIX			
(Bar-Tender's)	6 fl. oz.	177	18.0
TONGUE (USDA):			
Beef, medium fat:			
Raw, untrimmed	1 lb.	714	1.4
Braised	4 oz.	277	.5
Calf:			
Raw, untrimmed	1 lb.	454	3.1
Braised	4 oz.	181	1.1
Hog:			
Raw, untrimmed	1 lb.	741	1.7
Braised	4 oz.	287	.6
Lamb:			
Raw, untrimmed	1 lb.	659	1.7
Braised	4 oz.	288	.6
Sheep:			
Raw, untrimmed	1 lb.	877	7.9
Braised	4 oz.	366	2.7
TONGUE, CANNED:			
(USDA):			
Pickled	1 oz.	76	Tr.
Potted or deviled	1 oz.	82	.2
(Hormel) cured	1 oz.	63	0.
TONIC WATER (See **SOFT DRINK**, quinine or tonic)			
TOOTIE FRUITIES, cereal			
(Malt-O-Meal)	1 cup (1-oz.)	113	24.7
TOPPING:			
Regular:			
Butterscotch (Smucker's)	1 T. (.7 oz.)	70	16.5
Caramel (Smucker's) hot	1 T.	75	14.0
Chocolate:			
(Hershey's) fudge	1 T.	50	9.0
(Smucker's):			
Regular	1 T.	65	13.5

Food and Description	Measure or Quantity	Calories	Carbo-hydrates (grams)
Fudge:			
Regular	1 T.	65	15.5
Hot	1 T.	55	9.0
Milk	1 T.	70	15.5
Marshmallow (Smucker's)	1 T.	60	14.5
Nut (Planters)	½ oz.	90	4.5
Peanut butter caramel (Smucker's)	1 T.	75	14.5
Pecans in syrup (Smucker's)	1 T.	65	14.0
Pineapple (Smucker's)	1 T. (.7 oz.)	65	16.0
Strawberry (Smucker's)	1 T.	60	15.0
Walnuts in syrup (Smucker's)	1 T.	65	13.5
Dietetic, chocolate (Smucker's)	1 T. (.6 oz.)	35	9.5
TOPPING, WHIPPED:			
Regular:			
Cool Whip (Birds Eye):			
Dairy	1 T.	16	1.2
Non-dairy	1 T.	13	1.0
Dover Farms, dairy	1 T. (.2 oz.)	17	1.2
(Johanna Farms) aerosol	1 T. (3 grams)	8	*1.0
Dietetic (Featherweight)	1 T.	3	.5
*Mix:			
Regular, *Dream Whip*	1 T. (.2 oz.)	9	.9
Dietetic (Estee)	1 T.	4	Tr.
TORTELLINI, frozen:			
(Armour) *Classics Lite*, with meat	10-oz. dinner	250	8.0
(Buitoni):			
Cheese filled:			
Regular	2.6-oz. serving	222	29.8
Tricolor	2.6-oz. serving	221	29.7
Verdi	2.6-oz. serving	220	29.8
Meat filled:			
Plain	2.4-oz. serving	212	21.9
Entree	2.5-oz. serving	223	32.4
(Green Giant):			
Cheese, marinara, One Serving	5½-oz. pkg.	260	37.0

(USDA) = United States Department of Agriculture
(HHS/FAO) = Health and Human Services/Food and Agriculture Organization
* = prepared as package directs

Food and Description	Measure or Quantity	Calories	Carbo-hydrates (grams)
Provencale, microwave Garden Gourmet	9½-oz. pkg.	210	36.0
(Le Menu) cheese, healthy style:			
Dinner	10-oz. dinner	230	35.0
Entree	8-oz. entree	250	34.0
(Stouffer's):			
Cheese:			
Alfredo sauce	8⅞-oz. meal	600	32.0
Tomato sauce	9⅝-oz. meal	360	37.0
Vinaigrette	6⅞-oz. meal	400	24.0
Veal, in Alfredo sauce	8⅝-oz. meal	500	32.0
TORTILLA (Old El Paso):			
Corn	1 piece	60	10.0
Flour	1 piece	150	27.0
TOSTADA SHELL:			
(Old El Paso)	1 shell (.4 oz.)	55	6.0
(Ortega)	1 shell (.4 oz.)	50	6.0
TOTAL, cereal (General Mills):			
Regular	1 cup (1 oz.)	110	22.0
Corn	1 cup (1 oz.)	110	24.0
Raisin bran	1 cup (1.5-oz.)	140	33.0
TOWEL GOURD, raw (USDA):			
Unpared	1 lb. (weighed with skin)	69	15.8
Pared	4 oz.	20	4.6
TRIPE:			
Beef (USDA):			
Commercial	4 oz.	113	0.
Pickled	4 oz.	70	0.
Canned (Libby's)	¼ of 24-oz. can	290	1.1
TRIPLE SEC LIQUEUR (Mr. Boston)	1 fl. oz.	79	8.5
TRIX, cereal (General Mills)	1 cup (1 oz.)	110	25.0

Food and Description	Measure or Quantity	Calories	Carbo-hydrates (grams)
TROPICAL CITRUS DRINK, chilled or *frozen (Five Alive)	6 fl. oz.	85	21.3
TROPIC QUENCHER DRINK, mix, dietetic, *Crystal Light*	8 fl. oz.	3	Tr.
TROUT (USDA):			
Brook, fresh:			
Whole	1 lb. (weighed whole)	224	0.
Meat only	4 oz.	115	0.
Lake (See **LAKE TROUT**)			
Rainbow:			
Fresh, meat with skin	4 oz.	221	0.
Canned	4 oz.	237	0.
TUNA:			
Raw (USDA) meat only:			
Bluefin	4 oz.	164	0.
Yellowfin	4 oz.	151	0.
Canned in oil:			
(Bumble Bee):			
Chunk, light, solids & liq.	½ of 6½-oz. can	265	0.
Solid, white, solids & liq.	½ cup (3.5 oz.)	285	0.
(Carnation) solids & liq.	6½-oz. can	427	0.
(Progresso) light, solid	⅓ cup	150	*1.0
(Sea Trader) chunk, light	3¼ oz.	230	0.
(Star Kist) solid, white, solids & liq.	7-oz. serving	503	0.
Canned in water:			
(Breast O'Chicken)	6½-oz. can	211	0.
(Bumble Bee):			
Chunk, light, solids & liq.	½ cup	117	0.
Solid, white, solids & liq.	½ cup	126	0.
(Sea Trader):			
Chunk, light	3¼ oz.	110	0.
White albacore	2 oz.	100	0.
(Star Kist) light	7-oz. can	220	0.

(USDA) = United States Department of Agriculture
(HHS/FAO) = Health and Human Services/Food and Agriculture Organization
* = prepared as package directs

Food and Description	Measure or Quantity	Calories	Carbo-hydrates (grams)
*TUNA HELPER			
(General Mills):			
Au gratin	⅕ of pkg.	280	30.0
Cheesy noodles 'n tuna	⅕ of pkg.	250	28.0
Creamy mushroom	⅕ of pkg.	220	28.0
Creamy noodles 'n tuna	⅕ of pkg.	300	30.0
Pot pie	⅙ of pkg.	420	31.0
Tetrazzini	⅕ of pkg.	240	27.0
TUNA NOODLES			
CASSEROLE, frozen			
(Stouffer's)	10-oz. meal	310	31.0
TUNA PIE, frozen			
(Banquet)	7-oz. pie	540	44.0
TUNA SALAD:			
Home recipe, (USDA) made with tuna, celery, mayonnaise, pickle, onion and egg	4-oz. serving	193	4.0
Canned (Carnation)	¼ of 7½-oz. can	100	3.3
TURBOT, GREENLAND			
(USDA) raw:			
Whole	1 lb. (weighed whole)	344	0.
Meat only	4 oz.	166	0.
TURKEY:			
Raw (USDA):			
Ready-to-cook	1 lb. (weighed with bones)	722	0.
Dark meat	4 oz.	145	0.
Light meat	4 oz.	132	0.
Skin only	4 oz.	459	0.
Barbecued (Louis Rich) breast, half	1 oz.	40	0.
Roasted (USDA):			
Flesh, skin & giblets	From 13½-lb. raw, ready-to-cook turkey	9678	0.
Flesh & skin	From 13½-lb. raw, ready-to cook turkey	7872	0.

Food and Description	Measure or Quantity	Calories	Carbo-hydrates (grams)
Flesh & skin	4 oz.	253	0.
Meat only:			
Chopped	1 cup (5 oz.)	268	0.
Diced	4 oz.	200	0.
Light	1 slice (4" × 2" × ¼", 3 oz.)	75	0.
Dark	1 slice (2½" × 1⅝" × ¼", .7 oz.)	43	0.
Skin only	1 oz.	128	0.
Giblets, simmered (USDA)	2 oz.	132	.9
Gizzard (USDA):			
Raw	4 oz.	178	1.2
Simmered	4 oz.	222	12.
Canned (Swanson) chunk	2½-oz. serving	120	0.
Packaged:			
(Carl Buddig) smoked:			
Regular	1 oz.	50	Tr.
Ham or salami	1 oz.	40	Tr.
Hebrew National, breast	1 oz.	37	*1.0
(Hormel) breast:			
Regular	1 slice	30	0.
Smoked	1 slice	25	0.
(Louis Rich):			
Turkey bologna	1-oz. slice	60	1.0
Turkey breast:			
Oven roasted	1-oz. slice	30	1.0
Smoked	.7-oz. slice	25	0.
Turkey cotto salami	1-oz. slice	50	Tr.
Turkey ham:			
Chopped	1-oz. slice	45	Tr.
Cured	1-oz. slice	35	Tr.
Turkey pastrami	1-oz. slice	35	Tr.
(Ohse):			
Oven cooked or smoked breast	1 oz.	30	1.0
Turkey bologna	1 oz.	70	2.0
Turkey salami	1 oz.	50	1.0
(Oscar Mayer) breast, smoked	¾-oz. slice	19	.2
Smoked (Louis Rich):			
Breast	1 oz.	35	0.

(USDA) = United States Department of Agriculture
(HHS/FAO) = Health and Human Services/Food and Agriculture Organization
* = prepared as package directs

Food and Description	Measure or Quantity	Calories	Carbo-hydrates (grams)
Drumsticks	1 oz. (without bone)	40	Tr.
Wing drumettes	1 oz. (without bone)	45	Tr.
TURKEY, POTTED (USDA)	1 oz.	70	0.
TURKEY DINNER OR ENTREE, frozen:			
(Armour) *Dinner Classics,* & dressing	11½-oz. dinner	320	34.0
(Banquet)	10½-oz. dinner	390	35.0
(Healthy Choice) breast of	10½-oz. dinner	290	39.0
(Le Menu):			
Regular	10½-oz. dinner	300	38.0
Healthy style:			
Dinner:			
Divan	10-oz. dinner	260	23.0
Sliced	10-oz. dinner	210	21.0
Entree:			
Glazed	8¼-oz. entree	260	18.0
Traditional	8-oz. entree	250	19.0
(Morton)	10-oz. meal	226	28.0
(Stouffer's):			
Regular:			
Casserole with gravy & dressing	9¾-oz. meal	360	29.0
Tetrazzini	10-oz. meal	380	28.0
Lean Cuisine:			
Breast, sliced, in mushroom sauce	8-oz. meal	240	20.0
Dijon	9½-oz. meal	270	22.0
Right Course, sliced, in mild curry sauce with rice pilaf	8¾-oz. meal	320	40.0
(Swanson):			
Regular	11½-oz. dinner	350	42.0
Homestyle Recipe, with dresssing & potatoes	9-oz. entree	290	30.0
Hungry Man	17-oz. dinner	550	61.0
(Weight Watchers) stuffed breast	8½-oz. meal	260	24.0
TURKEY NUGGET, frozen (Empire Kosher)	¼ of 12-oz. pkg.	255	14.0

Food and Description	Measure or Quantity	Calories	Carbohydrates (grams)
TURKEY PATTY, frozen			
(Empire Kosher)	¼ of 12-oz. pkg.	188	12.0
TURKEY PIE, frozen			
(Banquet)	7-oz. pie	510	39.0
(Empire Kosher)	8-oz. pie	491	50.0
(Morton)	7-oz. pie	420	27.0
(Stouffer's)	10-oz. pie	540	35.0
(Swanson):			
Regular	7-oz. pie	380	36.0
Hungry Man	16-oz. pie	650	57.0
TURKEY SALAD, canned			
(Carnation)	¼ of 7½-oz. can	110	31.1
TURNIP (USDA):			
Fresh:			
Without tops	1 lb. (weighed with skins)	117	25.7
Pared, diced	½ cup (2.4 oz.)	20	4.4
Pared, slices	½ cup (2.3 oz.)	19	4.2
Boiled, drained:			
Diced	½ cup (2.8 oz.)	18	3.8
Mashed	½ cup (4 oz.)	26	5.6
TURNIP GREENS, leaves & stems:			
Fresh (USDA):	1 lb. (weighed untrimmed)	107	19.0
Boiled (USDA):			
In small amount water, short time, drained	½ cup (2.5 oz.)	14	2.6
In large amount water, long time, drained	½ cup (2.5 oz.)	14	2.4
Canned:			
(USDA) solids & liq.	½ cup (4.1 oz.)	21	3.7
(Allen's) chopped, with diced turnips	½ cup	20	1.0
(Stokely-Van Camp) chopped	½ cup (4.1 oz.)	23	3.5

(USDA) = United States Department of Agriculture
(HHS/FAO) = Health and Human Services/Food and Agriculture
Organization
* = prepared as package directs

Food and Description	Measure or Quantity	Calories	Carbo-hydrates (grams)
(Sunshine) solids & liq.:			
Chopped	½ cup (4.1 oz.)	19	2.5
& diced turnips	½ cup (4.1 oz.)	21	3.2
Frozen:			
(Bel-Air) chopped	3.3-oz.	20	4.0
(Birds Eye):			
Chopped	⅓ of 10-oz. pkg.	20	3.0
Chopped, with sliced turnips	⅓ of 10-oz. pkg.	20	3.0
(Frosty Acres)	3.3-oz. serving	20	4.0
TURNIP ROOT, frozen (McKenzie) diced	1 oz.	4	1.0
TURNOVER:			
Frozen (Pepperidge Farm):			
Apple	1 turnover	300	34.0
Blueberry	1 turnover	310	32.0
Cherry	1 turnover	310	22.0
Peach	1 turnover	310	34.0
Raspberry	1 turnover	310	36.0
Refrigerated (Pillsbury)	1 turnover	170	23.0
TURTLE, GREEN (USDA):			
Raw:			
In shell	1 lb. (weighed in shell)	97	0.
Meat only	4 oz.	101	0.
Canned	4 oz.	120	0.

Food and Description	Measure or Quantity	Calories	Carbo-hydrates (grams)

U

ULTRA DIET QUICK
(TKI Foods):

Bar	1.2-oz. piece	130	17.0
*Mix:			
Dutch chocolate:			
Lowfat milk	8 fl. oz.	200	37.0
Water	8 fl. oz.	220	40.0
Strawberry	8 fl. oz.	100	19.0
Vanilla	8 fl. oz.	100	19.0

(USDA) = United States Department of Agriculture
(HHS/FAO) = Health and Human Services/Food and Agriculture
                    Organization
* = prepared as package directs

Food and Description	Measure or Quantity	Calories	Carbo-hydrates (grams)

V

V-8 JUICE (See **VEGETABLE JUICE COCKTAIL**)

Food and Description	Measure or Quantity	Calories	Carbo-hydrates (grams)
VANDERMINT, liqueur	1 fl. oz.	90	10.2
VANILLA EXTRACT (Virginia Dare) pure, 35% alcohol	1 tsp.	10	DNA
VEAL, medium fat (USDA):			
Chuck:			
Raw	1 lb. (weighed with bone)	628	0.
Braised, lean & fat	4 oz.	266	0.
Flank:			
Raw	1 lb. (weighed with bone)	1410	0.
Stewed, lean & fat	4 oz.	442	0.
Foreshank:			
Raw	1 lb. (weighed with bone)	368	0.
Stewed, lean & fat	4 oz.	245	0.
Loin:			
Raw	1 lb. (weighed with bone)	681	0.
Broiled, medium done, chop, lean & fat	4 oz.	265	0.
Plate:			
Raw	1 lb. (weighed with bone)	828	0.
Stewed, lean & fat	4 oz.	344	0.
Rib:			
Raw, lean & fat	1 lb. (weighed with bone)	723	0.
Roasted, medium done, lean & fat	4 oz.	305	0.

Food and Description	Measure or Quantity	Calories	Carbo-hydrates (grams)
Round & rump:			
Raw	1 lb. (weighed with bone)	573	0.
Broiled, steak or cutlet, lean & fat	4 oz. (weighed with bone)	245	0.
VEAL DINNER, frozen:			
(Armour) *Dinner Classics,* parmigiana	11¼-oz. meal	400	34.0
(Banquet) parmigiana:			
Cookin' Bags	4-oz. meal	230	20.0
Family Entree, patties	¼ of 2-lb. pkg.	370	33.0
(Le Menu) parmigiana	11½-oz. dinner	390	36.0
(Morton) parmigiana	10-oz. dinner	260	35.0
(Swanson) parmigiana:			
Regular, 4-compartment	12¾-oz. dinner	430	42.0
Homestyle Recipe	10-oz. entree	330	33.0
Hungry Man	18¼-oz. dinner	590	57.0
(Weight Watchers) patty, parmigiana	8¹/₁₆ meal	220	8.0
VEAL STEAK, frozen (Hormel):			
Regular	4-oz. serving	130	2.0
Breaded	4-oz. serving	240	13.0
VEGETABLE (See specific variety such as **CAULI-FLOWER; SQUASH;** etc.)			
VEGETABLE, MIXED:			
Canned, regular pack:			
(Chun King) chow mein, drained	½ of 8-oz. can	32	6.3
(La Choy) drained:			
Chinese	⅓ of 14-oz. can	12	2.0
Chop suey	½ cup (4.7 oz.)	9	2.0
(Town House)	½ cup	45	7.0
(Veg-all) solids & liq.	½ cup	35	8.0

(USDA) = United States Department of Agriculture
(HHS/FAO) = Health and Human Services/Food and Agriculture Organization
* = prepared as package directs

Food and Description	Measure or Quantity	Calories	Carbo-hydrates (grams)
Canned, dietetic pack:			
(Featherweight) low sodium	½ cup (4 oz.)	40	8.0
(Larsen) *Fresh-Lite*, no added salt	½ cup	35	8.0
Frozen:			
(Bel-Air):			
Regular	3.3 oz.	65	13.0
Chinese	3.3 oz.	30	6.0
Hawaiian	3.3 oz.	50	14.0
Japanese	3.3 oz.	35	8.0
Winter mix	3.3 oz.	40	5.0
(Birds Eye):			
Regular:			
Broccoli, cauliflower & carrot in butter sauce	⅓ of 10-oz. pkg.	51	5.7
Broccoli, cauliflower & carrot in cheese sauce	⅓ of 10-oz. pkg.	72	7.9
Broccoli, cauliflower & red pepper	⅓ of 10-oz. pkg.	31	4.7
Carrot, pea & onion, deluxe	⅓ of 10-oz. pkg.	52	10.0
Medley, in butter sauce	⅓ of 10-oz. pkg.	62	9.7
Mixed	⅓ of 10-oz. pkg.	68	13.3
Mixed, with onion sauce	⅓ of 8-oz. pkg.	103	11.7
Pea & potato in cream sauce	⅓ of 8-oz. pkg.	164	15.6
Farm Fresh:			
Broccoli, carrot & water chestnut	⅕ of 16-oz. pkg.	36	6.5
Broccoli, cauliflower & carrot strips	⅕ of 16-oz. pkg.	30	5.3
Broccoli, corn & red pepper	⅕ of 16-oz. pkg.	58	10.9
Broccoli, green bean, onion & red pepper	⅕ of 16-oz. pkg.	31	5.4
Brussels sprout, cauliflower & carrot	⅕ of 16-oz. pkg.	38	6.5
Cauliflower, green bean & carrot	⅕ of 16-oz. pkg.	42	8.1
Green bean, corn, carrot & pearl onion	⅕ of 16-oz. pkg.	49	10.1
Green bean, cauliflower & carrot	⅕ of 16-oz. pkg.	32	6.1

Food and Description	Measure or Quantity	Calories	Carbo-hydrates (grams)
Pea, carrot & pearl onion	⅓ of 16-oz. pkg.	59	10.7
International:			
Bavarian style beans & spaetzle	⅓ of 10-oz. pkg.	112	11.5
Chinese style	⅓ of 10-oz. pkg.	85	8.4
Far Eastern style	⅓ of 10-oz. pkg.	84	8.4
Italian style	⅓ of 10-oz. pkg.	114	11.4
Japanese style	⅓ of 10-oz. pkg.	102	10.4
Mexican style	⅓ of 10-oz. pkg.	133	16.1
New England style	⅓ of 10-oz. pkg.	129	14.2
San Francisco style	⅓ of 10-oz. pkg.	99	10.9
Stir Fry:			
Chinese style	⅓ of 10-oz. pkg.	36	6.9
Japanese style	⅓ of 10-oz. pkg.	32	5.9
(Green Giant):			
Regular:			
Broccoli, carrot fanfare	½ cup	25	5.0
Broccoli, cauliflower & carrot in cheese sauce	½ cup	60	8.0
Broccoli, cauliflower supreme	½ cup	20	4.0
Cauliflower, green bean festival	½ cup	16	3.0
Corn, broccoli bounty	½ cup	60	11.0
Mixed, butter sauce	½ cup	80	12.0
Mixed, polybag	½ cup	50	10.0
Pea, pea pod & water chestnut in butter sauce	½ cup	80	10.0
Pea & cauliflower medley	½ cup	40	7.0
Harvest Fresh	½ cup	60	13.0
Harvest Get Togethers:			
Broccoli-cauliflower medley	½ cup	60	10.0
Broccoli fanfare	½ cup.	80	14.2
Cauliflower-carrot bonanza	½ cup	60	7.0
Chinese style	½ cup	60	7.0

(USDA) = United States Department of Agriculture
(HHS/FAO) = Health and Human Services/Food and Agriculture Organization
* = prepared as package directs

Food and Description	Measure or Quantity	Calories	Carbohydrates (grams)
Japanese style	½ cup	45	8.0
(Frosty Acres):			
Regular	3.3-oz. serving	65	13.0
Dutch style	3.2-oz. serving	30	5.0
Italian	3.2-oz. serving	40	8.0
Oriental	3.2-oz. serving	25	5.0
Rancho Fiesta	3.2-oz. serving	60	13.0
Soup mix	3-oz. serving	45	11.0
Stew	3-oz. serving	42	10.0
Swiss mix	3-oz. serving	25	5.0
(La Choy) stir fry	4-oz. serving	40	7.9
(Larsen):			
Regular	3.3-oz. serving	70	13.0
California or Italian blend	3.3-oz. serving	30	6.0
Chuckwagon blend	3.3-oz. serving	70	16.0
Midwestern blend	3.3-oz. serving	40	8.0
Oriental or winter blend	3.3-oz. serving	25	5.0
Scandinavian blend	3.3-oz. serving	45	9.0
For soup or stew	3.3-oz. serving	50	11.0
Wisconsin blend	3.3-oz. serving	50	12.0
(Ore-Ida) medley, breaded	3 oz.	160	17.0
VEGETABLE BOUILLON:			
(Herb-Ox):			
Cube	1 cube	6	.6
Packet	1 packet	12	2.2
(Knorr)	1 packet	16	.9
(Wyler's) instant	1 tsp.	6	1.0
VEGETABLE FAT (See **FAT**)			
VEGETABLE JUICE COCKTAIL:			
Regular:			
(Mott's)	6 fl. oz.	30	7.0
(Smucker's)	8 fl. oz.	58	13.0
V-8, regular or hot	6 fl. oz.	35	8.0
Dietetic, V-8, low sodium	6 fl. oz.	35	8.0
"VEGETARIAN FOODS":			
Canned or dry:			
Chicken, fried (Loma Linda) with gravy	1½-oz. piece	70	2.0

Food and Description	Measure or Quantity	Calories	Carbo-hydrates (grams)
*Chicken, supreme (Loma Linda)	¼ cup	50	4.0
Chili (Worthington)	½ cup (4.9 oz.)	177	13.2
Choplet (Worthington)	1 choplet (1.6 oz.)	50	1.7
Dinner cuts (Loma Linda) drained:			
Regular	1 piece (1.8 oz.)	55	2.0
No salt added	1 piece (1.8 oz.)	55	2.0
Dinner loaf (Loma Linda)	¼ cup (.6 oz.)	50	4.0
Franks, big (Loma Linda)	1.8-oz. frank	100	4.0
Franks, sizzle (Loma Linda)	1.2-oz. frank	85	1.5
FriChik (Worthington)	1 piece (1.6 oz.)	75	2.5
Granburger (Worthington)	1 oz.	96	5.8
Linkettes (Loma Linda)	1.3-oz. link	75	2.5
Little links (Loma Linda) drained	.8-oz. link	40	1.0
Non-Meatballs (Worthington)	1 meatball (.6 oz.)	32	1.9
Numete (Worthington)	½" slice (2.4 oz.)	145	7.1
Nuteena (Loma Linda)	½" slice (2.4 oz.)	160	5.0
*Ocean platter (Loma Linda)	¼ cup	50	5.0
*Patty mix (Loma Linda)	¼ cup	50	4.0
Peanuts & soya (USDA)	4 oz.	269	15.2
Prime Stakes	1 slice	171	7.8
Proteena (Loma Linda)	½" slice	144	6.5
Protose (Worthington)	½" slice	140	5.0
Redi-burger (Loma Linda)	½" slice (2.4 oz.)	130	5.0
Sandwich spread (Loma Linda)	1 T. (.5 oz.)	23	1.3
Savorex (Loma Linda)	1 tsp.	16	1.0
*Savory dinner loaf (Loma Linda)	1 slice (¼ cup dry)	110	4.0
Skallops (Worthington) drained	½ cup (3 oz.)	89	3.0
Soyagen (Loma Linda):			
All purpose or no sucrose	½ cup	65	7.0
Carob	½ cup	70	8.0

(USDA) = United States Department of Agriculture
(HHS/FAO) = Health and Human Services/Food and Agriculture Organization
* = prepared as package directs

Food and Description	Measure or Quantity	Calories	Carbo-hydrates (grams)
Soyameat (Worthington):			
Beef, sliced	1 slice (1 oz.)	44	2.6
Chicken, diced	1 oz.	40	1.4
Soyamel, any kind (Worthington)	1 oz.	120	12.2
Stew pack (Loma Linda) drained	2 oz.	70	4.0
Super Links (Worthington)	1 link (1.9 oz.)	110	3.7
Swiss steak with gravy (Loma Linda)	1 steak (2¾ oz.)	140	8.0
Taystee cuts (Loma Linda)	1 cut (1.3 oz.)	35	1.0
Tender bits (Loma Linda) drained	1 piece	20	1.0
Tender rounds (Loma Linda)	1-oz. piece	20	1.2
Vege-burger (Loma Linda):			
Regular	½ cup	110	4.0
No salt added	½ cup	140	4.0
Vegelona (Loma Linda)	½" slice (2.4 oz.)	100	6.0
Vega-links (Worthington)	1 link (1.1 oz.)	55	2.8
Veg-scallops (Loma Linda)	1 piece (.5 oz.)	12	.3
Vita-Burger (Loma Linda)	1 T. (¼ oz.)	23	2.3
Wheat protein (USDA)	4 oz.	170	10.8
Worthington 209	1 slice (1.1 oz.)	58	2.2
Frozen:			
Beef pie (Worthington)	8-oz. pie	278	41.8
Bologna (Loma Linda)	1 oz.	75	2.5
Bolono (Worthington)	¾-oz. slice	23	1.0
Chicken (Loma Linda)	1-oz. slice	46	2.1
Chicken, fried (Loma Linda)	2-oz. serving	180	2.0
Chicken pie (Worthington)	8-oz. pie	346	37.5
Chic-Ketts (Worthington)	1 oz.	53	2.2
Chik-Nuggets (Loma Linda)	1 piece (.6 oz.)	45	3.4
Chik-Patties (Loma Linda)	1 patty (3 oz.)	226	15.0
Corn dogs (Loma Linda)	1 piece (2.6 oz.)	250	7.0
Corned beef, sliced (Worthington)	1 slice (.5 oz.)	32	1.9
Fillets (Worthington)	1½-oz. piece	90	4.6
FriPats (Worthington)	1 patty	204	5.2
Griddle steak (Loma Linda)	1 piece (2 oz.)	190	5.0
Meatballs (Loma Linda)	1 meatball (.3 oz.)	63	.8
Meatless salami (Worthington)	¾-oz. slice	44	1.2

Food and Description	Measure or Quantity	Calories	Carbohydrates (grams)
Ocean fillet (Loma Linda)	1 piece (2 oz.)	160	5.0
Olive loaf (Loma Linda)	1 slice (1 oz.)	59	2.7
Prosage (Worthington):			
Links	1 link	60	1.5
Patty	1.3-oz. piece	96	2.8
Roll	⅜″ slice (1.2 oz.)	86	2.0
Roast beef (Loma Linda)	1 oz.	53	2.6
Salami (Loma Linda)	1 slice (1 oz.)	49	2.8
Sizzle burger (Loma Linda)	1 burger (2.5 oz.)	210	13.0
Smoked beef, slices (Worthington)	1 slice	14	1.1
Stakelets (Worthington)	3-oz. piece	164	9.4
Tuno (Worthington)	2-oz. serving	81	3.4
Turkey (Loma Linda)	1 slice (1 oz.)	47	2.3
Wahm roll (Worthington)	1 slice (.8 oz.)	36	1.9
VENISON (USDA) raw, lean, meat only	4 oz.	143	0.
VERMOUTH:			
Dry & extra dry (Lejon; Noilly Pratt)	1 fl. oz.	33	1.0
Sweet (Lejon; Taylor)	1 fl. oz.	45	3.8
VICHY WATER (Schweppes)	Any quantity	0	0.
VINEGAR:			
Cider:			
(USDA)	1 T. (.5 oz.)	2	.9
(USDA)	½ cup (4.2 oz.)	17	7.1
(Town House)	1 T.	0	0.
(White House) Apple	1 T.	2	1.0
Distilled:			
(USDA)	1 T. (.5 oz.)	2	.8
(USDA)	½ cup (4.2 oz.)	14	6.0
Red, red with garlic or white wine (Regina)	1 T. (.5 oz.)	Tr.	Tr.

(USDA) = United States Department of Agriculture
(HHS/FAO) = Health and Human Services/Food and Agriculture Organization
* = prepared as package directs

Food and Description	Measure or Quantity	Calories	Carbo-hydrates (grams)
VINESPINACH OR BASELLA (USDA) raw	4 oz.	22	3.9
VODKA, unflavored (See **DISTILLED LIQUOR**)			

Food and Description	Measure or Quantity	Calories	Carbohydrates (grams)

W

WAFFLE:
Home recipe (USDA)	7" waffle (2.6 oz.)	209	28.1
Frozen:			
(Aunt Jemima) jumbo	1 waffle	86	14.5
(Eggo):			
Regular	1 waffle	120	16.0
Apple cinnamon	1 waffle	130	18.0
Blueberry	1 waffle	130	18.0
Buttermilk	1 waffle	120	16.0
Home style	1 waffle	120	16.0
(Roman Meal):			
Regular	1 waffle	140	16.5
Golden Delight	1 waffle	131	15.1

WAFFLE BREAKFAST, frozen
(Swanson) *Great Starts*:
Regular, with bacon	2.2-oz. meal	230	19.0
Belgian:			
& sausage	2.85-oz. meal	280	21.0
& strawberries with sausage	3½-oz. meal	210	31.0

WAFFLE MIX (See also
**PANCAKE & WAFFLE
MIX**) (USDA):
Complete mix:			
Dry	1 oz.	130	18.5
*Prepared with water	2.6-oz. waffle	229	30.2
Incomplete mix:			
Dry	1 oz.	101	21.5
*Prepared with egg & milk	2.6-oz. waffle	206	27.2

(USDA) = United States Department of Agriculture
(HHS/FAO) = Health and Human Services/Food and Agriculture
            Organization
* = prepared as package directs

Food and Description	Measure or Quantity	Calories	Carbo-hydrates (grams)
*Prepared with egg & milk	7.1-oz. waffle (9″ × 9″ × ⅝″, 1⅛ cups)	550	72.4

WAFFLE SYRUP (See **SYRUP**)

WALNUT:
(USDA):
Black, in shell, whole	1 lb. (weighed in shell)	627	14.8
Black, shelled, whole	4 oz. (weighed whole)	712	16.8
Black, chopped	½ cup (2.1 oz.)	377	8.9
English or Persian, shelled, whole	1 lb. (weighed in shell)	1327	32.2
English or Persian, shelled, whole	4 oz.	738	17.9
English or Persian, halves	½ cup (1.8 oz.)	356	6.5
(California) halves & pieces	½ cup (1.8 oz.)	356	6.5
(Fisher):			
Black	½ cup (2.1 oz.)	374	8.8
English	½ cup (2.1 oz.)	389	9.5

WATER CHESTNUT, CHINESE:
Raw (USDA):
Whole	1 lb. (weighed unpeeled)	272	66.5
Peeled	4 oz.	90	21.5
Canned:			
(Chun King) drained:			
Sliced	½ of 8-oz. can	89	21.5
Whole	½ of 8-oz. can	85	22.9
(La Choy) drained, sliced	½ of 8-oz. can	32	7.8

WATERCRESS, raw (USDA):
| Untrimmed | ½ lb. (weighed untrimmed) | 40 | 6.2 |
| Trimmed | ½ cup (.6 oz.) | 3 | .5 |

WATERMELON, fresh (USDA):
| Whole | 1 lb. (weighed with rind) | 54 | 13.4 |

Food and Description	Measure or Quantity	Calories	Carbo-hydrates (grams)
Wedge	4″ × 8″ wedge (2 lb. measured with rind)	111	27.3
Diced	½ cup	21	5.1
WAX GOURD, raw (USDA):			
Whole	1 lb. (weighed with skin & cavity contents)	41	9.4
Flesh only	4 oz.	15	3.4
WEAKFISH (USDA):			
Raw, whole	1 lb. (weighed whole)	263	0.
Broiled, meat only	4 oz.	236	0.
WELSH RAREBIT:			
Home recipe	1 cup (8.2 oz.)	415	14.6
Frozen (Stouffer's)	5-oz. serving	350	8.0
WENDY'S:			
Bacon, breakfast	1 strip	55	Tr.
Bacon cheeseburger on white bun	1 burger	460	23.0
Breakfast sandwich	1 sandwich	370	33.0
Buns:			
Wheat, multi-grain	1 bun	135	23.0
White	1 bun	160	28.0
Chicken sandwich on multi-grain bun	1 sandwich	320	31.0
Chili:			
Regular	8 oz.	260	26.0
Large	12 oz.	390	39.0
Condiments:			
Bacon	½ strip	30	Tr.
Cheese, American	1 slice	70	Tr.
Ketchup	1 tsp.	6	1.0
Mayonnaise	1 T.	100	Tr.
Mustard	1 tsp.	4	Tr.
Onion rings	.3-oz. piece	4	Tr.

(USDA) = United States Department of Agriculture
(HHS/FAO) = Health and Human Services/Food and Agriculture Organization
* = prepared as package directs

Food and Description	Measure or Quantity	Calories	Carbo- hydrates (grams)
Pickle, dill	4 slices	1	Tr.
Relish	.3-oz. serving	14	3.0
Tomato	1 slice	2	Tr.
Danish	1 piece	360	44.0
Drinks:			
Coffee	6 fl. oz.	2	Tr.
Cola:			
Regular	12 fl. oz.	110	29.0
Dietetic	12 fl. oz.	Tr.	Tr.
Fruit flavored drink	12 fl. oz.	110	28.0
Hot chocolate	6 fl. oz.	100	17.0
Milk:			
Regular	8 fl. oz.	150	11.0
Chocolate	8 fl. oz.	210	26.0
Non-cola	12 fl. oz.	100	26.0
Orange juice	6 fl. oz.	80	17.0
Egg, scrambled	1 order	190	7.0
Frosty dairy dessert:			
Small	12 fl. oz.	400	59.0
Medium	16 fl. oz.	533	78.7
Large	20 fl. oz.	667	98.3
Hamburger:			
Double, on white bun	1 burger	560	24.0
Kids Meal	1 burger	220	11.0
Single:			
On wheat bun	1 burger	340	20.0
On white bun	1 burger	350	27.0
Omelet:			
Ham & cheese	1 omelet	250	6.0
Ham, cheese & mushroom	1 omelet	290	7.0
Ham, cheese, onion & green pepper	1 omelet	280	7.0
Mushroom, onion & green pepper	1 omelet	210	7.0
Potato:			
Baked, hot stuffed:			
Plain	1 potato	250	53.0
Bacon & cheese	1 potato	570	57.0
Broccoli & cheese	1 potato	500	54.0
Cheese	1 potato	590	55.0
Chicken à la king	1 potato	350	59.0
Chili & cheese	1 potato	510	63.0
Sour cream & chives	1 potato	460	53.0
Stroganoff & sour cream	1 potato	490	60.0
French fries	regular order	280	35.0

Food and Description	Measure or Quantity	Calories	Carbo-hydrates (grams)
Home fries	1 order	360	37.0
Salad bar, *Garden Spot:*			
Alfalfa sprouts	2 oz.	20	2.0
Bacon bits	⅛ oz.	10	Tr.
Blueberries, fresh	1 T.	8	2.0
Breadstick	1 piece	20	2.0
Broccoli	½ cup	14	2.0
Cantaloupe	1 piece (2 oz.)	4	1.0
Carrot	¼ cup	12	3.0
Cauliflower	½ cup	14	3.0
Cheese:			
American, imitation	1 oz.	70	1.0
Cheddar, imitation	1 oz.	90	1.0
Cottage	½ cup	110	3.0
Mozzarella, imitation	1 oz.	90	Tr.
Swiss, imitation	1 oz.	80	Tr.
Chow mein noodles	¼ cup	60	6.0
Cole slaw	½ cup	90	3.0
Cracker, saltine	1 piece	11	2.0
Crouton	1 piece	2	.2
Cucumber	¼ cup	4	1.0
Eggs	1 T.	14	Tr.
Mushroom	¼ cup	6	Tr.
Onions, red	1 T.	4	Tr.
Orange, fresh	1 piece	5	1.4
Pasta salad	½ cup	134	17.0
Peas, green	½ cup	60	9.0
Peaches, in syrup	1 piece	8	2.0
Peppers:			
Banana or mild pepperoncini	1 T.	18	4.0
Bell	¼ cup	4	1.0
Jalapeño	1 T.	9	2.0
Pineapple chunks in juice	½ cup	80	20.0
Sunflower seeds & raisins	¼ cup	180	12.0
Tomato	1 oz.	6	1.0
Turkey ham	¼ cup	46	1.0
Watermelon, fresh	1 piece (1 oz.)	1	Tr.

(USDA) = United States Department of Agriculture
(HHS/FAO) = Health and Human Services/Food and Agriculture
Organization
* = prepared as package directs

Food and Description	Measure or Quantity	Calories	Carbo-hydrates (grams)
Salad dressing:			
Regular:			
Blue cheese	1 T.	60	Tr.
Celery seed	1 T.	70	3.0
French, red	1 T.	70	5.0
Italian, golden	1 T.	45	3.0
Oil	1 T.	130	Tr.
Ranch	1 T.	80	Tr.
1000 Island	1 T.	70	2.0
Dietetic:			
Bacon & tomato	1 T.	45	2.0
Cucumber, creamy	1 T.	50	2.0
Italian	1 T.	25	2.0
1000 Island	1 T.	45	2.0
Wine vinegar	1 T.	2	Tr.
Salad; side, pick-up window	1 salad	110	5.0
Salad, taco	1 salad	390	36.0
Sausage	1 patty	200	Tr.
Toast:			
Regular, with margarine	1 slice	125	17.5
French	1 slice	200	22.5
WESTERN DINNER, frozen:			
(Banquet)	11-oz. dinner	630	40.0
(Morton)	10-oz. dinner	290	29.0
(Swanson):			
Regular, 4-compartment dinner	11½-oz. dinner	430	43.0
Hungry Man	17¾-oz. dinner	820	73.0
WHEAT GERM:			
(USDA)	1 oz.	103	13.2
(Elam's) raw	1 T. (.3 oz.)	28	3.2
(Kretschmer)	1 oz.	110	13.0
WHEAT GERM CEREAL			
(Kretschmer):			
Regular	¼ cup (1 oz.)	110	13.0
Brown sugar & honey	¼ cup (1 oz.)	110	17.0
WHEAT HEARTS, cereal			
(General Mills)	1 oz. dry	110	21.0
WHEATIES, cereal			
(General Mills)	1 cup (1 oz.)	100	23.0

Food and Description	Measure or Quantity	Calories	Carbo-hydrates (grams)
WHEAT PUFF, cereal			
(Post)	7/8 cup	104	26.0
WHEAT, ROLLED (USDA):			
Uncooked	1 cup (3.1 oz.)	296	66.3
Cooked	1 cup (7.7 oz.)	163	36.7
WHEAT, SHREDDED, cereal (See **SHREDDED WHEAT**)			
WHEAT, WHOLE GRAIN			
(USDA) hard red spring	1 oz.	94	19.6
WHEAT, WHOLE-MEAL, cereal (USDA):			
Dry	1 oz.	96	20.5
Cooked	4 oz.	51	10.7
WHEY (USDA):			
Dry	1 oz.	99	20.8
Fluid	1 cup (8.6 oz.)	63	12.4
WHIPPED TOPPING (See **TOPPING, WHIPPED**)			
WHISKEY (See **DISTILLED LIQUOR**)			
WHISKEY SOUR COCKTAIL:			
(Mr. Boston) 12½% alcohol	3 fl. oz.	120	14.4
*Mix (Bar-Tender's)	3½ fl. oz.	177	18.0
WHITE CASTLE:			
Bun	.8-oz. bun	74	13.9
Cheeseburger	1 serving	200	15.5
Chicken sandwich	2¼-oz. sandwich	186	20.5
Fish sandwich without tartar sauce	2.1-oz. serving	155	20.9

(USDA) = United States Department of Agriculture
(HHS/FAO) = Health and Human Services/Food and Agriculture Organization
* = prepared as package directs

Food and Description	Measure or Quantity	Calories	Carbo-hydrates (grams)
French fries	3.4-oz. serving	301	37.7
Hamburger	1 burger	161	15.4
Onion chips	1 serving	329	38.8
Onion rings	1 serving	245	26.6
Sausage & egg sandwich	1 sandwich	322	16.0
Sausage sandwich	1 sandwich	196	13.3
WHITEFISH, LAKE (USDA):			
Raw, meat only	4 oz.	176	0.
Baked, stuffed, home recipe, with bacon, butter, onion, celery & breadcrumbs	4 oz.	244	6.6
Smoked	4 oz.	176	0.

WHOPPER (See **BURGER KING**)

WIENER (See **FRANKFURTER**)

WILD BERRY DRINK, canned (Hi-C)

	6 fl. oz.	92	22.5

WINE (See individual listings)

WINE, COOKING (Regina):			
Burgundy or sauterne	¼ cup	2	Tr.
Sherry	¼ cup	20	5.0
WINE COOLER (Bartles & Jaymes):			
Light berry	6 fl. oz.	71	15.0
Premium berry	6 fl. oz.	107	16.8
Premium black cherry	6 fl. oz.	104	16.1
Premium blush	6 fl. oz.	94	11.1

Food and Description	Measure or Quantity	Calories	Carbo-hydrates (grams)

Y

YAM (USDA):
Raw:
  Whole

	1 lb. (weighed with skin)	394	90.5
Flesh only	4 oz.	115	26.3

Canned & frozen (See **SWEET POTATO**)

YAM BEAN, raw (USDA):

Unpared tuber	1 lb. (weighed unpared)	225	52.2
Pared tuber	4 oz.	62	14.5

YEAST:
Baker's:
  Compressed:

(USDA)	1 oz.	24	3.1
(Fleischmann's)	1 cube	15	2.0

  Dry:

(USDA)	1 oz.	80	11.0
(USDA)	7-gram pkg.	20	2.7
(Fleischmann's)	1 packet	20	3.0

YOGURT:
Regular:
  Plain:

(Bison)	8-oz. container	160	16.8
(Borden) *Lite-Line*	8-oz. container	140	18.0
(Dannon):			
Low fat	8-oz. container	140	16.0
Non-fat	8-oz. container	110	16.0
(Friendship)	8-oz. container	150	17.0

(USDA) = United States Department of Agriculture
(HHS/FAO) = Health and Human Services/Food and Agriculture Organization
* = prepared as package directs

Food and Description	Measure or Quantity	Calories	Carbo-hydrates (grams)
(Johanna Farms) sundae style	8-oz. container	150	17.0
(La Yogurt)	6-oz. container	140	12.0
(Lucerne):			
Gourmet	6-oz. container	130	12.0
Lowfat	8-oz. container	160	17.0
Nonfat	8-oz. container	130	18.0
(Mountain High)	8-oz. container	200	16.0
(Whitney's)	6-oz. container	150	13.0
Yoplait, regular	6-oz. container	130	13.0
Apple:			
(Dannon) Dutch, Fruit-on-the-Bottom	8-oz. container	240	43.0
(Lucerne) spice, lowfat	8-oz. container	260	46.0
(Sweet'n Low) Dutch	8-oz. container	150	33.0
Apple-cinnamon, *Yoplait*, Breakfast Yogurt	6-oz. container	220	38.0
Apricot (Lucerne) lowfat	8-oz. container	260	46.0
Apricot-pineapple (Lucerne) lowfat	8-oz. container	260	46.0
Banana (Dannon) Fruit-on-the-Bottom	8-oz. container	240	43.0
Berry:			
(Whitney's) wild	6-oz. container	200	33.0
Yoplait:			
Breakfast Yogurt	6-oz. container	210	40.0
Custard Style	6-oz. container	180	30.0
Blackberry (Lucerne)	8-oz. container	260	46.0
Blueberry:			
(Breyers)	8-oz. container	260	44.0
(Dannon):			
Fresh Flavors	8-oz. container	200	34.0
Fruit-on-the-Bottom	4.4-oz. container	130	23.0
Fruit-on-the-Bottom	8-oz. container	240	43.0
(Lucerne):			
Gourmet	6-oz. container	190	32.0
Lowfat	8-oz. container	260	46.0
Nonfat	8-oz. container	180	10.0
(Mountain High)	8-oz. container	220	31.0
(Whitney's)	6-oz. container	200	33.0
Yoplait:			
Regular	6-oz. container	190	32.0
Custard Style	6-oz. container	190	32.0
Light	6-oz. container	90	14.0

Food and Description	Measure or Quantity	Calories	Carbo-hydrates (grams)
Boysenberry:			
(Dannon) Fruit-on-the-Bottom	8-oz. container	240	43.0
(Lucerne) lowfat	8-oz. container	260	46.0
(Whitney's)	6-oz. container	200	33.0
Yoplait	6-oz. container	190	32.0
Caramel pecan (Lucerne)	8-oz. serving	260	46.0
Cherry:			
(Breyers) black	8-oz. container	270	47.0
(Dannon) Fruit-on-the-Bottom	8-oz. container	240	43.0
(Sweet'n Low)	8-oz. container	150	33.0
(Whitney's)	6-oz. container	200	33.0
Yoplait:			
Breakfast Yogurt, with almonds	6-oz. container	200	38.0
Custard Style	6-oz. container	180	30.0
Cherry-vanilla, (Bordon)			
Lite-Line	8-oz. container	240	45.0
Coffee:			
(Dannon) Fresh Flavors	8-oz. container	200	34.0
(Friendship)	8-oz. container	210	35.0
(Johanna Farms) sundae style	8-oz. container	220	17.0
(Whitney's)	6-oz. container	200	28.0
Exotic fruit (Dannon) Fruit-on-the-Bottom	8-oz. container	240	43.0
Lemon:			
(Dannon) Fresh Flavors	8-oz. container	200	34.0
(Johanna Farms) sundae style	8-oz. container	220	17.0
(Lucerne) lowfat	8-oz. container	260	46.0
(Whitney's)	6-oz container	200	28.0
Yoplait:			
Regular	6-oz. container	190	32.0
Custard Style	6-oz. container	190	30.0
Lime (Lucerne) lowfat	1 cup	260	46.0
Mixed Berries (Dannon):			
Extra Smooth	4.4-oz. container	130	24.0
Fruit-on-the-Bottom	4.4-oz. container	130	23.0
Fruit-on-the-Bottom	8-oz. container	240	43.0

(USDA) = United States Department of Agriculture
(HHS/FAO) = Health and Human Services/Food and Agriculture Organization
* = prepared as package directs

Food and Description	Measure or Quantity	Calories	Carbo-hydrates (grams)
Peach:			
(Borden) *Lite-Line*	8-oz. container	230	42.0
(Breyers)	8-oz. container	270	46.0
(Dannon) Fruit-on-the-			
Bottom	8-oz. container	240	43.0
(Lucerne):			
Gourmet	6-oz. container	190	32.0
Lowfat	8-oz. container	260	46.0
Nonfat	8-oz. container	180	34.0
(Whitney's)	6-oz. container	200	33.0
Yoplait	6-oz. container	190	32.0
Pina colada:			
(Dannon) Fruit-on-the-			
Bottom	8-oz. container	240	43.0
(Lucerne) lowfat	1 cup	260	46.0
Yoplait	6-oz. container	190	32.0
Pineapple:			
(Breyers)	8-oz. container	270	45.0
(Light n' Lively)	8-oz. container	240	48.0
Yoplait	6-oz. container	190	32.0
Pineapple-grapefruit			
(Lucerne)	8-oz. container	260	46.0
Raspberry:			
(Breyers) red	8-oz. container	260	44.0
(Dannon):			
Extra Smooth	4.4-oz. container	130	24.0
Fresh Flavors	8-oz. container	200	34.0
Fruit-on-the-Bottom	4.4-oz. container	130	23.0
Fruit-on-the-Bottom	8-oz. container	240	43.0
(Light n' Lively) red	8-oz. container	230	43.0
(Lucerne):			
Regular or red	8-oz. container	260	46.0
Gourmet, red	6-oz. container	190	32.0
(Meadow-Gold) sundae			
style	8-oz. container	250	42.0
(Whitney's)	6-oz. container	200	33.0
Yoplait:			
Regular	6-oz. container	190	32.0
Custard Style	6-oz. container	190	32.0
Light	6-oz. container	90	14.0
Strawberry:			
(Borden) *Lite-Line*	8-oz. container	240	46.0
(Breyers)	8-oz. container	270	46.0

Food and Description	Measure or Quantity	Calories	Carbo-hydrates (grams)
(Dannon):			
Extra Smooth	4.4-oz. container	130	24.0
Fresh Flavors	8-oz. container	200	34.0
Fruit-on-the-Bottom	4.4-oz. container	130	23.0
Fruit-on-the-Bottom	8-oz. container	240	43.0
(Whitney's)	6-oz. container	200	33.0
Yoplait:			
Regular	6-oz. container	190	32.0
Breakfast Yogurt, with almonds	6-oz. container	200	38.0
Custard Style	6-oz. container	190	32.0
Light	6-oz. container	90	14.0
Strawberry-banana:			
(Dannon):			
Fresh Flavors	8-oz. container	200	34.0
Fruit-on-the-Bottom	4.4-oz. container	130	23.0
Fruit-on-the-Bottom	8-oz. container	240	43.0
(Light n' Lively)	8-oz. container	260	52.0
(Sweet'n Low)	8-oz. container	190	33.0
(Whitney's)	6-oz. container	200	33.0
Yoplait:			
Breakfast Yogurt	6-oz. container	240	43.0
Custard Style	6-oz. container	190	32.0
Strawberry colada (Colombo)	8-oz. container	230	36.0
Tropical, *Yoplait, Breakfast Yogurt*	6-oz. container	230	41.0
Tropical fruit (Sweet n' Low)	8-oz. container	150	33.0
Vanilla:			
(Breyers)	8-oz. container	230	31.0
(Dannon):			
Fresh Flavors	4.4-oz. container	110	20.0
Fresh Flavors	8-oz. container	220	34.0
(Lucerne) lowfat	1 cup	260	46.0
(Whitney's)	6-oz. container	200	28.0
Yoplait, Custard Style	6-oz. container	180	30.0
Wild berries (Whitney's)	6-oz. container	200	33.0
Frozen, hard:			
Banana (Dannon)			
Danny-in-a-Cup	8-oz. cup	210	42.0

(USDA) = United States Department of Agriculture
(HHS/FAO) = Health and Human Services/Food and Agriculture Organization
* = prepared as package directs

Food and Description	Measure or Quantity	Calories	Carbohydrates (grams)
Boysenberry (Dannon)			
Danny-On-A-Stick, carob coated	2½-fl.-oz. bar	140	15.0
Boysenberry swirl (Bison)	¼ of 16-oz. container	116	24.0
Chocolate:			
(Colombo) bar, chocolate coated	1 bar	145	17.0
(Dannon):			
Danny-in-a-Cup	8-fl.-oz. cup	190	32.0
Danny-On-A-Stick:			
Uncoated	2½-fl.-oz. bar	60	10.0
Chocolate coated	2½-fl.-oz. bar	130	12.0
Pina colada:			
(Colombo)	4-oz. serving	110	20.0
(Dannon):			
Danny-in-a-Cup	8-oz. cup	230	44.0
Danny-On-A-Stick, uncoated	2½-fl.-oz. bar	65	14.0
Raspberry, red (Dannon):			
Danny-in-a-cup	8-oz. container	210	42.0
Danny-On-A-Stick, chocolate coated	2½-fl.-oz. bar	130	15.0
Raspberry swirl (Bison)	¼ of 16-oz. container	116	24.0
Strawberry:			
(Colombo):			
Regular	4-oz. serving	110	20.0
Bar	1 bar	80	14.0
(Dannon):			
Danny-in-a-Cup	8-fl.-oz. container	210	42.0
Danny-On-A-Stick, chocolate coated	2½-fl.-oz. bar	130	15.0
Vanilla:			
(Bison)	¼ of 16-oz. container	116	24.0
(Colombo):			
Regular	4-oz. serving	110	20.0
Bar, chocolate coated	1 bar	145	17.0
(Dannon):			
Danny-in-a-Cup	8 fl. oz.	180	33.0
Danny-On-A-Stick	2½-fl.-oz. bar	60	11.0

Food and Description	Measure or Quantity	Calories	Carbo-hydrates (grams)
Frozen, soft-serve (Baskin-Robbins):			
Banana, cheesecake, Jamocha, orange, peach, pineapple, raspberry, strawberry or vanilla	1 fl. oz.	31	6.0
Chocolate	1 fl. oz.	35	6.1
Coconut	1 fl. oz.	36	5.5
Peanut butter	1 fl. oz.	37	5.8
YOGURT BAR, frozen (Dole):			
Cherry	1 bar	80	17.0
Chocolate	1 bar	70	13.0
Mixed berry or strawberry	1 bar	70	17.0
Strawberry-banana	1 bar	60	13.0

Food and Description	Measure or Quantity	Calories	Carbo-hydrates (grams)

Z

ZINFANDEL WINE (Louis M. Martini):
Red, 12½% alcohol	3 fl. oz.	64	Tr.
White, 11% alcohol	3 fl. oz.	55	1.5

ZINGERS (Dolly Madison):
Devil's food or white	1¼-oz. piece	140	23.0
Raspberry	1¼-oz. piece	130	20.0

ZWEIBACK:
(USDA)	1 oz.	120	21.1
(Gerber)	7-gram piece	30	5.1
(Nabisco)	1 piece	30	5.0